RESPIRATORY CARE
IN ALTERNATE SITES

To Kathy, my beloved,

who encouraged me to see this project through.

To my children, Ken Jr., Becky and Chris,

who kept me on track by monitoring the progress of this book

every step of the way.

To Mom and Dad,

who would have been proud of their son's accomplishment.

RESPIRATORY CARE IN ALTERNATE SITES

Kenneth A. Wyka, MS, RRT
Director of Marketing and Clinical Respiratory Services
for Jarvis & Jarvis Home Health Care,
Hasbrouck Heights, New Jersey;
Respiratory Care Consultant,
Berkeley Heights, New Jersey
and
Former Associate Professor of Clinical Cardiopulmonary Sciences
and Director of Respiratory Clinical Education
at the University of Medicine and Dentistry of New Jersey,
School of Health Related Professions, Newark, New Jersey

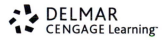

Australia • Brazil • Japan • Korea • Mexico • Singapore • Spain • United Kingdom • United States

DELMAR
CENGAGE Learning™

Respiratory Care in Alternative Sites
Kenneth A. Wyka, MS, RRT

Acquisitions Editor: Dawn Gerrain

Development Editor: Debra Flis

Project Editor: Coreen Rogers

Production Coordinator: John Mickelbank

Art and Design Coordinator: Vincent S. Berger

Editiorial Assitant: Donna L. Leto

Marketing Manager: Katherine Slezak

Cover Design: Bruice Rosche

For product information and technology assistance, contact us at
Cengage Learning Customer & Sales Support, 1-800-354-9706

For permission to use material from this text or product,
submit all requests online at **cengage.com/permissions**
Further permissions questions can be emailed to
permissionrequest@cengage.com

Library of Congress Control Number: 97-20039

ISBN-13: 978-0-8273-7679-3

ISBN-10: 0-8273-7679-0

Delmar
3 Columbia Circle,
PO Box 15015, Albany, NY 12212-0515
USA

Cengage Learning is a leading provider of customized learning solutions with office locations around the globe, including Singapore, the United Kingdom, Australia, Mexico, Brazil, and Japan. Locate your local office at:
international.cengage.com/region

Cengage Learning products are represented in Canada by Nelson Education, Ltd.

For your lifelong learning solutions, visit **delmar.cengage.com**

Visit our corporate website at **www.cengage.com**

Notice to the Reader

Publisher does not warrant or guarantee any of the products described herein or perform any independent analysis in connection with any of the product information contained herein. Publisher does not assume, and expressly disclaims, any obligation to obtain and include information other than that provided to it by the manufacturer. The reader is expressly warned to consider and adopt all safety precautions that might be indicated by the activities described herein and to avoid all potential hazards. By following the instructions contained herein, the reader willingly assumes all risks in connection with such instructions. The publisher makes no representations or warranties of any kind, including but not limited to, the warranties of fitness for particular purpose or merchantability, nor are any such representations implied with respect to the material set forth herein, and the publisher takes no responsibility with respect to such material. The publisher shall not be liable for any special, consequential, or exemplary damages resulting, in whole or part, from the readers' use of, or reliance upon, this material.

Printed in the United States of America
18 19 20 21 22   15 14 13 12 11

FD164

CONTENTS

FOREWORD

The health-care delivery system in the United States is changing rapidly from a system that relegated the cost of and access to care to second-tier values. Over the past few years, we've witnessed a reform movement that seeks to rein in what some consider to be uncontrolled health-care spending.

The changes throughout either reform movement include work force re-engineering, challenges to traditional hospital organizations, and a renewed emphasis on the importance of both clinical and economic outcome measures. Health-care providers and health-care provider employers must now search for ways to provide an acceptable quality of care while balancing costs for that care.

Market-driven reforms have brought about, among other things, the managed-care movement. While managed care in and of itself may not provide a solution to the problem of balancing care with cost, it is almost certain that one facet of managed care is here to stay. That component is risk contracting, or prospective payment. You may recall an early move to prospective payment was made in the early 1980s by the Health Care Financing Administration when it developed a diagnosis-related group by providing payment on a prospective basis. Risk shifted from the payer to the provider. We now see a scramble on the provider side of the equation to control the utilization or frequency of care, whether it be hospital admissions, length of stay, or respiratory care treatments. We also see the results of the foregoing efforts to de-emphasize acute care facilities as the primary health-care setting. Use of alternate care settings, that is to say, settings that act as an alternative to hospitals, is growing and will continue to grow in the future. Home care expenditures are estimated to almost triple by the year 2007, according to the Congressional Budget Office. It must also be noted that the amount of care provided in the most expensive setting—hospitals—will continue to decrease. As mentioned earlier, admissions are down, length of stay shorter, and utilization of support services is decreasing as well. This is in spite of the fact that the average hospital patient is experiencing a higher acuity level than in previous years. Therefore, there exists a strong trend that only the sickest of patients will be treated in hospitals. All others will receive care and services in other venues.

Provider organizations that share the financial risk for care required by patients now recognize that a large number of patients can be treated without compromising quality of care in other care settings such as skilled nursing, subacute, and the home.

It now becomes imperative for health-care providers, and especially respiratory care practitioners, to acquire the expertise necessary not only to work in a cost-conscious, market-driven health care delivery system, but also to be successfully positioned to provide respiratory care services in a multitude of settings which possess very different corporate cultures and with much more reliance on the providers to balance cost and clinical outcomes.

It is no longer enough to pursue excellence when treating patients who are ill. Successful practitioners, under the reformed system, must possess knowledge of the cost of care, a far broader skills inventory in order to improve efficiency, excellent communication skills, a sound knowledge of health-care financing, and an improved ability to empower consumers to take more responsibility for their health, and, in the case of the chronically ill, for their treatment.

The system can no longer afford to wait for consumers to become ill and then become involved with their care. If we are to achieve the goal of assuring quality health care at a reasonable cost, we must do more to keep consumers out of the system. Then we will tie into the values of managed-care organizations and other providers who enage in risk contracting. We must become disease state managers if we are to add value. We must guard against inappropriate utilization and assist physicians and other gatekeepers by assuming responsibility for demand engineering, especially within the context of patients with chronic pulmonary diseases.

In the past, employment in acute-care settings allowed respiratory care practitioners the luxury of specialization. We now see that the respiratory care generalist enjoys high value in alternate care settings. In order to function properly in alternate care settings, the respiratory care practitioner must become more holistic in philosophy. Roles and responsibilities, by comparison, are usually not as tightly controlled in alternate care settings as they are in acute-care settings, where politics and turf issues provide negative incentives for role expansion in hospitals. A demand for improved efficiency and greater responsibility in care planning result in appreciation of the value added by respiratory care practitioners when they're able to provide services that run the clinical gamut from ventilator care to patient instruction for self care and periodic evaluation. Respiratory care practitioners who are able to assist a wide variety of patients have been, and continue to be, in great demand in alternate care settings. We must, therefore, obtain more knowledge about the patient populations we serve. Special emphasis should be placed on gerontology given the dynamic growth forecast for this group as postwar baby boomers reach 65. But respiratory care practitioners can add further value by becoming more conversive in the business aspects of health care. After all, isn't that where the emphasis now resides in the system? But let's not stop there. Let's add organizational skills, communication skills, and education programs that empower patients and family caregivers, through increased knowledge and awareness of the disease state, to monitor physical condition, and when to call a professional health-care provider.

Respiratory care practitioners who possess all these attributes and skills will then be ideally positioned to work in all care settings, including physician group practices that require the services of qualified professionals to assist them in managing down the demand for the physician's time.

There has been a great deal of discussion about the need for seamless care, yet truly seamless care has eluded us thus far. Perhaps the best opportunity to remove some of the seams in the health-care system is provided in alternate care settings. Given the move toward prospective payment by virtue of growth-managed care and preliminary discussions by the Health Care Finance Administration to develop prospective payment in these areas, it would seem that the reimbursement systems, in effect, encourage care provider organizations in alternate sites to undertake responsibility for all care, education, and disease management outside the hospital. Such bundling of services is already beginning to take shape. This movement further emphasizes the need for respiratory care practitioners, among others, to expand their knowledge base in order to provide more value for their employers and assume more responsibility for treatment in managing patients with

employers and assume more responsibility for treatment in managing patients with chronic pulmonary diseases.

The changes in the health-care system have, in my opinion, liberated us from almost a half century of captivity in hospitals by virtue of the fact that adequate reimbursement for our services outside the hospital was not available. With the advent of managed care and prospective payment, the limitations of the fast-disappearing indemnity insurance programs are dissolving. We, however, must face the new challenges of acquiring the additional knowledge and skills necessary, and undertaking efforts to document our effectiveness from both clinical and economic standpoints. *Respiratory Care in Alternate Sites* will help you acquire the information you will need to succeed in alternate care settings.

Sam P. Giordano, MBA, RRT
Executive Director
American Association for Respiratory Care

PREFACE

Whether it was simply coincidence or just good timing, I began writing this book during my twenty-fifth anniversary as a respiratory-care practitioner (RCP). In 25 years I rose through the professional ranks, from staff technician and therapist, to program director, to department head and, finally, to consultant. In addition, I had the good fortune of having been involved with pulmonary rehabilitation since 1972 and respiratory home care since 1973. I have witnessed respiratory care evolve into a responsive, dynamic health-care profession. However, a number of recent events and changes in the heath-care industry have forced respiratory care to redirect itself to care in alternate sites. These events include health-care reform, managed care, and hospital restructuring.

Can respiratory care as a profession survive the trials of these changes? It can, simply because others in health care will begin to realize no one can replace RCPs or do what RCPs have done for so long given their resources and constraints. However, it will help if respiratory care as a profession realizes this first.

This is why I decided to write *Respiratory Care in Alternate Sites*. I also wanted to relay my experiences and knowledge of this subject to my students and colleagues in respiratory care. There is a need for a text that addresses the involvement of RCPs in pulmonary rehabilitation, home care, subacute care, and patient education. This text can serve as a reference, as course material for respiratory-care courses in home care or rehabilitation, or as part of an integrated fundamentals curriculum.

The fifteen chapters cover the broad spectrum of respiratory-care delivery in alternate sites. Chapter 1 serves as an introduction by examining how health-care reform and managed care are impacting health-care delivery, as well as the role respiratory care plays as a health-care profession. Chapters 2 through 6 look at pulmonary rehabilitation in terms of concept, patient selection, program components and design, program implementation, outcomes assessment, and reimbursement. Chapters 7 through 12 discuss respiratory home care as it relates to concept, patient-discharge planning, therapy and related equipment, protocols, accreditation, and reimbursement. Chapters 13 and 14 consider the defintion, delivery and monitoring of care, regulation, and reimbursement of subacute care. Finally, Chapter 15 looks closely at patient education and the roles RCPs can play in this increasingly important area. A glossary and index conclude the text.

It is my hope that *Respiratory Care in Alternate Sites* will encourage my fellow practitioners to become more actively involved in areas like pulmonary rehabilitation, respiratory home care, subacute care, and patient education. Hospital downsizing and a shift in health-care focus have caused many RCPs to seek employment in these areas. Other RCPs are taking a more proactive approach by selecting alternate-site care as part of their careers. As a profession, respiratory care will be better positioned to direct its future by becoming actively involved in the changes that are occurring and by assuming many facets of patient care.

ACKNOWLEDGMENTS

I would like to recognize and thank the following individuals for their assistance in making this book a reality:

- William F. Clark and David A. Gourley, my contributing authors, for the sacrifices they made during the past year to write their chapters and for their expertise, time, and effort
- Sam P. Giordano, MBA, RRT, Executive Director, American Association for Respiratory Care (AARC), Dallas, Texas
- Cheryl West, AARC Director of Government Affairs, Arlington, Virginia
- Jill Eicher, AARC Director of State Government Affairs, Arlington, Virginia
- Joint Commission on Accreditation of Healthcare Organizations (JCAHO), Oakbrook Terrace, Illinois
- HealthScan Products, Inc., Cedar Grove, New Jersey
- James M. Jarvis, BS, RRT, President, Jarvis & Jarvis Home Health Care, Inc., Hasbrouck Heights, New Jersey
- Mark Endicott, CRTT, President, Pulmonary Homecare, Inc., Newton, New Jersey
- Jack H. Dadaian, MD, Medical Director, Lung Diagnostics, Glen Ridge, New Jersey
- Barbara Kerns, CRTT, RPFT, Technical Director, Lung Diagnostics, Glen Ridge, New Jersey
- Donna Porcelli, Office Manager, Lung Diagnostics, Glen Ridge, New Jersey
- Debra Lea Bilotta, Office Manager, Respiratory Disease Associates, Glen Ridge, New Jersey
- JoAnn Sansone, Business Office Manager and Medical Claims Specialist, Respiratory Disease Associates, Glen Ridge, New Jersey
- Lori-Ann Mallack, RRT, Director, Nicholas Martini Pulmonary Center at St. Mary's Hospital, Passaic, New Jersey
- Carolyn Baranowski, MS, RRT, Administrative Director, Comprehensive Outpatient Rehabilitation Center, St. Barnabas Medical Center, Livingston, New Jersey
- Craig L. Scanlan, EdD, RRT, Director Respiratory Care Programs, University of Medicine and Dentistry of New Jersey—School of Health Related Professions, Newark, New Jersey
- Bruce Wyka, for his photography
- The reviewers, who provided valuable suggestions:
  - Beth Brown, Instructor, Respiratory Care, Macon College, Macon, Georgia
  - Daniel V. Cleveland, BS, RRT, Chairperson, Health Professions, Director, Respiratory Care Program, Onondaga Community College, Syracuse, New York
  - Jean Fisher, MBA, RRT, Assistant Professor, Respiratory Care, University of Charleston, Charleston, West Virginia
  - Janet H. Radcliff, BS, RRT, Instructor, Respiratory Care, Harrisburg Area Community College, Harrisburg, Pennsylvania
  - Mark Strausbaugh, BS, Ed, RRT, Program Director of Respiratory Care, Bryman College North, San Jose, California

CONTRIBUTORS

William F. Clark, MEd, RRT
Assistant Professor and Director, Respiratory Clinical Education
Department of Cardiopulmonary Sciences
University of Medicine and Dentistry of New Jersey
School of Health Related Professions
Newark, New Jersey

David A. Gourley, BA, RRT
President, Horizon Health Services
Riverdale, New Jersey
HME/Respiratory Surveyor
Joint Commission on Accreditation
of Healthcare Organizations (JCAHO)
Oakbrook Terrace, Illinois

CHAPTER ONE

HEALTH-CARE REFORM AND ITS IMPACT ON RESPIRATORY CARE

KEY TERMS

alternate site
cross-training
health-care reform
hospital restructuring

managed care
multicompetency or
multiskilling

patient-focused or
patient-centered care
seamless care

OBJECTIVES

Upon completing this chapter, the reader will be able to:

- List and describe the three major reasons for health-care reform.
- Define *hospital restructuring,* and describe its impact on respiratory care.
- Explain what *managed care* means, and describe its impact on health-care delivery in general.
- Identify and briefly describe at least four different managed-care organizations.
- Differentiate between *integrated health-care delivery* and *seamless patient care.*
- Explain what *patient-centered care* means, and describe its effect on the delivery of respiratory care.
- List three alternate-care sites where respiratory care is being administered, and identify the roles respiratory-care practitioners are assuming at each site.
- Differentiate between *multicompetency* and *cross-training,* and discuss their importance to the respiratory-care profession.

INTRODUCTION

To say the health-care system in the United States is in a state of change is an understatement at best. At worst, we might say that these changes were predictable and perhaps long overdue. Regardless of its timing, **health-care reform** in terms of delivery and payment is here to stay. This chapter examines the radical changes in health care and their impact on health care in general, but specifically on the respiratory-care profession. **Hospital restructuring** was one attempt to curb escalating health-care costs.

Patient-focused or **patient-centered care** models have been introduced and implemented in response to the changes, and health care, including respiratory care, has shifted to more cost-effective **alternate sites** like skilled nursing facilities (SNFs), nursing homes, extended-care facilities and subacute care facilities, not to mention the home. This book, beginning with this chapter, focuses on this shift to alternate-site care and the events and societal conditions that are responsible for the American health-care system upheaval.

HISTORICAL PERSPECTIVE

Today, the "watch words" in health care are **managed care,** patient-centered care, and reengineering. Terms like these frighten many health-care providers and managers, including those in respiratory care. For example, hospital decentralization, a process that involves distributing functions and powers from one central authority to several regional or local (unit) levels within an organization, could seriously affect many hospital-based respiratory-care departments. This downsizing or rightsizing, has led to hospital-wide layoffs in an effort whose goal was to better patient care. In an attempt to maintain some professional viability, many respiratory-care practitioners (RCPs), as part of a patient-centered care movement, have accepted assignments in specific hospital units and areas and have become members of those units and areas. Other respiratory-care departments have expanded to other care settings or have taken on diverse clinical services.

Efforts to restructure, reengineer, and downsize hospitals have been taking place since the early 1990s, but they have increased significantly since President Clinton's proposed health-care reform measures in 1994. While Congress never passed Clinton's proposed reforms, the health-care industry, namely health-insurance companies or payors and hospitals, instituted reform measures on their own, fueled by consulting firms eager to take an active role in the process.

The history of health-care reform goes back over 80 years, beginning in 1910 when the American Medical Association (AMA) expressed an interest in the area. In 1916 the AMA recommended the country institute some form of national health insurance. A cooperative health plan for farmers in Oklahoma was started in 1929, and a prepaid contract plan for California water-company employees followed in 1934, signaling the beginning of health maintenance organizations (HMOs) (see following Health Maintenance Organizations section) and managed care (Kongstvedt, 1995). In 1935, the Social Security Act was passed with Title V, which established Crippled Children Grants, and Title VI, which created state grants for public health.

Other prepaid group practice plans were initiated between the 1930s and 1960s, including Kaiser-Permanente in 1942. The first preferred provider organization (PPO) was established in the late 1970s. The PPO type of health-care plan contracts with independent providers for delivered services at a discount (Kongstvedt, 1995). The PPOs have grown considerably and are discussed later in this chapter. Given that Medicare and Medicaid legislation passed in 1965, prospective payments using diagnostic related groups (DRGs) were implemented in 1983, and President Clinton proposed health-care reform measures in 1994, it becomes easy to understand how and why the delivery of and payment for health-care services continue to change.

RESPIRATORY CARE PERSPECTIVE

Fighting to survive in the health-care milieu is the respiratory care profession. Since the late 1940s, respiratory care has fought to achieve an identity and recognition, not only from physicians and other health-care providers, but from insurance payors and the public as well. The American Association for Respiratory Care (AARC), based in Dallas, Texas, has over 35,000 members representing over one third the total practitioners within the United States. With representation in Washington, DC, and at the grassroots, state level, respiratory care is working hard to become a major player in the health-care arena.

Health-care reform, in the guise of managed care and **hospital restructuring,** will present opportunities of which the respiratory-care profession would like to take advantage if it is to continue growing. For example, changes in health-care delivery will give the respiratory-care profession a chance to demonstrate the versatility of its practitioners and the cost-effectiveness of care its practitioners provide. Specific opportunities will involve care offered at alternate sites like SNFs, outpatient rehabilitation centers, extended-care facilities, and the home. Practitioners will be more involved with their patients and able to follow patients from beginning to end, which is part of the **seamless-care** concept of caring for patients with little or no disruption from one care setting to another.

As Shakespeare noted in *The Tempest*, "What's past is prologue." In health care, as in many other industries, a long line of events have set the stage for today's evolutionary, perhaps revolutionary, health-care climate. In the midst of these changes and events, the respiratory-care profession is growing. Besides providing care at alternate sites, respiratory-care practitioners are using newer modes of mechanical ventilation and moving toward **multicompetency** or **multiskilling.** The impact of all these changes and events on respiratory care is only beginning to be felt, and they will continue to influence the profession well into the next century.

ESSENTIAL VOCABULARY AND CONCEPTS

Health-care reform and managed care seem to be creating a unique vocabulary, rich with terms and concepts that depict the activity and direction health-care administration and delivery are taking. The following section covers some of the more important terms and concepts associated with health care and its delivery. In most cases, a thorough description or explanation is offered rather than a simple one.

HEALTH-CARE REFORM

Health-care reform is a broad term that bridges several issues and concepts. Its roots are economical (ever-escalating health-care costs) and societal (access to health care for all citizens). *Managed care, patient-centered care*, and *hospital reengineering* or *restructuring* are all terms used today as health care heads into the twenty-first century. The terms are the result of a health-care reform movement that all levels of society have felt. This market-driven health-care reform is taking place because of several major forces in society, including:

- Increases in health-care spending continue to be out of control and unsustainable.
- The economics of health care are becoming unmanageable for government, businesses, providers, and individuals.
- Risk is deteriorating private health insurance.
- Increases in cost shifting are destabilizing the health-care system.
- The number of uninsured individuals continues to rise.

Many changes have taken place recently to make health-care services more available and affordable and health-care delivery more effective and efficient. While acutely ill patients will continue to be cared for in hospitals, the trend is to search for increased cost effectiveness while providing other levels of patient care at less expensive alternate-care sites. Nursing homes, SNFs, extended-care facilities, rehabilitation centers, physician offices, and the home have become, and will continue to be, major sites of noncritical or subacute patient care. The move toward more affordable alternate care has led to a need for more multiskilled or multicompetent practitioners. Managed care has made it more apparent that assimilating health-care services into a continuum of seamless care that can carry patients uninterrupted from one care setting to another is the primary goal of health-care reform.

Related to the growing need for seamless care is the need for health-care workforce reform, which is taking on added significance because state and federal health-care reform measures appear unlikely to be enacted. As the 1995 Pew Foundation Health Professions Commission Report outlined, health-care workforce reform is becoming more necessary because provider shortages and cost and access problems continue to trouble the health-care system. All states have considered the workforce issue and enacted some form of workforce-reform legislation. While most of the states' legislative activity has been centered on physician training, more emphasis is now being placed on other health-care provider programs as well (Eicher, 1995a).

In terms of workforce reform, licensure and reimbursement remain two areas of interest to the respiratory-care profession. The nonrestrictive nature of many state respiratory-care licensure laws, along with the multicompetency of many RCPs, allows the profession to expand its scope while preserving the flexibility of its workforce. However, the profession's nonrestrictive nature has also allowed practitioners in other health disciplines to perform respiratory-care procedures. Other state actions that will affect workforce reform are reimbursing for rural outpatient respiratory care under Medicaid, including respiratory care in any data-collection or planning projects, and demonstrating projects to emphasize the cost-effectiveness of respiratory care at alternate sites (Eicher, 1995b).

All this, including decreased hospital use and increased use of other care settings, is significantly impacting the respiratory job marketplace. Employment opportunities at alternate sites continue to increase and, at times, appear more plentiful at subacute facilities, rehabilitation centers, and home-care companies than in traditional hospital departments (Figure 1–1). Practitioners, both experienced and new graduates, are beginning to take advantage of the employment opportunities being created by health-care and health-care workforce reform. Many RCPs have come to realize the value and importance of multiskilling and becoming multicompetent.

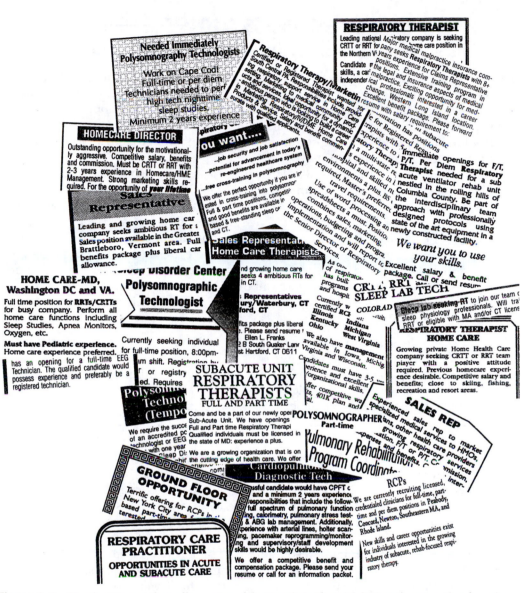

Figure 1–1 *Handwriting on the wall or a sign of the times? As these job listings from a national respiratory newsmagazine show, hospital positions are still advertised, but there are increasing employment opportunities at alternate sites or for those with multiskilling.*

The following case study addresses a unique concern facing many respiratory-care graduates. While it appears that fewer hospital staffing positions are available, employment opportunities at alternate sites seem to be increasing. Graduates must be aware of this change in the job marketplace and prepare accordingly.

CASE STUDY

Respiratory-Care Graduates Address the Changing Job Marketplace

Several 1995 graduates of respiratory-care programs in New Jersey found full-time hospital employment to be virtually nonexistent. As a result, one graduate found employment at a pulmonary diagnostic center performing arterial blood gases, pulmonary function tests, exercise evaluations, and rehabilitation classes. Another graduate was employed at an extended-care facility for long-term ventilator patients, and a third was employed by a respiratory home-care company.

Upon graduating, these three students expected to find hospital-based positions, but the changing job market in respiratory care, and in health care in general due to managed care, health-care reform, and hospital restructuring, changed their expectations. The shift is away from hospital-based care toward less expensive care at alternate-care sites, like subacute and extended-care facilities, specialized outpatient centers, and the home. The respiratory-care graduates sought employment where there were opportunities. They were fortunate to find positions at alternate-care sites, but they required significant orientation and additional training. Presently, all three are doing well in their respective positions and taking advantage of the opportunity to practice their profession outside the traditional hospital setting.

1. Based on the standard respiratory-care curriculum, were these graduates prepared for their positions at alternate sites?
2. What changes in the respiratory-care curriculum would prepare graduates for employment outside the hospital?
3. What role does multicompetency play in the respiratory-care job market?

Other recent trends are the proliferation of integrated delivery systems (IDSs) (see following Integrated Delivery Systems section), organized systems of health-care providers delivering a wide range of services, and the consolidation or closing of smaller hospitals (those with fewer than 100 beds). A number of smaller hospitals have been subsumed by larger conglomerates. Larger hospitals and medical centers have formed consortia to provide more extensive, cost-effective health care on all levels, which in turn have consolidated respiratory-care departments and reduced department size and staffing needs. The RCPs have sought employment outside the hospital setting, where employment opportunities have increased. This trend toward outside care has prompted some hospital departments to become involved with home and subacute care (Bunch, 1995a).

Managed care, with insurance reform and hospital restructuring, is a key element that will produce sweeping changes in the health-care industry well into the twenty-first century. Will more people have access to quality health care? Will patients receive better care? Will escalating health-care costs be contained? These are some important questions that must be addressed, specifically as they relate to respiratory care. The future of respiratory care depends on how the profession handles today's challenges and issues. Respiratory care's response will in part determine its role in health-care delivery in the next century.

ECONOMICS OF HEALTH CARE

Health-care expenditures are continuing to increase (Figure 1–2). Relating national health spending to the gross domestic product (GDP) paints a different picture of this trend, however (Figure 1–3). After rising continually in the 1960s and 1970s, national health spending plateaued in the 1990s. Measures like prospective payments through DRGs were enacted in 1983 to help curtail its rise. Health care now accounts for one eighth the nation's productivity. Almost 13 cents of every dollar of the gross national product (GNP) goes to financing health care (Prospective Payment Assessment Commission, 1994).

The continual rise in national health-care spending, fueled by economic inflation, rapidly developing technology, population increases, cost shifting by providers to pay for care rendered, and increasing frequency and intensity of services, has impacted traditional indemnity insurance plans, which reimburse providers on a fee-for-service basis. To control rising health-care expenditures, more people are enrolling in plans offered through managed care organizations (MCOs) like HMOs and PPOs. Many employers, in an effort to keep their operating budgets in line, are also opting for these more cost-effective plans.

According to the Congressional Budget Office (1994), health-care expenditures related to Medicaid, Medicare, and other entitlement and mandatory programs account for more than one half total spending in the federal budget (Figure 1–4). This figure has significantly impacted the federal deficit.

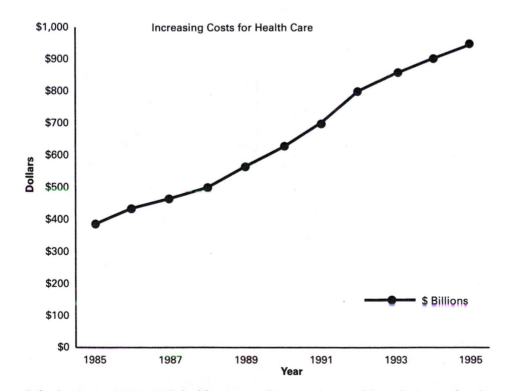

Figure 1–2 *In 10 years (1985–1995), health-care expenditures in the United States have more than doubled, and health-care costs are continuing to escalate.*

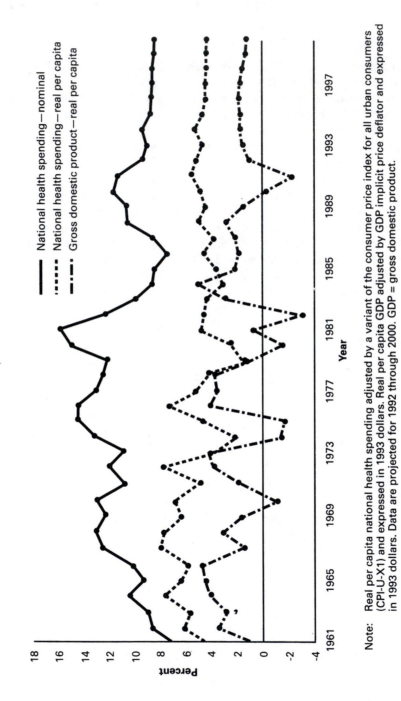

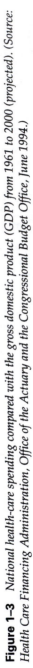

Note: Real per capita national health spending adjusted by a variant of the consumer price index for all urban consumers (CPI-U-X1) and expressed in 1993 dollars. Real per capita GDP adjusted by GDP implicit price deflator and expressed in 1993 dollars. Data are projected for 1992 through 2000. GDP = gross domestic product.

Figure 1–3 *National health-care spending compared with the gross domestic product (GDP) from 1961 to 2000 (projected). (Source: Health Care Financing Administration, Office of the Actuary and the Congressional Budget Office, June 1994.)*

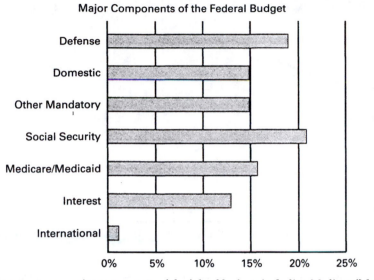

Figure 1–4 *There are seven major components of the federal budget, including Medicare/Medicaid, Social Security, and other mandatory programs that account for more than half total spending. (Source: Congressional Budget Office,* The Economic and Budget Outlook for Fiscal Years 1995–1999, *1994.)*

While the economics of health care bear on society and the nation as a whole, accessing health care remains more of a societal concern. *Health-care access* is an individual's ability to enter the health-care system independent of changes in overall health status and is characterized by "those dimensions which describe the potential and actual entry of a given population group to the health-care delivery system" (Aday, Anderson, & Fleming, 1980). Because health-care access had deteriorated for some, particularly the poor and some rural and minority populations, health-care reform was deemed necessary to provide health care for the approximately 30 to 40 million, or roughly 15 percent of the U.S. population, without health-care coverage. Figure 1–5 shows the trend of Americans with no health insurance; Figure 1–6 shows those who do.

President Clinton initiated the Health Security Act in 1994, to provide individuals with health-care coverage and Congress debated the issue feverishly. Although no legislation was passed, the health-care industry, namely hospitals and health-insurance companies, acted to protect their own interests and caused widespread changes in health-care services delivery and reimbursement, as well as health-care access for those with little or no health insurance. Health-care reform is not seen as one massive overhaul of the system, but in terms of these changes and the impact these changes have had on the continually changing health-care industry.

HOSPITAL RESTRUCTURING OR REENGINEERING

To help contain spiralling health-care costs while maintaining quality patient care, in 1991 the Pew Foundation initiated a grant to select hospitals to study hospital restructuring. *Hospital restructuring* has since become part of every hospital's vocabulary, whether the

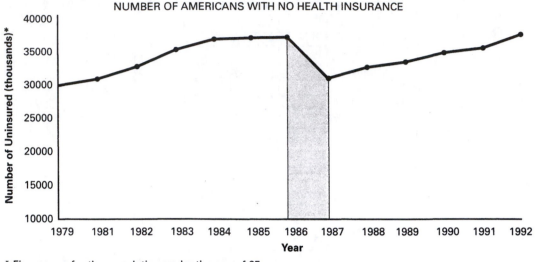

* Figures are for the population under the age of 65.
  Shaded area highlights the period in which the Census Bureau changed the wording of questions asked about insurance coverage.

Figure 1–5 *From 1979 to 1992 the number of Americans with no health insurance has steadily increased. (Source: U.S. Department of Commerce, Bureau of the Census, 1993.)*

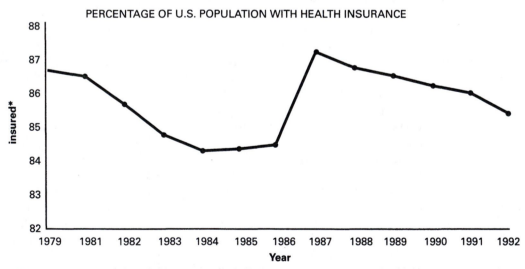

* Figures are for the population under the age of 65.

Figure 1–6 *From 1987 to now, the percentage of Americans with some type of health insurance coverage has steadily declined. (Source: U.S. Department of Commerce, Bureau of the Census, 1993.)*

TABLE 1–1 **Major health-care consultants involved in hospital restructuring or patient-centered care**

American Practice Management	E. C. Murphy	Methodist Healthcare
Anderson Consulting	Ernst & Young*	Peat-Marwick
Avatar Prognosis	Hay Consulting	Patient Focused Care Association
Axielrod	Health System Design	Primary Management
Booz-Allen & Hamilton	Hunter Group	Prism
CLC	Juran Associates	Pritchett Group
Compass Group	Larry Donnelly & Associates	Quorum Health Resources
Cooper & Lybrand	McFoul & Lyons	Sweetland-Northland Group
Deloitte-Touche	Mecon	West Hudson
DSA, Inc.	Medical Management Planning	XYDRA Corporation

---

*Most widely used consultant according to survey respondents.
(Source: *AARC Chartered Affiliate Restructuring Survey,* 1995a.)

hospital is restructuring, redesigning, or reengineering (Bunch, 1995b). *Restructuring* usually indicates the hospital must reexamine and redefine every department or position by role or function. *Restructuring* and *reengineering* are terms that do not necessarily reflect ways to downsize or decentralize hospital departments. Instead, they have a much broader meaning.

Health-care consultants are often contracted to study the delivery of medical and health care within an institution. After careful analysis, these consultants recommend approaches to staff size, departmental and related employee functions, and overall hospital operation. Table 1–1 lists major health-care consultants specializing in hospital restructuring. To make patient care more cost effective, patient-centered care models are often recommended and implemented. These models have had a far-reaching effect on hospital departments, health-care delivery, and the RCP.

Hospital restructuring can have a far-reaching impact on the viability and mere existence of the respiratory-care department. However, the outcome can be very positive, as the following case study illustrates.

CASE STUDY

Impact of Hospital Restructuring on the Respiratory-Care Department

The director of a respiratory-care department at a midwest regional medical center confronted the challenges health-care reform posed. The director's hospital had been recently restructured, and facing potential staff reductions, she worked with her administrator to develop an alternate-site respiratory-care service.

The hospital had recently acquired a nursing home as an extended-care facility. The director convinced hospital administration it would be expedient for RCPs to care for long-term, mechanically ventilated patients at that site. In addition, the director involved some of her staff in providing home-care visits to respiratory patients the hospital discharged. Consequently, the director added job diversity at the subacute and home-care levels. Because of the director's efforts, the hospital maintained its staffing levels, and was even allowed to budget for additional positions.

1. The director proactively dealt with her potential staffing cuts. How important is it for a director to have an administration that is proactive and willing to listen to suggestions for patient care and related services?
2. What additional training would be appropriate or necessary to prepare department staff for functions and responsibilities at alternate-care sites?
3. How should respiratory-care management and staff perceive hospital restructuring?

Restructuring efforts have caused nursing staff and other health-care providers to take over many general respiratory floor-care procedures, like low-flow oxygen therapy, hyperinflation therapy, and small-volume nebulizer treatments. Restructuring's impact on utilization, overall patient care, and sustainable cost savings remains to be seen. The RCPs have been reassigned to hospital departments or locations and, in many instances, laid off. In several states some layoffs have raised questions about licensure. State respiratory licensure laws, including Department of Health regulations, may require a credentialed manager to head the respiratory-care department. Hospitals appear to be avoiding the issue by promoting from within the department when department heads are relieved. In other cases, because of the responsibility realignment resulting from patient-centered care, respiratory-care department staffs have been cut substantially.

The employment at many hospitals may be in a state of flux, but the shift to care at alternate sites has produced new, exciting, and challenging job opportunities for the RCP. The job opportunities at specialty centers, physician offices, subacute facilities, and home-care companies are increasing. By the year 2000, medicine will be delivering about 55 percent of its care on an outpatient basis. Multiskilled or multicompetent practitioners are best suited to these roles outside the traditional hospital setting (Hall, 1995).

To survive any restructuring attempt, respiratory department managers are urged to become involved with the administrative process and the consultants at the onset. If managers are unaware of their departments' cost benefits, then others, namely the consultants, will claim the restructuring can be done more economically and better. Managers who take active roles and become major players in the restructuring process help to ensure their respiratory-care services remain active and viable, even though their jobs may be at stake (Daus, 1995).

Three questions respiratory care managers should address are:

1. What is the consulting firm's mission?
2. What activities and practices has the consulting firm been involved in?
3. Where has the firm consulted, and what were the outcomes?

By answering these questions, department managers better prepare and equip themselves to help guide the restructuring process and ensure more workable and positive outcomes. It is important that department managers become involved in the process early, understand their roles and functions, avoid being defensive or disruptive, and when possible, educate the consultants about the roles, functions, and services of respiratory care.

To support the restructuring process, the AARC has created a management section and appointed a director who is involved with collecting and sharing data between institutions, addressing managers' concerns, and helping address restructuring issues. The AARC has implemented several initiatives to better prepare its members for hospital restructuring and the market-driven changes occurring in the health-care industry, including:

- publishing of white papers on hospital restructuring;
- developing a restructuring network through a computerized information system that promotes communication between those who have undergone restructuring and those who are about to begin restructuring;
- creating programs that promote the RCP's uniqueness to hospital administrators, physicians, and MCOs;
- conducting studies and conferences promoting respiratory-care protocols and restructuring strategies; and
- offering educational opportunities focused on restructuring.

In addition, in September 1995 the AARC surveyed acute-care hospitals to characterize the work environment for RCPs and the operational environment of their institutions. Figure 1–7 illustrates the results of this survey. Restructuring's impact on the respiratory-care profession is powerful, but these survey results are only preliminary. Much work remains to be done before the final survey results are available (Dubbs & Weber, 1995).

The final impact hospital restructuring will have on curtailing spiralling health-care costs is still unclear. Initial studies indicate that cost savings have been realized for the first 2 to 3 years. The result after 5 to 10 years is debatable. Some preliminary findings suggest that cost savings are only short term and that health-care costs begin to increase again after 5 years. If this is true, the value of hiring consultants and restructuring an institution is questionable. Predicting the outcomes and the impact of restructuring on the health-care industry in general is premature.

DECENTRALIZATION

Decentralization distributes or reassigns staff to other departments or areas in an attempt to establish a more cost-effective method of patient care. Decentralizing hospital departments often causes downsizing by shifting lines of responsibility and function. Often, but not always, decentralization causes employee layoffs. Decentralization distributes functions from one central authority to regional or local authorities, in the case of a hospital, to units and/or patient floors. For example, an RCP may be permanently assigned to the emergency room or the intensive-care unit.

While the concept, especially that of patient-centered care models, is good, problems exist. Patient acuity and overall patient census within a unit or a department may shift, necessitating either fewer or more practitioners to meet therapeutic needs. Staffing

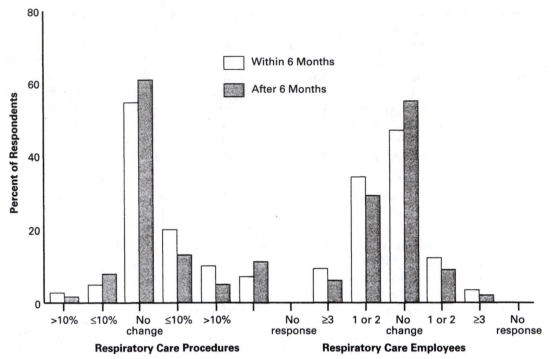

Figure 1–7 *This bar graph illustrates the relative number of respondents who perceived changes in the number of RCPs and services due to restructuring. (Source: "Quantitating the Impact of Restructuring: Results of the AARC Chartered-Affiliate Restructuring Survey," by W. H. Dubbs and K. Weber,* Convention Gazette, *December 3, 1995, 6. Copyright 1995 by the American Association for Respiratory Care. Reprinted with permission.)*

vacancies may occur because of illness, termination, or special leaves of absence. In these instances, finding replacements is a special problem for those managing the departments. There are no easy solutions. There are reports that hospitals that have tried patient-centered care models have abandoned them and returned to more traditional forms of patient care.

INDEMNITY PLANS

Indemnity plans, which are more traditional, usually involve an insurance company that offers coverage within a structure of fee schedules, service limitations, or exclusions as specified for the subscriber groups. Insured individuals are reimbursed a percentage of the billed amount (usually 70 to 80 percent) assuming an annual deductible has been satisfied and the carrier has reviewed and processed the claim.

MANAGED CARE

Like health-care reform, *managed care* is a vague term that describes a planned and coordinated system of health-care delivery that is trying to manage health-care costs, quality, and access. The goal of managed care is to provide quality health care at a lower cost by emphasizing preventive care. It is the market's response to burgeoning, market-driven health-care costs. Managed care accomplishes cost savings through associations with different MCOs or plans ranging from HMOs, PPOs, and point of service (POS) plans. MCOs use contracted providers with a benefits limitation to subscribers who use noncontracted providers, unless so authorized, and an authorization mechanism. Managed care is viewed as an organized system of health-care delivery in which primary-care providers control the use of, and referrals to, specialty care. It works by attempting to align payors' and providers' incentives to make the best use of available resources.

In other words, managed care attempts to control providers of health-care services and to what frequency and extent they provide these services. Its overall goal is to reduce volume while ensuring services are used appropriately. The health-care industry realizes that hospitals and specialists, the major providers, account for the greatest portion of today's health-care costs. Managed care allegedly spurs competition, causing providers to lower their costs, which downsizes health care and its delivery. Proponents of managed care tout several key features or characteristics that they contend enable it to reduce health-care costs (Table 1–2).

Opponents of managed care, namely physicians and other health-care providers not contracted by managed-care plans, remain skeptical. They feel managed care is not all it claims to be and cite numerous concerns regarding its intent, goals, operation, and management (Table 1–3).

Unfortunately, consumers on the receiving end of the managed-care debate are often unfamiliar with the complexities of the health-care delivery system and their choices.

TABLE 1–2 Proponents of managed care assert that the following features are responsible for the program's appeal to the health-care industry and public in general

---

Attempts to align incentives of payors and providers to make the best use of available resources	Reduces inpatient use, demand for specialty services, and the use of more expensive testing
Directs patients to use primary-care physicians	Substitutes lower-cost services for more expensive care
Changes the health-care financing system from fee-for-service to capitation	Stimulates the development of innovative methods of diagnosis and treatment
Promotes the use of nurse practitioners, physician assistants, and nurse midwives for routine primary care	Encourages the use of specialists as consultants, thereby reducing inappropriate specialist use
Advances the definition and dissemination of best practices	Requires primary-care physicians to manage the entire health-care delivery system
Requires providers to compete on the basis of prices, services, and outcomes	Encourages trials of conservative therapy rather than more aggressive approaches
Challenges hospitals to reduce operating costs	Encourages a greater focus on disease prevention
Stimulates the formation of integrated health-care delivery systems	

(Based on data from Terrill, *Health Care Delivery Systems,* 1995.)

TABLE 1–3   Opponents of managed care contend that the following characteristics diminish managed care's impact on the scope and quality of health-care delivery

---

Patients cannot choose who will provide their health and medical care

Some services and care are deemed to be less than adequate

Authorizations from primary-care physicians unnecessarily delay health-care delivery

Cost savings are achieved only by shifting costs and denying services

Managed-care executives receive a percentage of the cost savings they produce and are therefore driven by profit motives

Emphasis is on cost, not on quality of care

Managed care does not understand what it is really buying in terms of health care

Physicians and other providers who use fewer tests or resources are rewarded, while those who use more are penalized

Health-care provider networks under managed care appear to be monopolistic

Medical specialization and education are being undermined

Patients commonly accept health-care plans and hope for the best coverage and care. To this end, managed care is an attempt by the health-insurance industry to contain rising health-care costs by providing an acceptable medical and health-care service at the "best price possible." Offering the best price involves shifting from hospital-based care to more cost-effective physician-centered and outpatient care at subacute care settings or in the home.

Of particular concern are allegations that some primary-care physicians may be receiving rewards or bonuses for not referring patients to specialists, or not referring as many, even when indicated or necessary. These doctors are allegedly reluctant to use the services of specialists because they are told they will share in the plan's profits. This reward system could compromise the quality of care a patient receives. In contrast to doctors who do not refer, primary-care physicians who refer patients to specialists excessively run the risk of being dropped from the provider network, which may also compromise a patient's health-care services. It may be safe to conclude that the issue of health-care delivery, the cost of care, and profit motive will continue to impact managed care, its direction, and the way the public and health-care providers view it.

Effects on Medicare and Medicaid.   Considering the financial difficulties Medicare has experienced and will continue to experience in the foreseeable future, the trend toward managed care raises an interesting question: Can managed care cure entitlement programs like Medicare? Congressional leaders continue to consider changes in Medicare. On the state level legislators are looking at Medicaid. Many states have encouraged or required Medicaid recipients to join managed-care programs. While changes in Medicare and Medicaid are still unclear, one thing is certain: Many members of Congress believe managed-care programs will save money and are therefore the best solution.

Managed-care programs for Medicaid recipients are provided through waivers from federal Medicaid requirements. The two most common features of a waiver are expanding the Medicaid program to include low-income individuals not eligible for Medicaid and requiring enrollment in a managed-care program. Medicaid managed care appears to be the principal state health-care reform measure of the future. The extent to which respiratory care will benefit depends on: (1) the number and type of patients enrolled, (2) the use of respiratory home care as a cost-effective option, and (3) the capabilities of states to scrutinize and meet the long-term health-care needs of their citizens.

Potential benefits for Medicare and Medicaid beneficiaries include likely significant cost savings, coverage for some form of preventive care (e.g., annual physical examinations and/or vaccinations), and elimination of paperwork like claim forms, documentation, and bills. Most of the nation's Medicaid population is already in managed care, while Medicare beneficiaries are not (Eicher, 1995b). However, it appears that more Medicare beneficiaries are examining the benefits of managed-care plans and are considering moves to managed care. Since its inception in 1965, Medicare has been a defined-benefit program, which means there are virtually no limits on the amount the federal government can spend to pay physician and hospital bills for the disabled and elderly, but this is changing. In 1995, the Republicans in Congress proposed a 6.5 percent cap on annual Medicare spending until 2002, well below the current spending rate of 10 percent. The goal is to reduce spending by $270 billion from 1995 to 2002. Medicare now spends an average of $4,900 per year for each beneficiary, a figure that would grow at the current rate to $9,500 per individual by 2002. The purpose of the proposed plan is to encourage more Medicare recipients to be covered by managed-care programs. The government allows HMOs to offer a variety of coverage benefits to Medicare beneficiaries as an alternative to the traditional fee-for-service Medicare plan. Increasing numbers of traditional Medicare beneficiaries will convert their coverage to that of managed care plans, such as an HMO or PPO, and more are changing their coverage every day (Rosenblatt, 1995). In fact, HCFA reports an 87 percent increase in managed Medicare enrollment, a growth rate of 141 percent since 1993. Currently, there are more than 16.1 million Medicare HMO risk plan beneficiaries out of the approximately 37 million Medicare recipients (Meade, 1997).

In addition to offering coverage for the benefits customarily available through the traditional program, Medicare HMOs may provide coverage for hearing and vision aids, prescription medications, annual physical examinations, and vaccinations. According to the Medicare Beneficiaries Defense Fund headquartered in New York City, Medicare HMOs are paid by the federal government on either a cost-based or risk-based contract. Under the cost-based system, the government pays the HMO based on actual incurred costs. Conversely, under the risk-based system, the government pays the HMO a flat fee for each beneficiary. This flat fee is based on the average expenses incurred by Medicare beneficiaries in the county in which the HMO operates. Therefore, government payments for each HMO Medicare beneficiary vary from area to area. Most Medicare HMOs operate under this risk-based system (Epstein, 1996).

The trend of traditional Medicare beneficiaries converting to Medicare HMOs will have an interesting impact on health-care delivery to the elderly because there are several disadvantages to Medicare HMOs or other managed-care plans. First, Medicare beneficiaries are covered only by providers who are members of the HMO network. Second, access to medical specialists is decided by the beneficiary's primary-care physician. Finally, Medicare beneficiaries who venture outside the HMO's geographic area are covered only for emergency services (Epstein, 1996). These disadvantages can affect the level and type of care afforded Medicare beneficiaries, particularly those receiving some form of respiratory home care.

The case study that follows considers a potential problem when patients enroll in a managed-care plan and then must change health-care providers. The problem becomes more complicated when provider networks are closed, because it denies individuals and companies the opportunity to render care to patients covered under specific plans.

————————CASE STUDY————————

Impact of Managed Care on the Delivery of Respiratory Home Care

Margaret White was a 78-year-old female chronic obstructive pulmonary disease (COPD) patient who was receiving home oxygen via a concentrator and portable cylinders from a local supply company for the past 4 years. She was extremely pleased with the service this company had been providing. After encouragement from her physician, Margaret converted her traditional Medicare coverage to managed-care coverage, specifically an HMO. She believed her coverage and providers would remain the same. While her physician was a member of this HMO's provider network, her home-care company was not. As a result, Margaret was able to continue consulting her physician, but to her surprise and dismay, she was forced to use the services of another home-care company that was a member of the provider network.

Margaret's former oxygen supplier tried to become a member of her HMO, but it was closed. At this point in the history of the provider network, the patient was required to use only providers who were members. Margaret was uncertain of the type of equipment and service she would receive from her new company.

1. When this patient switched from her traditional Medicare carrier to the HMO, what were the implications for health-care providers?
2. What impact does a closed HMO provider network have on competition and free market trade?
3. Providers enroll in managed-care provider networks based on cost savings they can produce. Could this impact the type of equipment and the level of services that are provided? How?

To help ensure consumer protection, many state health departments and legislatures, like those in New Jersey, are updating regulations concerning the operation of HMO programs. Many of these HMO regulations took effect in the late 1970s. New regulations will provide consumers with information about the operation and policies of HMOs and other managed-care programs. The focus will be on the quality of care and financial stability (Epstein, 1995).

On the federal level, Medicare reform proposed by the Republicans in Congress would provide Medicare beneficiaries a pamphlet offering a choice of ten to twelve government-approved health care plans that would include HMOs and PPOs, plus innovative approaches like medical savings accounts and employer health plans. Another option would be "Medisave," which allows private insurance companies to charge deductibles as high as $10,000 to beneficiaries who switch to a catastrophic-only Medicare plan. In all cases, Medicare recipients could only enroll in health-care programs certified by the federal government for financial solvency and quality care. The recipients would complete a form and be assigned to the plans they selected. Enrollees would be allowed to switch plans every 30 days for the first 2 years, but afterward they would have to remain with the plan they chose for 12 months. Medicare payments from the government would go directly to the selected plans (Espo, 1995).

Other aspects of the federal proposal would increase Medicare premiums to $93 a month by the year 2002. In 1995, the monthly premium was $46.10, and it was intended to climb to $60 a month by 2002. Recommendations to limit lawsuit awards to a maximum $250,000 for punitive damages and $250,000 for pain and suffering have also been made. Additional savings would be realized by increasing annual deductibles to $200 a year per beneficiary by 2002 (Espo, 1995). Finally, payments to physicians and other providers would be reduced under the proposal. In particular, up to a 40 percent reduction in the reimbursement for home oxygen is being proposed. If enacted, this cut would devastate the level of services provided home-oxygen patients, as well as the jobs of RCPs employed in home care (Brown, 1995). However, the Clinton Administration in 1996 was leaning toward a more tolerable 10 percent reduction in home-oxygen reimbursement (Clark, 1996).

Medicare reform is an emotionally charged and highly politicized issue. Proponents of the Republican plan, who call the proposal "Medichoice," believe it will help keep Medicare solvent (Beck, Thomas, & Hager, 1995). However, opponents of the plan, like the Democrats and the elderly, believe otherwise. By tackling Medicare, opponents see Congress as challenging the basis of the entitlement problem, namely spending on the elderly. Specifically, opponents see a generational war beginning in which a diminutive younger population will have to support an ever-increasing senior population. The cost of supporting the elderly, in the form of Social Security and Medicare, now one third of federal spending, is becoming oppressive. By 2011, when many baby boomers become 65, Social Security and Medicare in their current forms are estimated to be unaffordable (Samuelson, 1995).

Critics claim that proposed reductions in Medicare spending will be used to fund tax cuts for large corporations and the wealthy. Critics also envision an era in which the elderly, because of spending cuts, will get less for their health-care dollar in a program they call "Mediscare" (Fineman, 1995). Health-care reform has occurred without legislative action. Medicare may follow a similar path. Medicare reform may occur whether or not Congress takes formal action. Time will tell what impact this reform will have on health-care delivery.

CAPITATION

Capitation, the per capita payment for health-care services delivered to a defined population over a set period, is usually calculated per member per month (PMPM). The primary objective of capitation is to limit costs. It reflects a set amount of money paid out based on the number of enrollees within a plan rather than on services delivered. It also represents a formal agreement in which a provider or a provider group has agreed to deliver a set of health-care services for a predetermined per capita cost. Physicians and other health-care providers usually receive in advance a negotiated monthly payment from the managed-care plan. This negotiated fee does not vary with the amount of service rendered.

HEALTH MAINTENANCE ORGANIZATIONS

The HMOs are an integral part of managed care and are the most popular of the managed-care plans that also include PPOs, independent practice associations (see following Independent Practice Associations) (IPAs), and POS plans. Traditionally HMOs are any legal for-profit or nonprofit organizations that provide and deliver a predetermined and agreed-upon set of health-care services and benefits to a voluntarily enrolled group in a specific geographical region for a fixed capitation or prepaid payment on a PMPM basis. However, with an increasing number of self-insured businesses and financial arrangements that are not prepayment, the HMO definition has changed. A more current definition describes the HMO as a health plan in which some of the health-care providers share some of the risk for medical expenses and primary-care physicians act as gatekeepers. Essential to the success of an HMO is the willingness of contracted physicians to accept financial risk in providing services to subscribers. If contracted physicians incurred expenses over budgeted costs, then they would have to absorb the shortfall. However, the participating physicians would also share any excess revenues. The focus is now on controlling escalating medical costs while still providing an acceptable level of care.

Historically, the prepaid group-practice plans that were the HMO prototypes started with the Group Health Association in Washington, DC, in 1937. The Kaiser-Permanente Medical Care Program, the largest and most widely known HMO prototype, followed in in 1942. Other, similar plans include the Group Health Cooperative of Puget Sound in 1947; the Health Insurance Plan of Greater New York, also in 1947; and the Group Health Plan of Minneapolis in 1957 (Kongstvedt, 1995). With the advent of managed care, HMOs have grown significantly. In 1990, HMOs were an over-$45 billion industry. In December 1991, there were 550 HMOs in the United States, representing 58 staff model plans, 67 group model plans, 86 networks, and 339 IPAs and serving a total enrollment of 38.6 million (Group Health Assocation of America [GHAA], 1992). By July 1994, close to 49 million or 19 percent of Americans were enrolled in HMOs (Figure 1–8) (Prospective Payment Assessment Commission, 1995). By the end of 1995, this figure reached 53.3 million, with an estimated 100,000,000 or 40 percent enrolled in some type of managed-care plan (Spragins, 1996).

PREFERRED PROVIDER ORGANIZATIONS

The PPOs are plans through which health-benefit plans and health-insurance companies contract with participating providers to purchase health-care services for their customers. Most PPOs contract directly with physicians, hospitals, and other health-care providers, including diagnostic facilities. These providers are selected based on their scopes of services, reputations, and cost efficiencies. Participating providers are required to accept, as full payment, payments made by the PPO. In return for these favorable payment rates, PPOs strive to ensure claims received are promptly paid. Most PPOs have implemented a utilization-management program to handle utilization and cost of services provided. PPOs also allow customers to use non-PPO providers when the need arises. However, the PPO reimburses at the contracted providers' discounted rate. The patient must pay the difference between the PPO's scheduled fee and the amount billed the

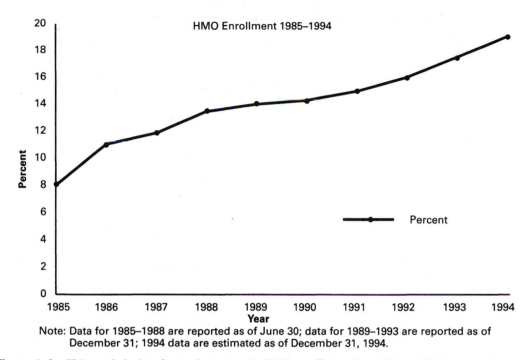

Figure 1–8 *This graph depicts the steady increase in HMO enrollment from 1985 to 1994 (expressed as a percent of the U.S. population). (Source: U.S. Department of Commerce, Bureau of the Census, 1994.)*

must pay the difference between the PPO's scheduled fee and the amount billed the patient.

The PPOs first appeared in the late 1970s. Many in the health-care profession consider PPOs to be evolving HMOs. However, PPOs do not incorporate many of the cost-control and quality-assessment features associated with HMOs. Like HMOs, PPOs have enjoyed a steady growth in enrollment rate. In fact, according to the 1992 *Directory of Operational PPOs*, employees covered by PPOs have increased from near zero in the late 1970s when they were first introduced to an estimated 37 million, not including dependents, by December 1991. Figure 1–9 illustrates the comparative market shares of traditional indemnity and the major managed-care plans.

POINT OF SERVICE PLANS

The POS plans might be called open-ended HMOs that offer features of both HMOs and PPOs. Some dual-choice POS plans involve enrolling a beneficiary in both an HMO and an indemnity plan. These plans provide different benefits based on whether the customer chooses to use providers within the plan and according to the authorization system or to go outside of the plan for health-care services. A triple-choice plan adds a PPO to the dual-choice option. Beneficiaries who decide to go outside the plan or network for services are responsible for the additional cost.

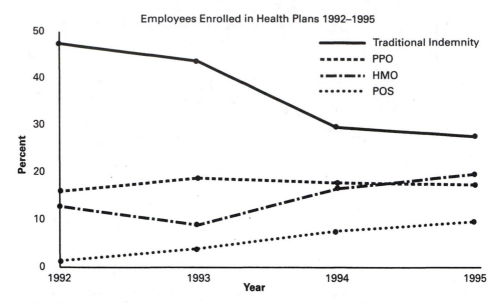

Figure 1–9 *Although most employees are still covered by traditional indemnity insurance, managed-care plans like POSs, PPOs, and HMOs are gaining popularity and, when combined, cover more employees than traditional indemnity. (Adapted from: Foster Higgins, 1995.)*

INTEGRATED DELIVERY SYSTEMS

The IDSs, also called *integrated health-care delivery systems*, are usually associated with health-care plans and combine the resources of physicians, hospitals, and other health-care/medical services to provide continuing and coordinated ambulatory and tertiary care to a defined portion of enrolled beneficiaries. The IDSs fall into three broad clusters: (1) systems that integrate only physicians, (2) systems that integrate physicians with hospitals or ancillary sites, and (3) systems that involve insurance functions. Examples of IDSs include IPAs, physician hospital organizations (PHOs), and management service organizations (MSOs) (for PHOs and MSOs see following sections).

In the same way managed care is advancing the development of alternate sites, integrated health-care delivery systems are being formed to provide greater continuity of care in the delivery of long-term patient services. In reality, alternate-site care is a component of integrated health care, which fosters the seamless-care concept of combining all patient-care settings to form one cohesive unit. The outcome enables patients to flow through the system with little or no disruption in their treatment and care (Bunch, 1995a).

The RCPs must aggressively set up respiratory-care services outside the traditional hospital setting. Department managers should look into establishing services in sub-acute units at SNFs, offering pulmonary rehabilitation at outpatient sites, or providing respiratory care in the home. Department managers must develop and sell business plans for respiratory care at alternate sites, then negotiate clinical-service contracts with these facilities. Integrated health-care delivery allows department heads to retain and even expand staffing levels, augment their scope of services, and **cross-train** their employees. Cross-training empowers employees to become multiskilled or competent, which helps them to maintain and perhaps ensure the integrity of their departments (Bunch, 1995a).

INDEPENDENT PRACTICE ASSOCIATIONS

The IPAs are legal entities or organizations established by physicians who have contracted with a managed-care plan to provide services for an agreed-upon capitation rate. The IPA acts as the bargaining unit for individual physicians who agree to provide services on a capitation or fee-for-service basis. The IPAs may also be thought of as medical-management groups that coordinate the delivery of health-care services to beneficiaries enrolled in an HMO.

PHYSICIAN HOSPITAL ORGANIZATIONS

The PHOs are informal but legal entities that bring hospitals and their attending medical staffs together. A PHO is usually developed to contract with a managed-care plan. At minimum, it allows a hospital and its physicians to negotiate with third-party payers. It is open to any member of the medical staff who applies, or it may be closed to those who fail to qualify.

The PHOs considered by the health-care industry as the earliest type of vertically integrated system, often form because of market forces brought on by managed care. They are actively involved with managing the relationship between providers and MCOs, or they may provide additional services, which brings them closer to being MSOs (Kongstvedt, 1995).

MANAGEMENT SERVICE ORGANIZATIONS

The MSOs are legally separate entities that are like service bureaus that provide practice-management services to physicians, hospitals, or physician-hospital organizations. The MSOs may own a medical facility or buy certain assets of a physician's practice, then provide services to the facility or physician at fair market rates. The MSOs, a form of integrated health-care delivery system, came about as a means to contract with managed-care organizations more effectively.

EXCLUSIVE PROVIDER ORGANIZATIONS

Exclusive provider organizations (EPOs) are managed-care plans that are like HMOs in that they use primary-care physicians as gatekeepers (except in emergencies, all care from providers other than the primary-care physician must be authorized before it is delivered), capitate services, and have limited provider networks. The EPOs require those enrolled in the plan to use the PPO-like provider network exclusively. Any care outside the network is the enrolled beneficiary's responsibility. The EPOs differ from HMOs in that physicians do not receive capitation but are reimbursed for the medical services they provide. As a result, EPOs are regulated under general insurance statutes instead of HMO regulations. Some states regard EPOs as HMOs.

MEDICAL SAVINGS ACCOUNTS

Medical savings accounts is one approach Congress has proposed to help curtail Medicare spending. Under this proposal, as of 2002, the federal government would pay beneficiaries choosing this method up to $5000 for a health-insurance plan with a deductible as high as $2000. Another $1700, the remainder of the government's $6700 contribution per recipient, would be placed in a tax-sheltered savings account each participant could use to pay medical bills or to save for future medical expenses. This proposal is currently in the planning stages and needs further consideration.

EMPLOYER HEALTH PLANS

Congress has also proposed employer health plans to reduce Medicare expenditures. Under this plan, beneficiaries would continue in the health-insurance plans their employers sponsored before they retired. The government would assume the first $6700 of the cost. Depending on the program, the employer or the recipient would assume any additional costs. Like medical savings accounts, employer health plans is only a proposal that Congress must approve before it can be implemented.

IMPACT ON RESPIRATORY CARE

The terms and concepts in this chapter describe some of the far-reaching effects health-care reform and managed care have had on the health-care industry. The effects health-care reform and managed care have had on respiratory care are just as profound. The respiratory-care profession must continually redefine and reestablish its role in the ever-changing health-care climate to remain viable. In March 1996 the AARC's Board of Directors voted to appropriate $1 million to document the economic and clinical impact of RCPs in traditional settings, as well as the impact of RCPs in their expanded roles in subacute care, SNFs, and home care. In a related area, the AARC's Task Force on Professional Direction will assume a number of research projects covering the 3-year period from 1996 to 1999 to document the role and value of RCPs. The Task Force's projects will focus on the:

- use of clinical practice guidelines (CPGs), especially by technical directors;
- RCP roles in primary care, case management, and demand management; and
- development of a skills inventory for successfully practicing respiratory care in managed health care (American Association for Respiratory Care [AARC], 1996).

Organizations are studying the RCP's role and value because positions in hospital-based respiratory-care departments have decreased while positions at alternate sites have increased both in number and in scope. It is safe to assume this trend will continue. The need for multicompetent or multiskilled practitioners will probably also continue to grow through cross-training, both inside and outside the hospital. Large companies and organizations worldwide may use the term *cross-training* with a negative connotation, but in respiratory care, cross-training is a way to survive the present economical and professional turmoil caused by health-care reform and managed care.

The following case study demonstrates how hospital-inspired changes can bring about profound and meaningful results that can enhance the value and effectiveness of respiratory care.

CASE STUDY

Downsizing Causes Respiratory Care Services to Be Provided at Alternate Sites

Because of changes in hospital reimbursement due to health-care reform and managed care, some hospitals throughout the country have considered downsizing to stay financially solvent. The director of respiratory care at a small community hospital in the southeastern United States had to adjust to the changes downsizing the hospital caused. Because this hospital was one of three within a small city, hospital administration believed downsizing was needed to keep the hospital in the community. Staffing cuts on all levels were discussed and planned.

The director of the respiratory-care department responded by deciding to institute a pulmonary rehabilitation program and involve a local respiratory-home-care company. As a result, department staffing remained intact and the hospital realized additional revenues. Activity in the pulmonary function laboratory increased, care for the chronic respiratory patient improved and expanded, and job satisfaction increased.

1. This respiratory-care department manager had to respond to threats to staffing and the department overall. How important is it for managers to do their "homework" on existing and possible respiratory-care services in a community or specific geographical area?
2. What specific training would the staff need to provide effective pulmonary rehabilitation and home-care services?
3. What would be the impact on the pulmonary function laboratory?

New opportunities are opening to the respiratory-care profession because of managed care and the hospital restructuring stemming from health-care reform. Some areas have been explored, while others are uncharted by most RCPs. The remainder of this chapter considers some of the RCP's professional paths, namely discharge planning, case management, patient-centered care, therapist-driven protocols (TDPs), and cross-training and multicompetency.

DISCHARGE PLANNING

Discharge planning, as defined by the AARC in its clinical practice guideline (CPG) on discharge planning for the respiratory care patient (1995b), is the development and implementation of a comprehensive plan for the safe discharge of the respiratory-care patient from a health-care facility and for the patient's continuing safe and effective care at an alternate site. Traditionally, the responsibility for discharge planning rested with social workers or registered nurses with the social-service department. These individuals would service the total needs of the patient, including respiratory needs. However, with advances in equipment and the levels of care, discharge planning has become more patient specific.

Because of this evolution, which was facilitated partly by managed care, the discharge-planning process has become one area of involvement for the RCP, particularly when patients with diagnosed cardiopulmonary dysfunction or disease are involved.

According to the CPG, the discharge plan guides a multidisciplinary effort to successfully transfer the patient from the health-care facility to the alternate site. The plan ensures the safety and efficacy of the respiratory-care patient's continuing care. Elements of the discharge plan include:

- evaluating the patient to ensure discharge is appropriate;
- determining the optimal site of care and identifying patient-care resources; and
- establishing that financial resources are adequate.

Discharge planning is indicated for all respiratory-care patients who are eligible for discharge or transfer to any alternate-site setting, including the home. Undesirable or unexpected outcomes may occur when early discharge occurs before the discharge plan is fully implemented. Planning and implementation should begin as early as possible. Plan complexity depends on the patient's condition, needs, and goals. Steps in the CPG discharge-planning process include:

- patient evaluation, which includes the need for ventilatory support, the patient's physical and functional capacity and need for other forms of respiratory care, the psychosocial conditions of the patient and his or her family, and goals of care from the perspective of the patient and the health-care team;
- site evaluation, which is dictated by the patient's goals and needs and must consider the resources available at the alternate site, like personnel, equipment, and physical environment;
- evaluation of financial resources (inadequate or nonexistent funding impacts the discharge plan and can determine the care site);
- development of the care plan;
- education and training of key personnel and demonstration of essential competencies; and
- consideration of limitations, which includes the patient's medical condition, the lack of a care site, the lack of resources, the lack of family cooperation, and the failure to identify all pertinent problems.

The CPG also addresses the importance of assessing need and outcome, identifying and acquiring all essential resources, and monitoring the progress of the plan by both the discharge-plan coordinator and the physician. The AARC discharge planning CPG presents specific criteria and guidelines for practitioners assuming the responsibility of planning the discharge of a respiratory patient to an alternate-care site (AARC, 1995b).

CASE MANAGEMENT

Case management is another area where RCPs can be involved and have an impact, especially when dealing with the ongoing care of chronic cardiorespiratory patients. Case management entails coordinating patient care through designated case managers to ensure the level of health care is appropriate and to reduce the costs of providing this care. Case management is practiced within the continuum of care that meets the ongoing needs of patients in environments that range from acute care to subacute care to the home. Case managers must interact effectively with all integral members of the patient's health-care team, including physicians, other health-care providers, family, and third-party payors. Frequently case management involves catastrophic or high-cost medical conditions.

A coalition of case-management organizations, which counts RCPs, nurses, social workers, and rehabilitation professionals among its 20,000 members, has defined specific duties of case managers to include:

- performing patient assessments and data collection;
- selecting the most appropriate site for care (e.g., acute, subacute, rehabilitation, or home); and
- determining the need for other health care and/or psychological services (Gibbons, 1995a).

Case managers are credentialed as certified case managers (CCM) through the Commission for Case Management Certification (CCMC). The credentialing examination is administered by the Certification of Insurance Rehabilitation Specialists Commission for the CCMC. Past eligibility standards made it difficult for non-nurses to qualify, because no respiratory licensure or credentialing examination had a bachelor-degree requirement. The selection criteria and certification process have been revised and now involve a three-step process.

Licensure or Certification. An applicant's license or certification must be based on the minimum educational requirements of a post-secondary program in a field that promotes the physical, psychological, or vocational well-being of the individuals served. This license or certificate is obtained by passing an examination in the applicant's area of specialization. In addition, through this license or certificate, candidates must be able to legally perform six patient-centered, core components of case management without the supervision of another licensed health-care professional. These six core components are: (1) assessing, (2) planning, (3) implementing, (4) coordinating, (5) monitoring, and (6) evaluating. Candidates applying for the certification examination must also be able to document the following for each core component:

- involvement in coordination and delivery of services;
- applicable physical and psychological factors;
- benefit systems and analysis of cost benefit;
- related case-management concepts; and
- related community resources.

Employment Experience. Candidates must be able to document acceptable employment experience as a case manager under one of the following work-related categories:

Category 1: 12 months of acceptable full-time employment under the supervision of a CCM or equivalent.

Category 2: 24 months of acceptable full-time employment or equivalent. Supervision by a CCM is not required.

Category 3: 12 months of acceptable full-time employment supervising the activities of individuals who provide direct case-management services or equivalent.

Certification Examination. Candidates who meet the licensure or certification and employment criteria established by the CCMC must sit for and achieve a passing score on the nationally administered examination to obtain the CCM designation (Bunch, 1996).

In addition to completing the three-step process, all candidates applying for the certification examination must be of good moral character, reputation, and fitness to practice case management. The fee for the examination is $125, and applications must be in by mid-January for the June exam (Gibbons, 1995a). Requirements for the CCM examination, including work-related criteria, are solid.

PATIENT-CENTERED CARE

In patient-centered care, all available resources are pooled to try to make patient care more efficient, cost effective, and responsive to patient needs. A patient-centered care hospital floor or unit would be staffed with nurses, X-ray technicians, physical therapists, lab personnel and RCPs to meet the daily needs of patients on that unit. Questions regarding staffing and coverage may arise when any of the following occur:

- members of the team or unit are ill, on vacation, or on leaves of absence;
- the patient census increases or decreases;
- the patient mix or acuity levels change(s); and
- emergencies arise requiring additional personnel.

Most of these problems can be avoided by budgeting appropriately, using optimal staffing patterns, and implementing contingency plans for emergencies. However, if staffing concerns are not properly addressed, they could adversely impact patient care and the delivery of related health-care services.

Another area of contention in patient-centered care is the training and use of unlicensed assistive personnel (UAP), who are also called patient care technicians (PCTs), patient care associates (PCAs) or clinical associates. The primary purpose of UAP is to relieve nurses and other practitioners of some of their duties and responsibilities. At some hospitals and medical centers throughout the country, UAP are noncredentialed nurse assistants or aides who perform phlebotomy, electrocardiograms, low-flow oxygen setups, incentive spirometry, and pulse oximetry (Brody, 1996). In these specific cases, units or floors are staffed by three-member teams caring for up to ten patients. The first member of the team is a registered nurse (RN) who functions as unit administrator. The second member is a UAP or PCT who is supervised by the RN and provides routine patient care. The third member of the team is a support associate who prepares patient rooms, keeps medical records in order, and performs other related duties (Gibbons, 1995b).

The training of UAP or clinical associates may be suspect. The first issue to be addressed relates to the individual's background and overall experience. The second relates to state licensure requirements. State licensure laws may be violated by the UAP's duties and scope of professional practice. Finally there are the issues of the length of training, usually 6 to 8 weeks, and the documentation of competency levels. Unless these issues are addressed properly, patient care may be less than adequate and at marginal cost savings.

In response to these concerns, Congress mandated the Institute of Medicine, a nonprofit research agency, to conduct a nationwide study on nurse staffing and its effect on hospital-based patient care. This study, completed in 1996, found no empirical evidence to back any claims that patient care was suffering as a result of the increasing use of UAP. Nonetheless, the study was "greatly concerned" about the lack of training standards, the testing and certification of ancillary nursing personnel as UAP, and the possible negative impact this practice might have on patient care (Brody, 1996).

Patient-centered care is collecting a growing number of critics, and its long-term impact on the delivery of health care is unknown. Implementing patient-centered care as part of hospital restructuring and decentralization, including managed care, is an ongoing issue and a source of concern for many health-care providers and the health-care industry in general.

THERAPIST-DRIVEN PROTOCOLS

Therapist-driven protocols (TDPs) or patient-driven protocols, which are a way to deliver patient care based on standards, are flourishing within the managed-care environment. When in place and used properly, TDPs can enhance and improve the quality of patient care, help lower operating costs, and create more job satisfaction (Gibbons, 1995b). However, TDPs require additional education and preparation through cross-training in the areas of patient assessment and the timing and quality of clinical decisions.

CROSS-TRAINING AND MULTICOMPETENCY

To meet the needs of the fluctuating job market and the restructuring of the health-care delivery system, formal educational programs will have to be redesigned. There will be a changing patient population, more cases of patient-centered approaches assessment and care, and greater emphasis on research (Barr, 1992). In addition, cross-training and multi-competency will become "watch words," and clinical experiences will include rotations in home care, nursing homes, rehabilitation centers, subacute and extended-care facilities, and perhaps even physician offices. Student practitioners' clinical skills and competencies will stress pulmonary function testing and cardiopulmonary stress evaluations. Bronchial provocation and sleep testing will also be covered, and greater emphasis will be placed on emergency airway management, fiberoptic bronchoscopy, hyperbaric oxygen delivery, and proficiency in A-line insertion, central venous pressure (CVP) lines, Swan-Ganz catheters, and balloon pump management. In neonatal intensive care units, required skills will include operating or working with high-frequency oscillators, neonatal monitors, patient transport, and surfactant delivery. Throughout the country, educational programs and hospital departments are already gearing up to provide students and staff with the training needed to perform these highly technical skills (Lesperance, 1995).

Other skills practitioners will have to acquire as a part of cross-training will include phlebotomy, intravenous (IV) insertion and maintenance, chest radiography, allergy testing, tuberculin skin testing, electrocardiography, holter monitoring, and other cardiovascular tests. Practitioners will also have to perform laboratory procedures like measuring theophylline levels via radio-immunoassay (RIA) techniques. These skills and procedures demand that respiratory-care curriculum and its structure and presentation change. In the past, multicompetency would have been on par with "jack of all trades, master of none," but today it means survival and potential for career growth and opportunity.

Some health-care practitioners believe the health-care market is evolving three levels of multiskilled practitioners:

1. *Low-level multiskilled practitioners* provide basic patient support services and requires 3 to 12 weeks of training. These practitioners are UAP or PCAs.
2. *Mid-level multiskilled practitioners* hold multiple credentials from formal training programs and can function competently at varied delivery settings. These practitioners are typically RCPs.
3. *High-level multiskilled practitioners* hold bachelors or higher degrees and can practice independently or semi-independently in at least two or more different competency areas. Nurse practitioners are examples (Scanlan, 1996).

Because of this evolution, respiratory-care programs must be able to address the career needs of RCPs, especially at the mid and high levels of multiskilling. This calls for curriculum redesign and additional course offerings, which will also make RCPs more marketable in any health-care facility or setting.

The following case study illustrates the need for curriculum redesign in the face of new job opportunities, both in and out of the hospital. Curriculum redesign is labor intensive but essential if practitioners are to be properly prepared for respiratory-care employment.

CASE STUDY

Restructured Job Market Calls for Curriculum Redesign

In light of the changing job marketplace, a respiratory-care program director at a community college in the Northeast decided to change the respiratory-care curriculum. All indicators, including the program's advisory committee, had demonstrated that full-time positions in local hospitals were scarce. To better prepare graduates for employment in the field, the program director and faculty placed greater emphasis on pulmonary rehabilitation, pulmonary function testing, home care, and subacute care. These curriculum changes were instituted both in the classroom and clinically.

In addition, college staff taught multicompetent skills that included phlebotomy, IV insertion and management, electrocardiograms, skin allergy and tuberculin testing, hemodynamic monitoring, and other related skills. Multiskilled graduates found they were better equipped to assume positions in pulmonary diagnostics, home care, subacute care, and pulmonary rehabilitation.

1. What are some of the key components to changing respiratory-care curricula that are described in this case study?
2. What added responsibilities are placed on the faculty when curricula are changed?
3. Why is it important to have an active and diverse respiratory-care program advisory committee? Who should sit on program advisory committees?

Change should not be perceived as negative. Change is the opportunity for growth. While some respiratory-care departments have relinquished simple oxygen and aerosol therapy for more highly technical and demanding responsibilities, others have continued simpler therapeutic modalities while assuming more complex and specialized regimens. Becoming an active player in this change will help to ensure the RCP remains viable in health-care delivery into the twenty-first century (Lesperance, 1995).

PEW FOUNDATION HEALTH PROFESSIONS COMMISSION

In October 1991, the Pew Foundation Health Professions Commission, a program of the Pew Charitable Trusts, published a document entitled, "Healthy America: Practitioners for 2005—An Agenda for Action for U.S. Health Professional Schools." Its purpose was to assist schools of allied health, dentistry, medicine, nursing, pharmacy, public health, and veterinary medicine to develop mission statements and related programs that responded to the changing needs of health care in America. The basic issue the Pew Commission addressed was ensuring today's students would be able to contribute and succeed in tomorrow's revolutionary and ever-changing health-care environment. It believed that health-care practitioners ought to be doing what they are not doing today (Sorbello, 1995).

In addition to the "Healthy America" document, the Commission published seventeen competencies it felt practitioners should develop and possess. These competencies included delivering contemporary clinical care, emphasizing primary care, participating in coordinated care, promoting healthy lifestyles and disease prevention, managing information, counseling on ethical issues, participating in a culturally diverse society, and continuing education. Some principles the Pew Commission identified involved improving curricula, expanding knowledge and skills, promoting inquiry skills, health, and disease prevention, developing faculty, and cross-training students with multiskilling or multicompetency levels. With these strategies, it is believed health professionals will learn to practice more effectively with greater patient and professional satisfaction (Sorbello, 1995).

While its ideas may be sound, the Pew Commission has encountered strong resistance to multiskilling. As a result, hospital administrators have been acting on their own to help ensure the workforce will meet the health-care needs of their patients. The second Pew Commission report was released toward the end of Phase One of the Pew Initiative. It was entitled "Health Professions Education for the Future: Schools in Service to the Nation," and it underscored the need for new attitudes and new approaches in health-professions education (Selker, 1993).

In November 1995, the Pew Commission released its third report, "Critical Challenges: Revitalizing the Health Professions for the Twenty-First Century." According to this report, health-care's organizational, financial, and legal framework has been transformed into a system of integrated care. This new system, which combines primary care, specialty care, and hospital services, has also produced the following difficulties for the health-care professions:

- closure of half the nation's hospitals, with a corresponding loss of 60 percent of hospital beds;
- expansion of primary care in ambulatory and community settings;
- surplus of up to 150,000 physicians as the demand for specialization shrinks, a surplus of up to 300,000 nurses as hospitals close, and a surplus of 40,000 pharmacists as the dispensing of drugs become automatized and centralized;
- consolidation of up to 200 allied-health professions into multiskilled professions;
- demands for public-health professionals to meet the needs of a market-driven health-care system; and
- alteration of health-professional schools and the ways in which those schools organize, structure, and frame their education, research, and patient-care activities.

This third report from the Pew Commission report concluded that restrictions imposed by accreditation, licensure, and professionalism limit the development of allied-health personnel as multiskilled practitioners. It also found that nonexclusionary state laws and regulations foster advanced practice. This characteristic will be essential to surviving in the changing health-care marketplace (Eicher, 1996).

SUMMARY

Health-care reform, although never formally passed by Congress, is having far-reaching effects on the health-care industry and specifically on health-care delivery. An integral component of the health-care reform movement is managed care, a dynamic and multifaceted concept that many believe is permanent. Escalating health-care costs and the need for all members of society to have access to quality health care have brought about these changes. The RCPs are seeing the impact of these changes in the forms of hospital restructuring, reimbursement for health-care services and delivery, and the virtual explosion of alternate-site care. Consequently, there will be new and even more demanding opportunities at alternate sites like diagnostic/rehabilitative centers, subacute and extended-care facilities, industry, and the home. Multicompetency or multiskilling will be required in the new job marketplace and formal educational programs will have to redesign their curricula to include cross-training if they are to prepare practitioners for new positions and responsibilities. Taking an active role is essential for surviving these changing and challenging times.

Review Questions

1. Which societal factors have brought about the need for health-care reform?
2. What is *managed care*, and how does it relate to the concept of health-care reform?
3. Name and briefly describe four types of managed-care organizations.
4. What factors in health-care delivery have caused the increase in alternate-site care, and what job opportunities exist for RCPs?
5. What is meant by *hospital restructuring?* What impact has hospital restructuring had on respiratory care?
6. What is meant by *patient-centered care*, and what role should respiratory care play?
7. Discuss the implications of an integrated health-care delivery system in today's' health-care market.
8. What is meant by *seamless patient care?*
9. Differentiate between multicompetency and cross-training, and state the importance of each to respiratory care.

References

Aday, L., Andersen, R., & Fleming, G. (1980). Health care in the U.S.: Equitable for whom? Beverly Hills: Sage.

American Association for Respiratory Care. (1995a). AARC chartered affiliate restructuring survey. Dallas, TX: AARC.

American Association for Respiratory Care. (1995b, December). AARC Clinical Practice Guideline. Discharge planning for the respiratory care patient. *Respiratory Care, 40*(12), 1308–1312.

American Association for Respiratory Care. (1996, April). $1,000,000 commitment announced. Task force to study RC under managed care. *AARC Report,* 1.

Barr, J. (1992, October 2–4). The restructuring of the American health care delivery system. Year 2001: Delineating the educational direction for the future respiratory care practitioner. *Proceedings of a National Concensus Conference on Respiratory Care Education,* 24–31. Dallas, TX: American Association for Respiratory Care.

Beck, M., Thomas, R., & Hager, M. (1995, September 18). The new fine print. *Newsweek, 126*(12), 42.

Brody, L. (1996, April 28). Aides taking on more nursing duties. *The Sunday Record, 101*(47), pp. A1, A6.

Brown, C. (1995, October 11). Memorandum to home care section members (AARC). Legislative alert. Washington, DC.

Bunch, D. (1995a, June). RCPs and integrated health care systems. *AARCTimes, 19*(6), 24–28.

Bunch, D. (1995b, July). Restructuring doesn't always mean downsizing: RC managers find positives in hospital redesign. *AARCTimes, 19*(7), 22.

Bunch, D. (1996, April). Eligibility criteria for taking the case manager certification examination are revised. *AARCTimes, 20*(4), 64–65.

Business Insurance Magazine. (1993, February 27).

Clark, L.J. (1996, Summer). Challenges of the home oxygen services coalition in 1996. *Home Care Section Bulletin, 2,* 7. American Association for Respiratory Care.

Congressional Budget Office. (1994, January). *The Economic and Budget Outlook,* 39.

Daus, C. (1995, June/July). Staffing in an era of change. *RT—The Journal for Respiratory Care Practitioners, 8*(4), 75–76.

Directory of Operational PPOs. (1992). Chicago: SMG Marketing Group.

Dubbs, W.H., & Weber, K. (1995, December 3). Quantitating the impact of restructuring. *Convention Gazette,* 1, 6–7. Dallas, TX. American Association for Respiratory Care.

Eicher, J. (1995a, January). Respiratory care under Medicaid managed care. *AARCTimes, 19*(1), 9.

Eicher, J. (1995b, February). The role of respiratory care in state health care workforce reform. *AARCTimes, 19*(2), 8, 62.

Eicher, J. (1996, February). Pew health professions commission releases report on workforce reform. *AARCTimes, 20*(2), 11–12.

Epstein, R. (1995, September 4). Is managed care the cure for Medicare? *The Record, 101*(79), p. H3.

Epstein, R. (1996, February 12). Medicare HMOs appear attractive. *The Record, 101*(217), p. H3.

Espo, D. (1995, September 22). Medicare under knife. *The Record, 101*(95), 1.

Fineman, H. (1995, September 18). Mediscare. *Newsweek, 126*(12), 38.

Foster Higgins and Company, Inc. [organization] (1995). New York: Consulting Firm.

Gibbons, M. (1995a, January/February). Revamping care. *Advance for Respiratory Care Managers, 4*(1), 19.

Gibbons, M. (1995b, October 16). RCPs open doors of opportunity for new roles as case managers. *Advance for Respiratory Care Practitioners, 8*(21), 5, 11.

Group Health Association of America. (1992, December). HMOs and managed care: The measure of health care reform. *HMO Fact Sheet.* Washington, DC: GHAA.

Hall, L. (1995, June/July). Cardiac rehabilitation in an era of managed care. *RT—The Journal for Respiratory Care Practitioners, 8*(4), 34.

The hospital of 2005 will use multi-skilled practitioners. (1995, September). *AARCTImes, 19*(9), 33.

Kongstvedt, P.R. (1995). *Essentials of managed health care.* Gaithersburg, MD: Aspen Publishers.

Leaperance, K. (1995, September 18). RCPs cross-train today to provide tomorrow's high tech respiratory care. *Advance for Respiratory Care Practitioners, 8*(19), 5.

Meade, K.M. (1997, April). Taking the risk out of Medicare HMOs. *Advance for Directors in Rehabilitation, 6*(4), 47.

Prospective Payment Assessment Commission. (1994, June). Medicare and the American health care system. *Report to the Congress.* Washington, DC.

Prospective Payment Assessment Commission. (1995, March 1). Medicare and the evolving health care system. *Report and Recommendations to the Congress.* Washington, DC.

Rosenblatt, R.A. (1995, September 10). GOP to unveil Medicare reforms. *The Sunday Record, 101*(14), p. A20.

Samuelson, R.J. (1995, September 18). Getting serious. *Newsweek, 126*(12), 40–41.

Scanlan, C.L. (1996, April). Using the Newark respiratory care programs as the base for training multiskilled health practitioners. *1996 Annual Report for Respiratory Care Programs* 1–2. Newark, NJ: UMDNJ-SHRP.

Selker, L.G. (1993, October 15–17). Health reform through educational reform—Strategies outlined by the Pew health professions commission. Year 2001: An action agenda. *Proceedings of the Second National Concensus Conference on Respiratory Care Education*, 20–28. Bethesda, MD: American Association for Respiratory Care.

Sorbello, J. (1995, Spring). Healthy America: Practitioners for 2005—The Pew Health Professions Commission. *Focus—Journal for Respiratory Care Managers and Educators*, 22–26.

Spragins, E. (1996, June 24). Does your HMO stack up? *Newsweek, 127*(26), 56–58.

Terrill, T.E. (1995, April 12). Health care delivery systems. *Compilation of Data* 56–58. Newark, NJ: UMDNJ.

Suggested Readings

Brook, R.H. (1994). Health care reform is on the way: Do we want to compete on quality? *Annals of Internal Medicine, 120*(1).

Bunch, D. (1995, May). Respiratory care career opportunities shift to alternate care sites. *AARCTimes, 19*(5).

Bunch, D. (1995, June). RCPs find opportunities in sleep diagnostics and monitoring. *AARCTimes, 19*(6).

Bunch, D. (1996, May). A look at restructuring in health care, corporate American. *AARCTimes, 20*(5), 41–43.

Eicher, J. (1995, December). Workforce regulation and cross-training. *AARCTimes, 19*(12), 29.

Gulliford, D.E. (1996, May). Middle-managers' survival guide: Career strategies under managed care. *AARCTimes, 20*(5), 50–52.

Lesperance, K. (1995, October 2). State-of-the-art equipment, therapies proliferate in non-traditional settings. *Advance for Respiratory Care Practitioners, 8*(20), 5, 38.

Marshall, K. (1995). Multiskilling: Re-engineering work process. *Healthcare Management Forum, 8*(2), 32–36.

O'Daniel, C. (1995, March). Health care skill standards and multiskilling: Implications for respiratory care education. *AARCTimes, 19*(3), 8–14.

Shrake, K.L. (1994, June). Strategies for developing the multicompetent respiratory care practitioner. *AARCTimes, 18*(6), 21–23.

Thomas-Payne, L. (1995, May). Government moves to managed care. *HomeCare, 17*(5).

U.S. Department of Health and Human Services. (1995). *Report of the National Commission on Allied Health.* Rockville, MD: U.S. Department of Health and Human Services, Public Health Service, Health Resources and Services Administration, Bureau of Health Professions, Division of Associated, Dental and Public Health Professions.

White, G. (1995, May). Retooling an educational program to meet the needs of the future. *AARCTimes, 19*(5), 76.

CHAPTER TWO

PAST AND CURRENT CONCEPTS OF PULMONARY REHABILITATION

KEY TERMS
---

activities of daily living
(ADL)
cardiac rehabilitation

Comprehensive
Outpatient Rehabilitation
Facility (CORF)
Health Care Financing
Administration (HCFA)

oxygen consumption
physical reconditioning
pulmonary rehabilitation

OBJECTIVES

Upon completing this chapter, the reader will be able to:

- Define *pulmonary rehabilitation.*
- Differentiate between pulmonary rehabilitation and cardiac rehabilitation.
- Discuss the rationale for pulmonary rehabilitation in terms of the interdependence of pulmonary function, cardiovascular status, and physical conditioning.
- State the major goal of pulmonary rehabilitation and its two principal objectives.
- Describe the impact comprehensive outpatient rehabilitation facilities (CORFs) have had on pulmonary rehabilitation.
- Explain the impact health-care reform has had on the growth and acceptance of pulmonary rehabilitation.

INTRODUCTION

The advent of health-care reform, managed care, and hospital restructuring in the 1990s have significantly shifted the delivery of respiratory care from the hospital to alternate sites like subacute and extended-care facilities, specialty centers, and the home. This shift in the delivery of care has also changed attitudes regarding how continuing respiratory care can be provided. Subacute care, home care, and **pulmonary rehabilitation** help make up the entity known as continuing care, which in turn has benefited from this change in attitude and renewed interest in alternate-site care.

Significant focus has been placed on the rehabilitation and reconditioning of the chronic lung patient, both in the hospital and at alternate sites. Many of these alternate sites, which cater to an ever-increasing outpatient population, now offer pulmonary-rehabilitation programs to help meet the needs of patients with chronic pulmonary disease. This chapter examines the past and current concepts of pulmonary rehabilitation and prepares for further study and discussion in subsequent chapters.

KEY DEFINITIONS AND CONCEPTS

In 1942, the Council on Rehabilitation defined *rehabilitation* as "the restoration of the individual to the fullest medical, mental, emotional, social, and vocational potential of which he/she is capable." This general definition depicted a process of returning individuals to particular levels or states of health. It did not imply the individuals had any particular dysfunctions or impairments. In 1974, the Committee on Pulmonary Rehabilitation of the American College of Chest Physicians (ACCP) became more specific and adopted the following definition:

> Pulmonary rehabilitation may be defined as an art of medical practice wherein an individually tailored, multidisciplinary program is formulated which, through accurate diagnosis, therapy, emotional support, and education, stabilizes or reverses both the physio- and psychopathology of pulmonary disease and attempts to return the patient to the highest possible functional capacity allowed by his/her pulmonary handicap and overall life situation (American Thoracic Society Executive Committee, 1981).

The key concepts in this definition are those of accurate diagnosis and patient evaluation, coupled with a multidisciplinary approach to stabilize and restore a patient's functional capacity. This ACCP definition formed the basis for an official statement on pulmonary rehabilitation, which was adopted by the American Thoracic Society (ATS) Executive Committee in 1981.

In 1977, AARC formed specialty sections, including one for rehabilitation and continuing care, now called the Continuing Care—Rehabilitation section. As with the other specialty sections, the Continuing Care—Rehabilitation section served as a consultant to the AARC, provided resource pools for primary and secondary research, served as a clearinghouse for information specific to the specialty, and helped play an integral role in communicating with and bringing people into the career of respiratory care (Eiserman, 1987). This specialty section has expanded the definition of pulmonary rehabilitation to include elements of patient education and an augmented role for the RCP. Because of increased specialization in this area, home care and subacute care, which were part of the Continuing Care—Rehabilitation section, formed separate specialty sections.

The many definitions of pulmonary rehabilitation that exist today encompass some very basic concepts and components, including:

- following a multidisciplinary approach in involving different health specialties;
- aiming to have pulmonary patients function as normally as possible;

- fostering medical direction and involvement; and
- tailoring multiple forms of treatment and approaches to patients' specific needs.

In most instances, pulmonary rehabilitation is aimed at chronic lung patients, especially those with asthma and COPD, but it is also a viable option for ventilator-dependent and quadriplegic patients. These special cases present enormous challenges to the RCPs who must work effectively within the health-care team on patients who cannot breathe on their own. Regardless of the type of patient in need of reconditioning, pulmonary rehabilitation involves education, breathing retraining, and physical conditioning through exercise.

PULMONARY VERSUS CARDIAC REHABILITATION

Pulmonary rehabilitation and cardiac rehabilitation differ based on which organ has diminished capacity. Pulmonary patients have exercise limitation due to dyspnea resulting from primary pulmonary impairment and dysfunction, a very low exercise tolerance, and, in most cases, pulmonary symptoms like cyanosis, desaturation, or wheezing with physical activity. In contrast, cardiac patients can perform greater amounts of work and are not limited solely by dyspnea.

Cardiac rehabilitation is a comprehensive education and exercise program designed to improve the cardiovascular fitness of patients with known cardiac dysfunction. Like pulmonary rehabilitation, cardiac rehabilitation requires a stress test to evaluate patient condition and status. Both programs are multidisciplinary, incorporate patient education and physical exercise, and are reimbursable by insurance. Basic equipment used during the exercise sessions of both programs, namely treadmills, exercycles, and arm ergometers, and space requirements are essentially the same. Differences between the two lie on patient focus and monitoring during exercise. Cardiac exercise programs are more concerned with patient pulse, blood pressure, and electrocardiogram via telemetry. Pulmonary patients are monitored for pulse rate, respiratory rate, oxygen saturation, and peak flow rates during exercise.

HISTORICAL PERSPECTIVE

Pulmonary rehabilitation has a rather poorly defined history and cannot be traced to one event or specific date. Its earliest roots can be tracked to the early 1950s when Alvan L. Barach, MD (the father of modern physiological therapy for COPD patients), commented that, "The progressive improvement in ability to walk without dyspnea suggested that a physiologic response similar to a training program in athletes may have been produced" (Barach, 1952). At that time, the clinical community was skeptical of any notion that lung patients should exercise and train to try to regain some degree of physical conditioning lost due to pulmonary dysfunction or impairment. It was not until 1962, only 10 years after Barach's observations, that the first study refuting the then-popular opinion that patients with COPD should rest and avoid stress was published (Hughes, 1983).

The study, by Dr. Alan Pierce and associates, demonstrated the now widely accepted concept that patients with COPD can undergo **physical reconditioning** to perform exercises with lower heart rates, respiratory rates, minute ventilation, and carbon dioxide production. The term *recondition* comes from Latin meaning, "to put back together." Studies by Paez and Christie confirmed that these positive changes were the result of improved efficiency of motion and oxygen use and could be achieved on an outpatient basis with minor supervision (Hughes, 1983).

Early rehabilitative measures and programs for patients with chronic lung disease were implemented in the hospital or at home with prescribed respiratory therapy and related home-care equipment. Such early attempts produced meaningful results and were promising enough for the medical profession to pursue the concept of pulmonary rehabilitation. Table 2–1 identifies some of the major studies published since the late 1960s involving pulmonary rehabilitation and documented patient outcomes.

PROFESSIONAL STANDARDS AND STATEMENTS

As discussed previously, the ACCP, AARC, and ATS have all adopted and/or published a definition or standard of pulmonary rehabilitation. To continue advancing pulmonary rehabilitation in terms of programs, services, professional practice, networking, and continuing education, the American Association of Cardiovascular and Pulmonary Rehabilitation (AACVPR) was incorporated in 1983. Headquartered in Middleton, Wisconsin, the AACVPR has developed a network of state affiliates. The AACVPR brings professional and public attention to the importance of pulmonary rehabilitation through its national pulmonary rehabilitation week celebrated in March every year and publications like the *Journal of Cardiopulmonary Rehabilitation* and the Association newsletter, *News and Views*. The AACVPR also maintains a directory of rehabilitation programs throughout the

TABLE 2–1 Some of the earlier clinical studies which have influenced the development and acceptance of pulmonary rehabilitation

Publication Date	Investigator(s)	Focus of Study
1967	Paez, Phillipson, Masangkay, and Sproule	Physiologic basis of training patients with emphysema
1968	Christie	Physical training in chronic obstructive lung disease
1970	Nicholas, Gilbert, Gabe, and Auchincloss	Evaluation of exercise therapy for patients with COPD
1971	Vyas, Banister, Morton, and Grzybowski	Response to exercise in patients with chronic airway obstruction
1977	McGavin, Gupta, Lloyd, and McHardy	Physical rehabilitation for the chronic bronchitic; results of controlled trial of exercises in the home
1980	Moser, Bokinsky, Savage, Archibald, and Hansen	Results of a comprehensive rehabilitation program

More detailed information about these studies, including sources, may be found in the Suggested Readings section at the end of this chapter.

The AACVPR also maintains a directory of rehabilitation programs throughout the United States.

In 1987, the AACVPR and AARC conducted the first joint national survey (discussed in detail in Chapter 4) to determine the extent of pulmonary rehabilitation programs in the United States in terms of numbers, design, and scope. Subsequent surveys continue to demonstrate steady growth in and acceptance of pulmonary rehabilitation as a viable therapeutic modality. A number of major developments have significantly contributed to this trend.

COMPREHENSIVE OUTPATIENT REHABILITATION FACILITIES

In December 1982, the **Health Care Financing Administration (HCFA)** released the regulations for **Comprehensive Outpatient Rehabilitation Facilities (CORFs).** As defined by the regulations, a CORF is "a nonresidential facility that is established and operated exclusively for the purpose of providing diagnostic, therapeutic, and restorative services to outpatients for the rehabilitation of injured, disabled, or sick persons, at a single fixed location, by or under the supervision of a physician." The facility and all personnel of a CORF must comply with all state and local laws or regulations, which means that both the facility and all practitioners must be licensed or credentialed according to state and local laws.

These CORF regulations expanded the benefits under Medicare—Part B to include services provided by CORFs. Specifically these regulations established the conditions these facilities must meet to participate in Medicare, defined specific facility services, and established reimbursement on a reasonable cost basis. It is important to note that these regulations defined personnel qualifications, including those of RCPs, and, more importantly, recognized the services rendered by RCPs in pulmonary-rehabilitation programs conducted at CORFs. Table 2–2 delineates these services.

TABLE 2–2 Respiratory-care services for a comprehensive outpatient rehabilitation facility (CORF)

Recognized respiratory-therapy services in a comprehensive outpatient rehabilitation facility (CORF) for the assessment, diagnostic evaluation, treatment, management, and monitoring of patients with deficiencies or abnormalities of cardiopulmonary function

Application of techniques for support of oxygenation and ventilation of the patient and for pulmonary rehabilitation	and patient education in the management of respiratory problems
Therapeutic use and monitoring of gases, mists, and aerosols and related equipment	Diagnostics tests like pulmonary function tests, spirometry, and blood-gas analysis, to be evaluated by a physician
Bronchial hygiene therapy	Periodic assessment of chronically ill patients and their need for respiratory therapy
Pulmonary rehabilitation techniques like exercise conditioning, breathing retraining,	

(Source: American Association for Respiratory Care [AARC], March 1983.)

The CORF regulations specified twelve services, including respiratory care, to be covered as CORF services and also described conditions when services would be excluded. Any of the following services are excluded from CORF coverage:

- services furnished to any hospital patient;
- services provided to a patient experiencing a temporary loss or reduction of function that is expected to improve spontaneously; and
- services provided as part of a maintenance program of repetitive activities that do not require the skilled services of nurses or therapists (AARC, 1983).

MANAGED CARE AND HEALTH-CARE REFORM

Managed care and health-care reform have brought about sweeping changes in how health care is delivered and reimbursed in America. Hospital restructuring is an offshoot of managed care and health-care reform. With hospital restructuring has come an increased focus on patient care outside the hospital at alternate sites. Since the mid-1980s in the United States, there has been a significant increase in the number of pulmonary-rehabilitation programs and the number of outpatient programs at specialty centers or clinics. Reasons for this include the need for respiratory-care departments to diversify by assuming other areas of responsibility, space limitations within hospitals, reimbursement available to CORFs, and the growing professional interest in pulmonary rehabilitation and physical reconditioning. These reasons have increased employment opportunities for RCPs.

REIMBURSEMENT

Payment for pulmonary rehabilitation has been, and continues to be, an issue of contention between providers and payors. Once this issue is resolved, it will be another stimulus for the growth of pulmonary rehabilitation. Presently, pulmonary rehabilitation is not reimbursed by Medicare or other insurance carriers as a blanket program. Instead, program elements like serial pulse oximetry determinations and breathing exercises are billed separately. Reimbursement is an important financial concern that is be discussed in greater detail in Chapter 6.

RATIONALE FOR PULMONARY REHABILITATION

It is estimated that over 10 percent of the U.S. population, or close to 26 million Americans, are living with some type of chronic pulmonary disease. Lung diseases, including COPD, now rank as the third leading cause of death in the United States, accounting for approximately 315,000 deaths annually. Direct and indirect expenditures for treating and managing lung disease each year total more than $56 billion (Cathcart, 1995). Asthma-related care alone accounts for over $6 billion (Kallstrom, 1995). In addition, COPD is ranked as the second leading cause of permanent disability in males over 40, resulting in Social Security disability payments of over $27 billion. Since 1979, the mortality rate for all lung diseases has increased steadily. This rate has increased faster than those of the other top ten causes of death, including heart disease and cancer. In fact, during the 1980s, deaths from COPD increased 60 percent, while deaths from heart disease decreased 30 percent (American Lung Association, 1996).

The budgetary constraints of the past few years have brought about many changes in the ways hospitals do business. In particular, hospitals have been working harder at releasing patients sooner and keeping them from hospital stays in the first place. Because patients with chronic lung disease tend to be admitted several times during any given year, they tend to become significant cost centers under DRGs and the proactive payment system. Keeping patients at home and improving their lifestyles has moved from being some unattainable goal to a necessity. To help make this a reality, hospitals now appear to be taking effective pulmonary-rehabilitation programs seriously.

Patients with chronic lung disease have a variety of physiologic and clinical manifestations that must be addressed as part of any pulmonary rehabilitation effort. These manifestations may include:

- increased airways resistance;
- hyperinflation with air trapping;
- decreased lung and chest wall compliance;
- disadvantaged respiratory muscles;
- decreased exercise capacity and endurance;
- significant arterial desaturation during exercise; and
- reduced oxygen consumption (the rate of oxygen uptake, which is a measure of a patient's work capacity).

The rationale for pulmonary rehabilitation is to control and perhaps reverse some of the processes that lead to decreased physical activity. A vicious cycle ensues in which dyspnea leads to inactivity, which leads to skeletal muscle atrophy, which leads to increased dyspnea and further physical inactivity (Figure 2–1). Patients eventually become prisoners in their homes, first confined to single rooms and then to their beds. Some type of intervention is essential to help break this cycle. Pulmonary rehabilitation can improve a patient's level of physical activity, reduce dyspnea, and return a patient to a more active lifestyle with fewer hospitalizations.

There is an integral relationship between pulmonary function, cardiovascular function, and skeletal muscle function. Each system depends upon and impacts the others when abnormalities or dysfunctions are evident. When one system falters, the others are affected and must compensate to the degree they are able. This is especially evident during any substantial physical activity like exercise.

One way of illustrating the relationship between lung (ventilation and gas exchange), heart (circulation), and muscle (physical performance) during exercise is shown in Figure 2–2. In cogwheel-like fashion, each component depends on the other when an individual, especially someone with cardiopulmonary impairment resulting in exercise intolerance, engages in any form of exercise or physical activity. Impaired lungs or ventilatory apparatuses do not properly oxygenate the blood or remove carbon dioxide. Cardiovascular problems result in reduced circulation with diminished oxygenation of the blood and body tissues. Poor physical conditioning affects oxygen consumption and the body's acid-base balance, which places additional demands on the cardiopulmonary system. Figure 2–2 alludes to the importance of a cardiopulmonary exercise evaluation (discussed in

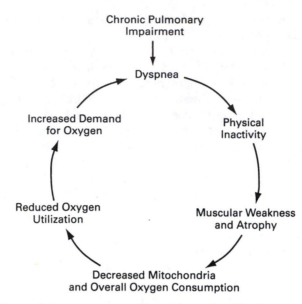

Figure 2–1 *This vicious cycle is a consequence of inactivity produced by dyspnea resulting from chronic pulmonary disease.*

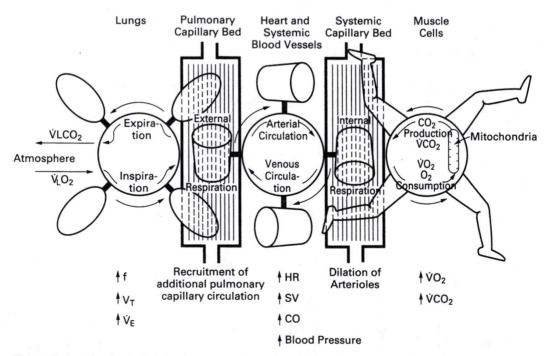

Figure 2–2 *The physical adaptation to exercise involves the interdependence of the pulmonary system, the cardiovascular system, and skeletal muscle. (Madama, 1993)*

Chapter 3) in differentiating between pulmonary, cardiac, and physical conditioning reasons for dyspnea and the inability to physically perform, thereby identifying the need for some type of rehabilitation program.

GOALS AND OBJECTIVES

The major goal of pulmonary rehabilitation is to restore the patient to the highest possible functional capacity allowed by the degree of pulmonary impairment and overall life situation. This goal implies each patient is an individual and suggests that pulmonary rehabilitation should be tailored to meet the needs of each patient. To help achieve this goal, pulmonary rehabilitation has two principal objectives: (1) control and alleviate the symptoms and pathophysiologic complications of respiratory impairment as much as possible, and (2) teach patients how to achieve optimal capability for carrying out their **activities of daily living (ADL)** (Hodgkin, Connors, & Bell, 1993).

Pulmonary-rehabilitation programs that are structured and administered properly can help reverse some of the problems associated with dyspnea and inactivity and thereby help patients cope with their overall pulmonary and physical impairment. The four major pillars of pulmonary rehabilitation, which help patients understand the concept of pulmonary rehabilitation, are:

1. Education (information to help patients comprehend the scope of their dysfunction and what measures can be employed to improve their conditions)
2. Breathing techniques (pursed-lip, diaphragmatic, and inspiratory resistive breathing)
3. Physical reconditioning (exercises to improve muscle tone, oxygen consumption, and overall exercise tolerance)
4. ADL (leading an active, productive lifestyle by conserving energy and pacing all activities)

While it may appear simple, in some ways pulmonary rehabilitation is analogous to an automobile tune-up. Before the tuneup, the car idles roughly, gives inferior performance, and has poor gas mileage. After the oil, filters, and spark plugs are changed, and the timing set, the car's performance and gas mileage improve. It is the same with pulmonary rehabilitation. A patient with poor conditioning has little or no exercise tolerance and reduced oxygen consumption. With proper breathing techniques and physical reconditioning, the patient improves like the automobile, with enhanced physical performance.

PROGRAM SEQUENCE AND STRATEGY

Sequencing involves a careful patient-selection process, patient evaluation with cardiopulmonary exercise testing, setting goals and objectives for patients, program implementation, periodic review and assessment of patient progress, and follow-up (Hodgkin, Connors, & Bell, 1993). This sequencing can take weeks or even months, depending on the length of the program. Strategies must be patient specific and should address the patient's condition, degree of pulmonary dysfunction, lifestyle, degree of family support, motivation, other related behavioral factors, and any special services. Strategies may consist of group sessions or a one-on-one approach involving one rehabilitation specialist with one patient, especially in ventilator-dependent or quadriplegic cases. Regardless of strategy, active patient participation is critical and leads to more successful outcomes than passive learning (Morgan & Hara, 1990).

REHABILITATION OUTCOMES

Outcomes are discussed in detail in Chapter 5, but a general comment is made here. Pulmonary rehabilitation enables patients to breathe effectively and attain a greater level of physical activity, reduces hospitalizations and medical costs, and allows patients to lead more active, productive lives. The rehabilitation goes beyond lung anatomy to skeletal and respiratory muscle conditioning, breathing techniques, pulmonary hygiene, and lifestyle changes. The success of pulmonary rehabilitation depends on a positive approach and attitude.

It is now accepted that blood oxygenation, maximal oxygen consumption, exercise tolerance, cardiovascular function, and overall physical conditioning will increase. It is here that patients will experience improvement in their conditions. Of course, some progress patients report is subjective, but an increasing number of studies now support the objective improvement many patients realize after breathing retraining and pulmonary rehabilitation (Celli, 1994).

SUMMARY

Pulmonary rehabilitation, although in existence for over 40 years, is actually in its infancy. Acceptance of this methodology of care for chronic lung patients is rapidly growing and becoming an integral part of continuing respiratory care, especially at alternate sites. Studies have indicated the potential benefits of pulmonary rehabilitation, but much more must be done. Practitioners must continue to document the benefits of rehabilitation to establish a more effective reimbursement mechanism and work closely with their colleagues to design and implement more patient specific and effective rehabilitation programs. With ever-increasing recognition, pulmonary rehabilitation seems to be headed on a course that will make it an essential part of long-term patient care.

Review Questions

1. What is the current definition of *pulmonary rehabilitation?*
2. Differentiate between pulmonary rehabilitation and cardiac rehabilitation.
3. State the major goal of pulmonary rehabilitation and its two principal objectives.
4. How are the functions of the lungs, the heart, and the skeletal muscles related in terms of a patient's ability to breathe and exercise?
5. What is a CORF, and what impact has it had on pulmonary rehabilitation?
6. How have health-care reform measures affected pulmonary rehabilitation?

References

American Association for Respiratory Care. (1983, March). CORF regulations released. *AARCTimes*, 7(3), 40–52.

American Lung Association. (1996). *Lung disease data 1996*. 1–3. American Lung Association. New York, NY.

American Thoracic Society Executive Committee. (1981, November). Pulmonary rehabilitation—An official statement of the American Thoracic Society. *American Review of Respiratory Disease, 124*, 663–666.

Barach, A.L., Bickerman, H.A., & Beck, G. (1952). Advances in the treatment of nontuberculous disease. *Bulletin of the NY Academy of Medicine, 28*, 353–384.

Cathcart, M. Other drivers of change deserve consideration. (1995, December). *AARCTimes, 19*(12), 36–37.

Celli, B.R. (1994, May). Physical reconditioning of patients with respiratory disease: Legs, arms, and breathing retraining. *Respiratory Care, 39*(5), 481–495.

Council on Rehabilitation. (1942). *Definition of rehabilitation*. Chicago: Council on Rehabilitation.

Eiserman, J. (1987, August). AARC specialty sections. *AARCTimes, 11*(8), 22–23.

Hodgkin, J.E., Connors, G.L., & Bell, C.W. (1993). *Pulmonary rehabilitation—Guidelines to success* (2nd ed.). Philadelphia, PA: J.B. Lippincott Company.

Hughes, R.L., & Davison, R. (1983, February). Limitations of exercise reconditioning in COLD. *Chest, 83*, 241–249.

Kallstrom, T. (1995, December). Asthma significantly affects health care expenditures. *AARCTimes, 19*(12), 38.

Madama, V. (1993). *Pulmonary function testing and cardiopulmonary stress testing*. Albany, NY: Delmar Publishers.

Morgan, E.J., & Hara, K. (1990). COPD: Rehabilitation guidelines. *Choices in Respiratory Management, 20*, 131–134.

Suggested Readings

Christie, D. (1968). Physical training in chronic obstructive lung disease. *British Medical Journal, 2*, 150–151.

McGavin, C.R., Gupta, S.P., Lloyd, E.L., & McHardy, G.J.R. (1977). Physical rehabilitation for the chronic bronchitic: Results of a controlled trial of exercises in the home. *Thorax, 32*, 307–311.

Moser, K.M., Bokinsky, G.E., Savage, R.T., Archibald, C.J., & Hansen, P.R. (1980). Results of a comprehensive rehabilitation program. *Archives of Internal Medicine, 140*, 1596–1601.

Nicholas, J.J., Gilbert, R., Gabe, R., & Auchincloss, J.H. (1970). Evaluation of an exercise therapy program for patients with chronic obstructive pulmonary disease. *American Review of Respiratory Disease, 102*, 1–9.

Paez, P.N., Phillipson, E.A., Masangkay, M., & Sproule, B.J. (1967). The physiologic basis of training patients with emphysema. *American Review of Respiratory Disease, 95*, 944–953.

Vyas, M.N., Banister, E.W., Morton, J.W., & Grzybowski, S. (1971). Response to exercise in patients with chronic airway obstruction. *American Review of Respiratory Disease, 103*, 390–400.

CHAPTER THREE

SELECTING PATIENTS FOR PULMONARY REHABILITATION

anaerobic threshold (AT)
carbon dioxide
production ($\dot{V}CO_2$)
cardiopulmonary
exercise (CPX) testing or
evaluation

functional status scales
or dyspnea indices
maximum oxygen
consumption ($\dot{V}O_{2max}$)

metabolic equivalents of
energy expenditure (METs)
respiratory quotient (RQ)
target heart rate

OBJECTIVES

Upon completing this chapter, the reader will be able to:

- List eight patient conditions for which pulmonary rehabilitation would prove beneficial.
- Define the role functional status scales or dyspnea indices play in patient evaluation.
- Identify three testing regimens used in evaluating patients for pulmonary rehabilitation.
- State the importance of cardiopulmonary exercise (CPX) testing in the patient-selection process.
- Identify five major components of the cardiopulmonary exercise (CPX) test, and state the importance or relevance of each.
- List three criteria for including a patient in a pulmonary-rehabilitation program.
- List three criteria for excluding a patient from a pulmonary-rehabilitation program.

INTRODUCTION

An essential component of the pulmonary-rehabilitation sequence is the patient selection and evaluation process. On the surface, this process appears to be relatively simple. Chronic-pulmonary patients physically incapacitated by their dyspnea would seem to be ideal candidates for breathing retraining and physical reconditioning. However, the process is complicated and involves issues related to patient diagnosis, overall evaluation of underlying conditions, baseline findings, potential for improvement, and patient safety.

Identifying and evaluating viable candidates for pulmonary rehabilitation is challenging for the physician and the RCPs involved in diagnostic testing and rehabilitation. Patient inclusion and exclusion must be addressed in the most objective fashion possible. Naturally, pulmonary function testing, blood-gas analysis and exercise evaluation all play important roles in patient assessment, because the specific reasons for dyspnea and exercise limitation must be ascertained. Dyspnea and exercise intolerance can result from pulmonary disease, cardiac disease, a combined cardiopulmonary problem, poor conditioning in general, or psychosomatic origins that also must be identified and addressed accordingly.

BASIS FOR PATIENT SELECTION

When the pulmonary system is impaired, there can be several reasons why exercise capacity is diminished. Four major reasons for exercise limitation are:

1. abnormal pulmonary mechanics, namely changes in compliance and airway resistance (R_{aw})
2. abnormal gas exchange resulting in hypoxemia and arterial desaturation
3. impaired cardiac output
4. sensation of dyspnea

Abnormal pulmonary mechanics often result in increased respiratory muscle work for a set level of ventilation. This increase in breathing work may be due to increased airway resistance (R_{aw}), hyperinflation, or decreases in lung or chest wall compliance. Because of this, respiratory muscle fatigue may occur, and the ability to ventilate adequately may be impaired. This results in a sensation of dyspnea and abnormalities in gas exchange.

Gas-exchange abnormalities are manifested in hypoxemia with arterial desaturation, reduced delivery of oxygen to the tissues, and lactic acidosis. Arterial desaturation also occurs during activity, especially exercise, in patients with COPD. In fact, hypoxemia during exercise is common in COPD patients. The work of breathing increases because of the higher level of ventilation required to compensate for the drop in pH. Patients sense this as dyspnea, which limits their levels of work or physical activity.

Cardiac dysfunction frequently follows chronic lung disease as a result of the effects of hypoxemia on the cardiovascular system. The COPD patients with normal cardiac function at rest may develop pulmonary hypertension and cor pulmonale or elevated right atrial pressures during exercise. This may lead to reduced cardiac output due to some of the following reasons. Elevated right atrial pressure can produce a drop in the gradient for venous return to the heart, which diminishes cardiac output. In addition, if right ventricular hypertrophy is present, elevations in left ventricular filling pressure or the pressure in the left ventricle during diastole will be evident, resulting in pulmonary vascular congestion and an interference with cardiac output. Finally, in patients with increased airway resistance, decreased compliance, or hyperinflation, pleural pressure can become more negative. This increases the pressure gradient against which the heart must pump with a limit on the amount of blood ejected from the left ventricle. Pulmonary vascular congestion and transvascular fluid filtration follow, resulting in dyspnea and tightness in the chest.

Because of these clinical manifestations, patients seek help from their physicians, and physicians often consider the potential benefits of pulmonary rehabilitation. The first step in the process is patient identification and evaluation using a testing regimen that includes chest X ray, arterial blood gas analysis, pulmonary function testing, and **cardiopulmonary exercise (CPX) testing.**

TESTING REGIMENS

Before any testing is performed, a complete patient workup should be completed. The workup includes:

- a complete patient history consisting of medical/surgical, occupational, family, and social (outside activities plus any smoking and/or alcohol consumption) components;
- physical examination;
- laboratory testing (complete blood count, blood chemistry, theophylline level, and alpha-1 antitrypsin titer);
- electrocardiogram; and
- chest X ray.

Self-assessment scores, patient evaluation tools, and COPD disability scales, all useful in classifying and categorizing a patient's level of physical activity and degree of dyspnea, should also be completed by both the patient and the health-care provider (Hodgkin, Zorn, & Connors, 1993). This information, in conjunction with appropriate cardiopulmonary function testing, enables the physician and the rehabilitation specialist to evaluate the type and degree of impairment and to tailor a pulmonary rehabilitation routine to each patient's needs.

Functional status scales or **dyspnea indices,** other relevant appraisals of a patient's condition, have also gained popularity as outcome measures for pulmonary rehabilitation. Because the major goal of pulmonary rehabilitation is to improve a patient's ability to function in daily life, indices like the Medical Research Council Dyspnea Index (MRCI), the Baseline and Transition Dyspnea Index, and the Modified Dyspnea Index (MDI) can provide valuable assessments of a patient's performance and level of dyspnea (Holden et al., 1990).

The MRCI grades dyspnea in the following way:

Grade I   Dyspnea on vigorous effort only

Grade II   Troubled by inclines or when hurrying on level ground

Grade III   Short of breath walking with others of similar age and physique, even on level ground, but can walk a mile slowly and do own shopping

Grade IV   Short of breath with mild activities, cannot walk one block or climb one flight of stairs without stopping for breath (Holman, 1966)

The second index, the MDI, has five rating criteria for levels of dyspnea. The first criteria for grade assignment examines functional impairment at work where:

Grade 4   No impairment
Grade 3   Slight impairment
Grade 2   Moderate impairment
Grade 1   Severe impairment
W   Impairment amount uncertain—patient is impaired by shortness of breath but amount cannot be specified due to insufficient details
X   Unknown—information unavailable
Y   Impaired for reasons other than shortness of breath, like chest pain or hip disease
Z   Patient has not had a job since before the symptoms of shortness of breath began and has not since sought work

The second criteria for grade assignment in the MDI examines functional impairment at home where:

Grade 4   No impairment
Grade 3   Slight impairment
Grade 2   Moderate impairment
Grade 1   Severe impairment
W   Impairment amount uncertain
X   Unknown
Y   Impaired for reasons other than shortness of breath

The third criteria for grade assignment in the MDI has instructions for assigning a composite functional grade for work and home. The fourth criteria for grade assignment looks at the magnitude of the task as:

Grade 4   Extraordinary—shortness of breath only with extraordinary activity
Grade 3   Major—shortness of breath only with major activities
Grade 2   Moderate—shortness of breath with moderate or average tasks
Grade 1   Light—shortness of breath with light activities
Grade 0   No task—shortness of breath with no activity
W   Amount uncertain
X   Unknown
Y   Impaired for reasons other than shortness of breath

The fifth and final criteria for grade assignment in the MDI assesses the magnitude of effort as.

Grade 4   Performed briskly without pausing or slowing
Grade 3   Performed slowly but without pausing or stopping

Grade 2   Performed slowly with rare pauses to catch breath

Grade 1   Performed slowly with many pauses and stops

Grade 0   Shortness of breath at rest

W   Amount uncertain

X   Unknown

Y   Impaired for reasons other than shortness of breath (Stoller, Ferranti, & Feinstein, 1986)

The MRCI and the MDI enable physicians and rehabilitation specialists to analyze patient status, set realistic performance goals for each patient, and more effectively evaluate the efficacy of pulmonary rehabilitation. However, the testing regimens provide more objective assessments of patient condition and overall physical ability. The three most frequently used regimens are the pulmonary function test, arterial blood gas analysis, and the CPX test.

PULMONARY FUNCTION TESTING

The standard pulmonary function test (PFT) consists of pre- and post-bronchodilator spirometry with a timed forced vital capacity (FVC) and flow volume loop, maximum voluntary ventilation (MVV) maneuver, lung volume and capacity determination using a helium equilibration or nitrogen washout technique, and diffusing capacity of the lung (DL_{CO}) using the single-breath method. The PFTs like these allow for differentiating between obstructive and restrictive disease, establishing a baseline for the patient, determining the extent of pulmonary impairment, and identifying the degree of reversal produced by bronchodilator therapy.

ARTERIAL BLOOD GAS ANALYSIS

The arterial blood gas (ABG) analysis commonly performed during the PFT identifies any hypoxemia, carbon dioxide retention, and/or acid-base imbalance. While the degree of improvement pulmonary rehabilitation has on a patient's overall pulmonary function is still uncertain, it is advisable to have PFTs and ABGs performed at the beginning of rehabilitation for patient tracking and determination of overall patient progress. Pulse oximetry is also used to determine a patient's level of oxygenation, but it is more useful in serial determinations to determine any degree of arterial desaturation with physical activities like walking or stair climbing.

CARDIOPULMONARY EXERCISE TEST OR EVALUATION

The most important aspect of patient evaluation and testing before any pulmonary rehabilitation effort is the stress or CPX test. This is the most complex test and the most important in terms of the patient data and information it provides. The CPX test might even be considered the "gold standard" when it comes to selecting patients for pulmonary reha-

considered the "gold standard" when it comes to selecting patients for pulmonary rehabilitation. The CPX test is indispensable in that it:

- Allows for differentiating between pulmonary and cardiac causes of dyspnea.
- Determines the degree of oxygen desaturation and/or hypoxemia that occurs with physical exertion.
- Establishes a baseline for each patient's level of physical conditioning.
- Determines each patient's **target heart rate,** which will be used in the exercise prescription and physical-reconditioning program. A target heart rate approximates the actual heart rate at an oxygen consumption 65 to 75 percent of the predicted ($\dot{V}O_{2max}$).
- Enables physicians and practitioners to track and document patient progress.
- Identifies possible patient problems and may be used to exclude patients from pulmonary rehabilitation.

The interdependency between lung, heart, and skeletal muscle establishes an essential basis for the CPX test (Figure 3–1). It also accounts for why individuals, especially

RELATIONSHIPS BETWEEN THE PHYSIOLOGICAL MECHANISMS THAT SUPPORT MUSCULAR WORK

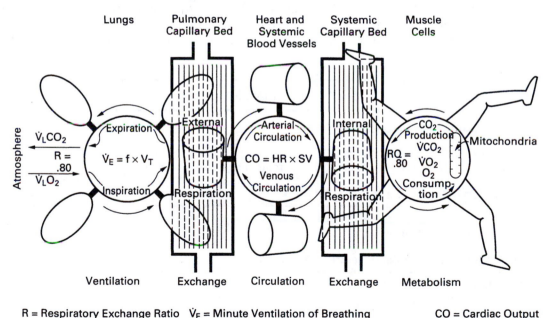

R = Respiratory Exchange Ratio	$\dot{V}_E$ = Minute Ventilation of Breathing	CO = Cardiac Output
RQ = Respiratory Quotient	f = Frequency of Breathing (Respiratory Rate)	HR = Heart Rate
	V_T = Tidal Volume of Breathing	SV = Stroke Volume

Figure 3–1 *This illustration depicts the relationship between the various physiologic mechanisms that support muscular work. It also represents the basis for the CPX evaluation. Note the reciprocating impacts pulmonary, cardiovascular, and muscular functions have on each other.*

cardiopulmonary patients, experience dyspnea during exercise. Patients experience dyspnea during minimal physical activity. When the physiologic mechanisms that support muscular work are impaired or dysfunctional to any appreciable degree, dyspnea results, and physical activity reduces or ceases. The CPX test is the best tool for testing the integrity of the vital relationship between the pulmonary system, cardiovascular system, and muscle performance. The AARC has published a CPG specifically outlining exercise testing for evaluating hypoxemia and/or desaturation. This CPG examines key components like definition and description; precautions and/or possible complications; procedural limitations; assessment of need and test quality; essential resources; recommendations regarding monitoring; and infection-control measures (American Association for Respiratory Care [AARC], 1992).

Indications and contraindications for a CPX test vary from general to specific, depending on the underlying pulmonary or cardiovascular condition. Major indications for testing include patient assessment/evaluation and facilitating the differentiation between pulmonary or cardiac dysfunction and overall poor physical conditioning. The main contraindications involve acute electrocardiographic changes associated with serious cardiac dysrhythmias and angina. Additional indications and contraindications for CPX testing are listed in Tables 3-1 and 3-2, or they may be found in the AARC's CPG on exercise testing (AARC, 1992).

Components of the Exercise Evaluation. The two basic components of the CPX test include regimens determining lung function and regimens measuring cardiovascular function. Another way of looking at testing components is to separate them into cate-

---

TABLE 3–1 General and specific indications for cardiopulmonary stress testing

---

General Indications for Stress Testing

- Assessment of general physical fitness
- Evaluation of dyspnea (with and without related chest pain and fatigue)

Evaluation of Certain Pulmonary Disorders

- COPDs, including exercise-induced asthma
- Interstitial lung disease

Evaluation of Certain Cardiovascular Disorders

- Pulmonary vascular disorders
- Coronary artery disease
- Other vascular disorders

Other General Disorders

- Neuromuscular disorders
- Obesity
- Anxiety-induced hyperventilation

TABLE 3–2 General and specific contraindications for cardiopulmonary stress testing

---

General Contraindications

- Limiting neurologic disorders
- Limiting neuromuscular disorders
- Limiting orthopedic disorders

Pulmonary Contraindications

- FEV_1 less than 30 percent of predicted
- PaO_2 less than 40 mm Hg with patient breathing room air
- $PaCO_2$ greater than 70 mm Hg
- Severe pulmonary hypertension

Cardiovascular Contraindications

- Acute pericarditis
- Congestive heart failure
- Recent myocardial infarction (within the last 4 weeks)
- Second- or third-degree heart blocks
- Significant atrial or ventricular tachyarrhythmias
- Uncontrolled hypertension
- Unstable angina
- Recent systemic or pulmonary embolism
- Severe aortic stenosis
- Thrombophlebitis or intracardiac thrombi

---

gories based on type of equipment and instrumentation needed, namely simple and complex. Components of the exercise evaluation to assess lung function include determining all the following:

- respiratory rate (RR or f)
- tidal volume and minute ventilation (V_T and $\dot{V}_E$)
- oxygen saturation via pulse oximetry (SpO_2)
- oxygen uptake or consumption ($\dot{V}O_2$ and $\dot{V}O_{2max}$)
- **carbon dioxide production ($\dot{V}CO_2$)**
- **respiratory quotient** or **RQ** (the ratio of carbon dioxide production to oxygen consumption)
- **metabolic equivalents of energy expenditure (METs)** or oxygen consumption during exercise (1 MET equals approximately 3.5 ml of oxygen consumption per kilogram of body weight per minute; at rest all patients are at 1.0 MET)
- **anaerobic threshold (AT)** where carbon dioxide production equals oxygen consumption
- deadspace to tidal volume ratio (V_D/V_T)
- breathing reserve determined as $1 - [\dot{V}_{Emax}/MVV]$

Components to assess or measure cardiovascular function include:

- heart rate (HR) or pulse,
- blood pressure (B/P),
- electrocardiogram (ECG),
- O_2 pulse (oxygen consumption per heart beat),
- cardiac output (CO or $\dot{Q}$),
- heart rate reserve determined as: $1 - [(HR_{max} - HR_{rest} / HR_{pred.max} - HR_{rest})]$.

When the components of a CPX evaluation are grouped based on equipment and instrumentation complexity, two major classifications that include pulmonary and cardiac testing components or parameters result. Testing components requiring simple equipment include:

- respiratory frequency and heart rate
- tidal volume and minute ventilation
- pulse oximetry
- blood pressure
- electrocardiogram

Testing components requiring complex equipment include:

- oxygen consumption
- carbon dioxide production
- respiratory quotient
- METs
- anaerobic threshold
- deadspace to tidal volume ratio
- O_2 pulse

Equipment and Personnel. A CPX test requires rather complex and sophisticated instrumentation, including a metabolic measurement cart with the capability to perform rapid breath-by-breath analysis of oxygen and carbon dioxide, a spirometer, or a pneumotachometer and computer; pulse oximeter; ergometer and/or treadmill; electrocardiographic monitor and recorder; blood-pressure-measuring equipment, and emergency crash cart with resuscitation equipment. Expenditures on equipment will exceed $100,000. In terms of personnel, an individual who is certified or registered in pulmonary function testing and technology (CPFT or RPFT credential) through the National Board for Respiratory Care (NBRC) with sufficient training and experience will be able to conduct this type of testing. A physician must also be present during testing, and there should be enough space to accommodate all necessary equipment and allow for a comfortable, nonclaustrophobic testing environment for both patient and staff.

Testing Procedure and Protocols. Patients being tested should fast for several hours before testing, because diet can influence test results in terms of CO_2 production. In addition, patients should not use inhaled bronchodilators at least 2 hours before testing, but much of this depends on the severity of the patient's condition. Some patients with very severe pulmonary disease may not be able to perform an exercise test unless they use an inhaled bronchodilator at the start of the evaluation. If the purpose or goal of the exercise test is to identify the presence of possible exercise-induced bronchospasm, then no traditional beta-adrenergic bronchodilators should be inhaled 6 to 8 hours prior to the examination. Serevent® (salmeterol xinofoate) should not be inhaled 12 to 24 hours before the test.

Because of the potential risks associated with the CPX test, a patient consent form must be completed before the patient proceeds with any test. This consent should describe basic aspects of the CPX test, mention possible complications associated with the procedure, indicate who will perform and monitor the test, and specify the test's approximate duration. Each patient should read, date, and sign the consent form, as should a witness, before any testing occurs. This consent should be designed clearly and concisely with the intent of informing and protecting the patient and the facility.

The CPX testing procedure begins with a preliminary spirometric evaluation to establish a baseline. Next, the patient undergoes a resting ECG, and blood pressure and oxygen saturation are determined. The patient interface with the metabolic measurement cart can be a mouthpiece with a nose clip or a mask that creates a tight seal around the nose and mouth. Use of a mouthpiece or a mask hinges on any anatomic abnormalities of the patient's mouth or nose and on patient tolerance and compliance. Mouthpieces are most commonly used. Hypoxemic patients may require supplemental oxygen during the test. The computer will have to correct these results and modify them to reflect an F_IO_2 of 0.21.

Depending on the patient's condition, stature, and overall physical ability, the stress test is performed with the patient on a treadmill, an ergometer, or a step test following specific protocols. These protocols determine at what workload the patient will begin and at what intervals the workload will increase. Selecting the correct testing protocol is important if the CPX evaluation is to test the patient properly and assess cardiopulmonary status and overall physical conditioning accurately. If the testing protocol is too difficult, the patient will not be able to perform or tolerate the testing regimen. If the protocol is too easy, the patient will not be stressed or challenged adequately. In either case, the testing will result in insufficient data and patient information. Table 3–3 examines some of the major exercise protocols in terms of number of stages, length of each stage, and incremental variations when a treadmill is used during exercise testing.

When an ergometer or electromechanical cycle is used in a stress test, a ramp or gradational/incremental format is employed in which the workload (measured in watts) is gradually increased at intervals of 1 or 2 minutes, depending on patient age, condition, and/or predicted exercise capacity. Patients usually start with a 2-minute warm-up period with no load or resistance. This freewheeling or unloaded pedalling allows the patient to adjust to the equipment. Patients are usually instructed to pedal at a rate of 50 to 60 revolutions per minute (rpm) as the workload on the cycle is increased gradually. Ergometers require proper handlebar and seat height for each patient. At proper seat height, the legs are almost extended at the bottom of the downstroke, and there is a slight bend in each knee (Zavala, 1985).

Ramp protocols range from 5- to 50-watt increments, with 15 to 25 watts being the average. The increment used depends on the reason for testing, the patient's overall condition, and the patient's predicted work-rate capacity. Workload is usually increased at 1- to 2-minute intervals. Forced expiratory volume in 1 second (FEV_1) multiplied by 35 yields the patient's approximate maximum minute ventilation ($\dot{V}_{Emax}$). Currently, some investigators are using 40 as a factor instead of 35, which results in a higher predicted

TABLE 3–3 **Depending on the nature and extent of each patient's disability, a number of treadmill protocols are routinely employed during cardiopulmonary stress testing. This table compares six major exercise protocols currently used**

Protocol	Description	Comments
Naughton	Uses ten stages or periods of 3 minutes each, separated by 3 minutes of rest. Test begins with level walking at 1, 1.5, and 2 mph. Incline is then increased to 3.5 percent, then to 7 percent at 2 mph. In the sixth stage, the incline is reduced to 5 percent, but the speed is increased to 3 mph. For the final four stages, the grade is increased by 2.5 percent for each period, but the speed is maintained at 3 mph.	None.
Bruce	Test begins with 3-minute periods of walking at 1.7 mph at a 0 percent, 5 percent, or 10 percent grade. The grade and speed are then increased 2 percent and 0.8 mph respectively every 3 minutes until an 18 percent grade and 5 mph speed are attained. Afterward, speed is increased by 0.5 mph every 3 minutes.	The 0 percent and 5 percent grades are omitted in more physically fit individuals.
Balke	Speed remains at 3.3 mph with a grade of 0 percent for the first minute, increasing by a 1 percent increment each succeeding minute.	Modification uses a 3 mph speed with an increase in grade of 2.5 percent every 2 minutes.
Fox	Speed remains at 3 mph with a 2 percent increase in grade every 2 minutes.	None.
Jones and Campbell	Speed remains constant at 2, 2.5, 3, or 3.5 mph with a 2.5 percent increase in grade every minute.	None.
Ellestad	Uses seven stages or periods, each 2 or 3 minutes long, at speeds of 1.7, 3, 4, 5, 6, 7, and 8 mph respectively. The grade is 10 percent for the first four stages with durations of 3, 2, 2, and 3 minutes. Each of the final three stages lasts 2 minutes using a 15 percent grade.	May be too difficult for most patients being tested.

(Based on data from *Manual on Exercise Testing: A Training Handbook* by D. C. Zavala and *Principles of Exercise Testing and Interpretation* by K. Wasserman et al., 1985.)

value for maximum minute ventilation. Regardless of the factor, approximating the $\dot{V}_{Emax}$ allows for predicting each patient's maximum work capacity, which in turn determines the appropriate watt increment. When a patient's predicted $\dot{V}_{Emax}$ is less than 30 liters per minute (LPM), a 10-watt ramp protocol is recommended; between 30 and 50 LPM, a 15-watt ramp protocol should be used; and between 50 and 75 LPM, a 20-watt ramp should be used. A $\dot{V}_{Emax}$ over 75 LPM requires 25-watt increments or more, depending on the patient. This is usually the case for patients who have no pulmonary disease and are being evaluated to ascertain their levels of physical conditioning. Athletes fall into this category.

The following example demonstrates how the proper ramp protocol would be determined for a COPD patient undergoing an exercise evaluation. Spirometry reveals an FEV_1 of 1.2 L. Using 35 as the factor, the predicted $\dot{V}_{Emax}$ is 42 LPM. In this case, a 15-watt ramp protocol would be used. The patient would start unloaded cycling at 0 watts, then go to 15 watts after 2 minutes. After another 2 minutes, the workload would be increased to 30 watts. The workload would be increased in 15-watt increments every 2 minutes until enough data had been collected or the patient was unable to continue testing for any reason. This type of approach enables the investigator to approximate a patient's ability and performance, which insures the test will collect the greatest amount of patient data possible.

Finally, exercise evaluations can be performed using a step test. The Harvard Step Test is one example. The step test is the least expensive and simplest way to assess a patient's level of conditioning. However, because it is both impractical and difficult to measure physiologic parameters like maximum oxygen consumption and minute ventilation, this type of testing is recommended for field experiments. Investigators have concluded that central exhaustion limited treadmill exercise during testing, while leg exhaustion limited cycling activity. A combination of central and leg exhaustion limited stepping. Of the three methods, treadmill testing is preferred for laboratory use, because the maximum oxygen consumption measured was higher and leg discomfort was less than with the cycle ergometer (Wasserman et al., 1987).

The CPX testing can be performed at constant workload, incremental to maximum workload, or ramp to maximum workload depending on a patient's condition and physical ability. Once in progress, testing continues until sufficient data is obtained or the patient demonstrates exercise to a maximum level by approaching 85 percent of the predicted maximum oxygen consumption, 70 percent of the calculated maximum ventilation, and/or 90 percent of the maximum predicted heart rate. The objective is to have testing last about 10 to 12 minutes, 6 minutes if the patient is elderly (Zavala, 1985). In most instances, patients exceed the anaerobic threshold (respiratory quotient [RQ] > 1.0). However, some very debilitated patients may start the exercise test with an RQ close to 1.0. Remember, the predicted maximum ventilation is determined by multiplying the patient's FEV_1 by a factor of 35 or 40, while predicted maximum heart rate may be determined by either of the following equations:

Maximum HR = 210 − (0.65 × age in years); or

Maximum HR = 220 − age in years

The CPX testing may be terminated for a number of other reasons, including equipment or monitoring-system failure, patient exhaustion or fatigue, clinical signs and symptoms of physiologic distress (dizziness, headache, sweating, cyanosis, pallor, angina, or severe dyspnea), signs of significant hypoxemia with a decrease in either PaO_2 or oxygen saturation, major cardiac arrhythmias, or blood pressure changes (Madama, 1993).

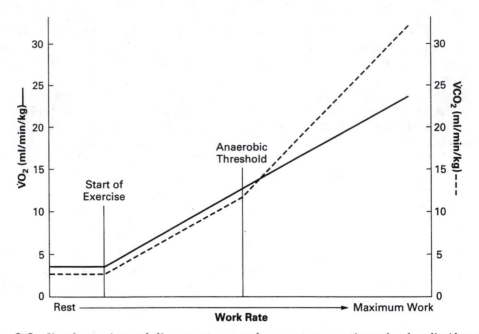

Figure 3–2 *Key changes in metabolic parameters, namely oxygen consumption and carbon dioxide production, take place during exercise. Observe what occurs when the anaerobic threshold is reached.*

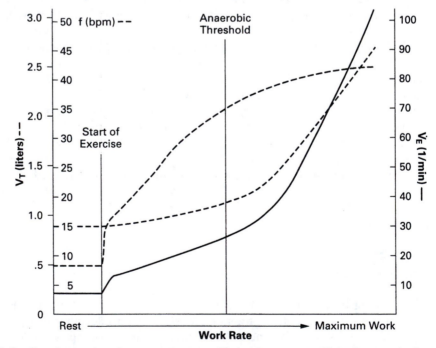

Figure 3–3 *Key changes in pulmonary parameters like respiratory rate, tidal volume, and minute ventilation occur during exercise*

Testing Results. During the test, all the previous components are measured and monitored constantly. In particular, metabolic, pulmonary, and cardiovascular parameters are analyzed both by computerized equipment and testing personnel. Changes in the patient's workload with regard to ventilation, oxygen consumption, carbon dioxide production, and cardiac output (HR and stroke volume) reflect a definite response to the exercise demands. Figures 3–2, 3–3, and 3–4 illustrate the changes in metabolic, pulmonary, and cardiovascular parameters produced during exercise testing. This invaluable data is then interpreted, allowing for a precise evaluation of the patient and a determination of the type and extent of reconditioning program needed.

Both lung and cardiac function must be properly and accurately assessed to evaluate a patient's overall condition and the underlying cause(s) of dyspnea and exercise intolerance. Table 3–4 compares exercise intolerance based on lung function, cardiac function, and poor conditioning as determined from CPX evaluations. Note the basic similarities and differences that must be considered when interpreting data and drawing conclusions as to the reasons behind a patient's inability to breathe while engaging in any level or

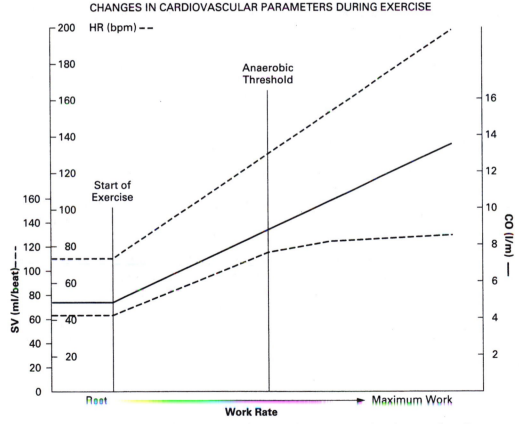

Figure 3–4 *Key changes in cardiovascular parameters, including HR, stroke volume, and cardiac output, occur during exercise*

TABLE 3-4 **Exercise intolerance may be attributed to pulmonary disorders, cardiovascular disorders, or poor physical conditioning. This table describes the general patterns these abnormalities have on key cardiopulmonary stress-testing parameters**

Parameters at Maximal Exercise	Poor Conditioning	Pulmonary Disorders	Cardiovascular Disorders
$\dot{V}O_{2max}$	Low	Low	Low
METS	Low	Low	Low
$\dot{V}_{Emax}/MVV$	Low	High	Low
O_2 saturated	N	Low	N
V_D/V_T	N	N or High	N
HR_{max}/workload	High	N	High*
O_2pulse	N	N	Low

Low = Measured value is less than normal
High = Measured value is greater than normal
N = Measured value is within the normal range
*In addition to the HR/workload values being elevated, there are corresponding ECG arrhythmias.

degree of physical activity. It is also important to note any degree of oxygen desaturation that may result from physical activity so that appropriate therapy can be instituted during the exercise portion of any pulmonary-rehabilitation program.

CRITERIA FOR INCLUSION

Patients should be placed in pulmonary rehabilitation programs for many subjective reasons. However, objective criteria are more reliable and more useful in substantiating the benefits and value of pulmonary rehabilitation and physical reconditioning. To be included in pulmonary-rehabilitation programs patients with primary respiratory limitation to exercise must fulfill one of the following criteria:

- demonstrate a respiratory limitation to exercise that results in termination of exercise stress testing at a level < 75 percent of the predicted $\dot{V}O_{2max}$;
- show significant, irreversible airway obstruction with an FEV_1 < 2.0 liters or an FEV_1/forced vital capacity (FVC) ($FEV_{1\%}$) < 60 percent;
- have significant restrictive lung disease with a total lung capacity (TLC) < 80 percent of predicted value and a single-breath DL_{co} of < 80 percent of predicted; or
- have pulmonary vascular disease in which the DL_{co} using the single-breath method is < 80 percent of predicted value or have exercise limited to < 75 percent of the predicted $\dot{V}O_{2max}$.

Using this type of criteria in the patient-selection process ensures patient safety during exercise sessions and provides a degree of objectivity when tracking patient progress or determining patient outcomes. The following case study describes a patient who successfully met the testing criteria for inclusion in a pulmonary-rehabilitation program.

───CASE STUDY───

Results of an Exercise Evaluation
Indicating the Need for Pulmonary Rehabilitation

William Hall was a fifty-two-year-old black male who was diagnosed with severe chronic obstructive airways disease and a ventilatory defect. The partial pressure of oxygen in arterial blood (PaO_2) was reduced, but the partial pressure of carbon dioxide in arterial blood ($PaCO_2$) and pH were within normal limits consistent with mild hypoxemia. The indication for the exercise study was to determine whether cardiac or pulmonary factors limit patient activities and to evaluate the level of physical fitness so that a safe and effective reconditioning program could be established.

A CPX test was performed using a cycle ergometer with a ramp protocol of 10-watt increments. The total duration of the study was 9:50 minutes. The study was terminated due to patient fatigue. The results exhibited a maximum power output, work rate capacity, and $\dot{V}O_{2max}$ reduced to 40 percent of predicted. The anaerobic threshold was not reached, and the maximum METs was 3.6. In addition, oxygen saturation remained within acceptable limits, and the respiratory rate at the end of the study was 40 with a reduction in the respiratory reserve. The HR reserve was within normal limits, the peak HR was 93 percent of the maximum predicted HR, and the blood pressure was normal and rose normally throughout the study. The HR at 65 percent of $\dot{V}O_{2max}$ was 116 beats per minute (BPM). The ECG showed a normal sinus rhythm with no ST-T wave changes or arrhythmias. The oxygen pulse was reduced.

These results demonstrated the limiting factor to the patient's physical activity was pulmonary disease with pulmonary vascular impairment. Hall was referred to pulmonary rehabilitation with a target HR during physical reconditioning of 116 BPM. Supplemental oxygen was recommended only on an as-needed basis, but metered dose bronchodilator was advised before exercise activity.

1. Because this exercise evaluation lasted almost 10 minutes and the patient did not achieve the anaerobic threshold, should a ramp protocol of 15- or 20-watt increments have been used instead? What are the possible consequences with this increase in ramp protocol?
2. Although the patient had mild hypoxemia at rest, his oxygen saturation remained within acceptable limits throughout the exercise study. How would you account for this?
3. The target HR prescribed for this patient during exercise was the HR at 65 percent of maximum oxygen uptake. Why 65 percent and not 85 percent or 100 percent?

CRITERIA FOR EXCLUSION

Objective criteria are also useful in excluding patients from pulmonary rehabilitation. Patients who are excluded are those who:

- do not fulfill the criteria for inclusion (see preceding Criteria for Inclusion section);
- have a significant cardiovascular component to exercise limitation (except those with pulmonary vascular disease); and
- demonstrate an adverse cardiovascular response to exercise, like major arrhythmias or significant changes in blood pressure, and require cardiovascular monitoring during rehabilitation.

Exclusionary criteria differentiate between primary cardiac and pulmonary defects and dysfunction. They also help to ensure patients are safe and that only patients who can benefit from the program are selected and permitted to participate. The following case study depicts a patient who did not meet the criteria for inclusion in a pulmonary-rehabilitation program based on results from a CPX test.

─────────────────CASE STUDY─────────────────

Results of an Exercise Evaluation
Excluding a Patient from Pulmonary Rehabilitation

John Knight was a sixty-nine-year-old white male diagnosed with chronic obstructive airways disease and exertional dyspnea. The ABGs were within normal limits with no hypoxemia evident. Spirometry revealed mildly advanced obstructive airways disease of the large-airway type. A CPX evaluation was performed to determine whether cardiac or pulmonary factors limit patient activities and to evaluate the level of physical fitness so that a safe and effective reconditioning program could be established.

The evaluation was performed using a cycle ergometer with ramp protocol at 15-watt increments. The test was terminated because of significant ST-T wave depression on ECG. Results demonstrated a reduction in maximum power output, work rate capacity, and $\dot{V}O_{2max}$ to 69 percent of predicted. Anaerobic threshold was reached, and the maximum METs was 4.5. The respiratory rate at the end of the study was 26, and the respiratory reserve was within normal limits. Oxygen saturation was normal and unchanged throughout. The peak HR was 90 percent of the predicted maximum HR, and the HR reserve was within normal limits. Blood pressure was normal and rose normally throughout the test. The O_2 pulse was reduced. The ECG demonstrated significant ST-T wave depression at maximum exercise, which led to the study's termination. The work rate capacity and $\dot{V}O_{2max}$ were reduced to 69 percent of predicted, but the limiting factor was cardiac impairment.

Because the limiting factor for the patient's exercise capacity was cardiac disease, further cardiac evaluation should be undertaken. Consequently, Knight was excluded from pulmonary rehabilitation.

1. What would the possible consequences have been if the patient had been referred to pulmonary rehabilitation without an exercise evaluation?

2. What significance, if any, did the O_2 pulse play in the patient's evaluation?
3. Why would a well-structured and well-implemented pulmonary-rehabilitation program have failed to help this patient?

SPECIFIC PATIENT CONDITIONS

After proper testing and evaluation, patients are prescribed by their physicians to attend pulmonary rehabilitation on an inpatient or outpatient basis. While any chronic-pulmonary patient may meet the inclusionary criteria, specific conditions appear to be more appropriate than others for pulmonary rehabilitation and physical reconditioning. These conditions are categorized as follows:

1. COPD
   Pulmonary emphysema
   Chronic bronchitis
   Bronchial asthma
   Bronchiectasis
   Cystic fibrosis

2. Restrictive lung diseases
   Sarcoidosis
   Pulmonary fibrosis
   Kyphoscoliosis
   Occupational lung diseases (pneumoconioses)
   Adult respiratory distress syndrome (ARDS)
   Obesity
   Poliomyelitis

3. Atypical conditions
   Lung resection
   Lung transplantation
   Pulmonary vascular disease
   Obstructive sleep apnea (OSA)

Of special interest is the group of patients with nonsurgical OSA who may meet the parameters for, and benefit from, pulmonary rehabilitation. Recent studies suggest that these patients have improved significantly after completing programs focused on weight loss (nutrition and exercise) and sleep position. Other aspects of pulmonary rehabilitation, including increased contact with health-care providers, behavior modification, and compliance with prescribed therapeutic regimens, should also help in the overall management of sleep apnea syndrome (Goren, 1996).

Finally, it is important to note that most of the current knowledge of physical reconditioning has been obtained from patients with the intrinsic lung diseases identified here. Very little data exists regarding rehabilitation and reconditioning in patients with degenerative neuromuscular diseases like amyotrophic lateral sclerosis (ALS), multiple sclerosis, or other similar conditions with symptomatic pump failure. In these patients, physical training and exercise may worsen, not improve, their overall conditions. Breathing retraining may help as long it does not increase the workload or burden already weakened respiratory muscles. Ventilatory assistance and rest may benefit the patient with pump failure more than exercise. More research is required in this area (Celli, 1994).

SUMMARY

This chapter covered patient evaluation and selection for pulmonary rehabilitation. Evaluation should include an extensive patient history and assessment; complete pulmonary function testing; blood gas analysis to measure and determine the level of oxygenation, ventilation, and acid-base balance; a laboratory workup; chest radiographs; electrocardiography; and, most importantly, a CPX evaluation. Testing and patient evaluation allow practitioners to differentiate between the primary pulmonary and cardiac causes of dyspnea and to establish a baseline of physical conditioning for each patient. Without this information, it is impossible to select patients for pulmonary rehabilitation properly, tailor programs and routines to each patient's needs, or track patient progress and outcomes properly. Patient evaluation and selection are labor-intensive but necessary tasks if pulmonary rehabilitation is to succeed.

Review Questions

1. What patient populations are best suited for pulmonary rehabilitation?
2. How are functional status scales or dyspnea indices used in patient evaluation?
3. What role(s) do pulmonary function testing, blood gas analysis, and other diagnostic studies play in patient evaluation before pulmonary rehabilitation?
4. Why is a CPX evaluation necessary for patients entering pulmonary-rehabilitation programs?
5. List and define five parameters measured during an exercise evaluation.
6. Identify the three criteria for including patients in pulmonary rehabilitation.
7. Identify the three criteria for excluding patients from pulmonary rehabilitation.

References

American Association for Respiratory Care. (1992, August). AARC Clinical Practice Guideline. Exercise testing for evaluation of hypoxemia and/or desaturation. *Respiratory Care, 37*(8), 907–912.

Celli, B.R. (1994, May). Physical reconditioning of patients with respiratory diseases: Legs, arms and breathing retraining. *Respiratory Care, 39*(5), 482.

Goren, S.M. (1996, February/March). Moving OSA patients into pulmonary rehabilitation. *RT—The Journal for Respiratory Care Practitioners, 9*(2), 25–26.

Hodgkin, J.E., Zorn, E.G., & Connors, G.L. (1993). *Pulmonary rehabilitation—Guidelines to success* (2nd ed.). Philadelphia, PA: J.B. Lippincott Publishers.

Holden, D.A., Stelmach, K.D., Curtis, P.S., Beck, G.J., & Stoller, J.K. (1990, April). The impact of a rehabilitation program on functional status of patients with chronic lung disease. *Respiratory Care, 35*(4), 332.

Holman, W.J. (1966). *Instructions for use of the questionnaire on respiratory symptoms.* Devon, England: Medical Research Council, Committee on Research into Chronic Bronchitis.

Madama, V.C. (1993). *Pulmonary function testing and cardiopulmonary stress testing.* Albany, NY: Delmar Publishers.

Stoller, J.K., Ferranti, R., & Feinstein, A.R. (1986). Further specification and evaluation of a new clinical index for dyspnea. *American Review of Respiratory Disease, 134,* 1129–1134.

Wasserman, K., Hansen, J.E., Sue, D.Y., & Whipp, B.J. (1987). *Principles of exercise testing and interpretation.* Philadelphia, PA: Lea & Febiger.

Zavala, D.C. (1985). *Manual on exercise testing: a training handbook.* Iowa City, IA: Press of the University of Iowa.

Suggested Readings

American College of Sports Medicine. (1995). *ACSM's guidelines for exercise testing and prescription* (5th ed.). Baltimore, MD: Williams & Wilkins.

Foster, C. (1990 June/July). Cardiopulmonary exercise testing. *RT—The Journal for Respiratory Care Practitioners, 3,* 13–17.

Jones, N.L. (1988). *Clinical exercise testing* (3rd ed.). Philadelphia, PA: W.B. Saunders Company.

Naughton, J. (1988). *Exercise testing: Physiological, biomechanical and clinical principles.* New York, NY: Futura Publishing Company.

Scanlan, C. (Ed.). (1995). *Egan's fundamentals of respiratory care* (Chapter 37, 6th ed.). St. Louis, MO: Mosby-Year Book, Inc.

Wanger, J. (1992, February/March). The role of the RCP in the exercise laboratory. *RT—The Journal for Respiratory Care Practitioners, 5,* 26–33, 72–74.

Weber, K.T., & Janicki, J.S. (1986). *Cardiopulmonary exercise testing: Physiologic principles and clinical applications.* Philadelphia, PA: W.B. Saunders Company.

CHAPTER FOUR

KEY ELEMENTS OF A PULMONARY- REHABILITATION PROGRAM

KEY TERMS

closed-format program
exercise prescription
open-ended program

patient-treatment
or care plan
overload

reversibility
specificity of training
ventilatory muscle endurance

OBJECTIVES

Upon completing this chapter, the reader will be able to:

- Identify five key components of a pulmonary-rehabilitation program.
- Differentiate between open-ended and closed pulmonary-rehabilitation programs.
- Describe the space and equipment needs of pulmonary rehabilitation.
- Identify the key personnel in pulmonary rehabilitation.
- Explain how ventilatory muscle endurance can be achieved through breathing-retraining techniques.
- Identify and discuss the importance of the three principles of exercise training.
- Identify key features of a patient-treatment plan.

INTRODUCTION

Patient selection is the first part of the pulmonary-rehabilitation process. The next step is to design and implement a rehabilitation program that addresses each patient's specific condition, life situation, and overall needs. Patients often have many needs, and those needs may be grouped as physiological, psychological, social, or financial. Designing and implementing a rehabilitation program may sound simple, but it is as labor intensive as patient selection. This chapter examines the many essential components of pulmonary rehabilitation, including location, space and equipment, personnel, program design, patient needs, and treatment plan.

PROGRAM FORMATS

Pulmonary rehabilitation may take several distinct forms or types. The following sections compare closed-format programs with open-ended programs and individual pulmonary rehabilitation sessions with group rehabilitation activities.

CLOSED-FORMAT PROGRAMS

Closed-format programs are traditional and use a set time period with a designated number of sessions and a specific end date. Sessions may be conducted once, twice, or three times a week, and the program may run from 6 to 16 weeks. Closed-format programs are usually introductory, addressing the key concepts of breathing retraining, physical conditioning, ADL, administration of medications, use of respiratory home care, and aspects of a healthy lifestyle. When the program concludes, patients are instructed to continue individually the breathing and exercise routines in which they were instructed. Follow-up, if any, depends on the program or the patient's condition and ability to comply with the **exercise prescription.**

OPEN-ENDED PROGRAMS

Open-ended programs, unlike their close-format counterparts, do not designate a number of class sessions or specific end dates. Open-ended programs are ongoing. Patients in open-ended programs continue in their programs and progress at their own paces until they achieve specific objectives and prescribed performance levels. Patients meet regularly, which may be one to three times a week. Practitioners are cautioned not to call this type of rehabilitation program a maintenance program, because Medicare and other payors do not reimburse for maintenance programs. According to Medicare, therapy services are only covered when performed with the expectation of restoring the level of function that was lost or reduced. Therapy performed repetitively to maintain a level of function is not eligible for reimbursement. Maintenance begins when the therapeutic goals of a treatment plan have been achieved or when no additional progress is expected. It consists of activities that preserve a patient's level of function and prevent further regression (Xact Medicare Services, 1995). Once a patient is at maintenance level, Medicare considers rehabilitation unnecessary. Instead, it reimburses only those who continually need rehabilitation. This issue of payment for rehabilitation services is discussed in greater depth in Chapter 6.

Open-ended programs recognize the continual need for physical reconditioning and patient care. Pulmonary rehabilitation is like substance-abuse programs where patients never fully recover but are constantly recovering. For example, unless there is a cure with full recovery, chronic lung patients, whose conditions seem to almost always change or fluctuate, always need some type of formal pulmonary rehabilitation. Table 4–1 examines the advantages and disadvantages of open-ended and closed-format pulmonary-rehabilitation programs.

TABLE 4–1   A comparison of the major advantages and disadvantages of open-ended and closed-format pulmonary-rehabilitation programs

	Advantages	Disadvantages
Open-ended	Provides for ongoing rehabilitative therapy and services	Patients do not know when their programs will end
	Allows personal rehabilitative objectives to be achieved	Need or reimbursement for program may be questioned
	Allows personal performance goals or targets to be attained	May exhaust the limits of available resources
	Allows patients to proceed at their own paces and levels of comfort	Patients may become bored with the routines of their programs
	Allows patients to drop or continue their programs on an as-needed basis	
	Allows for continual reinforcement of key concepts	
Closed-format	Establishes a definite time frame for the program	May not allow enough time for rehabilitation objectives to be achieved
	Patients know what to expect from their programs	May not allow enough time for performance goals to be attained
	Allows for more effective budgeting and resource use	Program may be too weak or strong for patients' needs
	Establishes an introduction or an orientation to rehabilitation	May not allow for patients to proceed at their own paces or levels of comfort
	At completion, patients may continue with reconditioning on their own or in an open-ended program	

INDIVIDUAL REHABILITATION SESSIONS

Pulmonary rehabilitation may be conducted individually or in groups. Individual sessions, which require less equipment and fewer personnel, may be conducted in the hospital, at home, or at the rehabilitation facility. Each patient receives individualized attention. The program is tailored to each patient's condition and needs, which makes implementation both easier and more effective.

Individual programs are especially effective for ventilator-dependent patients who are being weaned from ventilatory support or for those with neurologic disorders. These programs also help patients with spinal-cord injuries who are learning to breathe on their own off the ventilator. One type of breathing-retraining method is glossopharyngeal or "frog" breathing, which enables patients to remain off ventilatory support from minutes to hours at a time. The RCPs involved in this type of rehabilitation must teach and coach each patient to gulp or swallow air into the lungs using the tongue, pharynx, and larynx in a breathing motion like that seen in frogs. Glossopharyngeal breathing allows for some increase in the vital capacity and a more forceful cough, resulting in more effective removal of secretions and less frequent infections (Burton, Gee, & Hodgkin, 1977).

The patient's home is another setting in which individualized programs may be implemented. Homebound patients include those with severe, chronic pulmonary disease; ventilator-dependent patients; and those who are so debilitated that out-of-house activities are simply not possible. Home programs can be designed to cover the same material and allow for similar breathing retraining and physical reconditioning as formal programs conducted at hospitals or outpatient centers. Home programs place greater emphasis on patient and family education, home-care equipment use, and infection-control measures. Home programs that include regular practitioner visits may contribute significantly to a patient's physical and psychological recovery by increasing the patient's physical ability, self-confidence, and self-esteem and decreasing his or her hospitalizations

TABLE 4–2   A comparison of the major advantages and disadvantages of individual and group pulmonary-rehabilitation programs

	Advantages	Disadvantages
Individual	Easier to implement and follow patient's progress	Not the most efficient use of resources
	Allows for personalized instruction and therapy	May require extensive travel to the patient's home
	Focuses on patient's specific rehabilitation objectives	Patient has no social interaction with other patients
	Meets patient's specific time and travel needs	Fewer patients are cared for daily or weekly
	Allows rehabilitation to be delivered in the home	May pose scheduling difficulties
	Is best for patients being weaned from ventilation or learning specialized breathing techniques	May decrease a department's or facility's revenue
	Less chance of spreading infection	
Group	Allows for more efficient use of resources	More difficult to tailor the program to individual needs
	Allows for social interaction between patients in the group	Requires a central location and adequate space for group sessions
	Enhances learning, reconditioning, and group support	Depending on group size, may need more equipment
	More patients can be rehabilitated daily or weekly	Scheduling difficulties may occur with larger groups
	Can increase a department's or facility's revenue	Greater chance of spreading infection

(McMahon, 1988). Patients may progress to points that allow them to continue their reconditioning processes as outpatients.

Other instances in which individual programs are implemented are those in which patients live in rural areas or have transportation difficulties. In these cases, one or two sessions can be given to initiate the reconditioning process. These sessions usually include breathing retraining and an exercise prescription to gradually enhance the patient's physical condition. These principles are followed up and reinforced as needed, often depending on the patient's ability to obtain transportation.

GROUP REHABILITATION ACTIVITIES

Group rehabilitation sessions, a more cost-effective way to offer pulmonary rehabilitation, involve classes with from four to twelve patients, depending on space, equipment, personnel, and enrollment. One of the major reasons patients attend rehabilitation programs is psychosocial in nature. Group support has always been an effective way to address psychologically any physical problem or handicap. Group members tend to strengthen, bolster, and sustain each other because they share a difficulty, namely dyspnea resulting from some degree of pulmonary impairment or dysfunction.

While groups can enhance the learning and rehabilitative process, they must remain focused and committed to the program's goals. In addition, while group sessions are more cost effective, it is not always possible to gather patients in one place at one time, and patients may not always relate positively and constructively. Table 4–2 lists the major advantages and disadvantages of group and individual rehabilitation.

PROGRAM COMPONENTS AND CONTENT

This section of the chapter is very important because it addresses the key elements of designing a pulmonary-rehabilitation program. Space, personnel, and equipment resources depend on program design and format. Group sessions conducted in closed-format or open-ended fashion require substantially more than individual sessions in terms of space and equipment. Regardless of the program's design or format, personnel are contingent on patient numbers and the level of detail of the sessions.

LOCATION AND SPACE

Location and space are the first concerns facing any administrator of a pulmonary-rehabilitation program. Several factors influence where a program will be conducted and how much space will be appropriated for its operation.

Location Options.   Pulmonary rehabilitation can be conducted as an inpatient function or an outpatient service. Most inpatient pulmonary rehabilitation is conducted in a hospital. Several residential rehabilitation centers, like the Burke Rehabilitation Hospital in White Plains, New York, and the National Jewish Center for Immunology and Respiratory Medicine in Denver, Colorado, offer inpatient and outpatient programs and cater to patients who are severely debilitated. Patients who can reside at these types of facilities for short or extended periods participate in daily rehabilitation and reconditioning routines.

However, most pulmonary rehabilitation is implemented on an outpatient basis with patients visiting the facility (hospital or center) weekly or more frequently. Facilities offering outpatient services must address patient needs in terms of accessibility, parking, and mass transit. It is easier for patients to attend regularly scheduled sessions at hospitals or centers that are centrally located and close to major access roads and mass transportation. In addition to being accessible by major routes, outpatient facilities must also be wheelchair accessible with ramps and elevators. It is difficult for patients to attend rehabilitation classes when a facility is too far from their homes, not near mass transportation or located where parking is too expensive or too far from the building.

Facilities have a number of options to address these concerns. When possible, parking should be adjacent the facility's entrance. If this is not feasible, valet parking should be considered. Finally, the services of any community or hospital-based coach service could be employed. Valet parking or a community-coach or van-transportation service not only attend to patients' transportation needs but can be used to market and advertise the program.

Space Considerations.   In addition to being suitably located, facilities must have adequate space allowances for patient seating and physical activities to ensure overall comfort and room for equipment and storage. If the only space available for a rehabilitation program is in the basement of a building, special care should be taken to ensure the basement is mold and mildew free. The ideal facility is on the ground floor of a building with a patient reception or waiting room and a television or music. The facility would have a secured area for coats and personal belongings, an office where appointments are made and records kept, a classroom with audiovisual aids, an exercise area, an equipment and supply storage space, and restrooms. Separate male and female showers with lockers for personal effects is ideal but not necessary. Figure 4–1 is a proposed layout for a pulmonary-rehabilitation facility.

Space in terms of square footage depends on the available space, projected patient population, and budgetary/financial considerations. For an average class of eight to twelve patients, a classroom that is 12 feet by 16 feet (192 square feet) is adequate, and an exercise area about twice this size (up to 400 square feet) should suffice. Ventilation in the space must be adequate. Windows and wall mirrors provide a sense of openness and roominess and reduce any claustrophobic sensations. Renovations can add to the comfort of most pulmonary-rehabilitation areas, but they can be expensive. Moving walls, adding a restroom, updating the electrical system, installing new heating and/or ventilation, laying new flooring, and installing lighting and ceilings can cost from approximately $50,000 to well over $100,000 depending on the contractor and materials.

When planning and renovating space, a hospital's engineering department should be involved to ensure compliance with local and state building and fire codes. Outpatient facilities should use a building contractor and safety inspector. Several specific areas require attention in this arena. The space and its restrooms must be wheelchair accessible to conform with the Americans with Disabilities Act (ADA). Restrooms should also have convenient grab bars and safety call bells. The entire area should be constructed with safe and proper building and flooring materials. Pile carpeting, which is difficult to keep clean

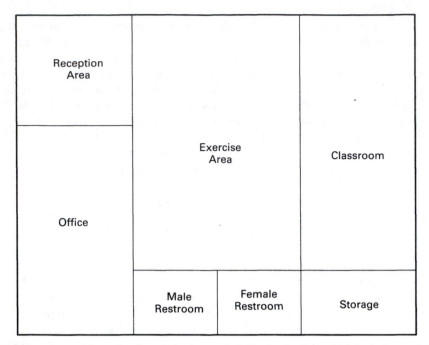

Figure 4–1 *A suggested floor plan for a pulmonary-rehabilitation facility, which includes space for patient instruction, exercise, and equipment storage*

and move equipment on and may trap dust, pollen, and mold, should be avoided. A bright, durable, nonskid vinyl surface is recommended for floors. The electrical system should have outlets with ground-fault interrupter (GFI) protector receptacles and be connected to an uninterrupted, battery-powered power supply (UPS). It would be disastrous to have patients walking on treadmills if a power outage occurs. Naturally, emergency call and sprinkler systems should also be in place.

In addition, the space must have adequate heating, ventilation, and air conditioning, (HVAC). The American Institute of Architects with the U.S. Department of Health and Human Services (USDHHS) has developed (HVAC) codes for hospitals and other medical facilities. The two departments recommend a ventilation rate of 20 cubic feet per minute (CFM) per person. Therefore, a rehabilitation class of twelve people (ten patients and two practitioners) would need at least 240 CFM (12 people × 20 CFM). In this case, more than 300 CFM would be advised to help ensure adequate ventilation and greater patient comfort. The number of air exchanges or the total volume of air in a room that is changed per hour should range between 6 and 10 to meet or exceed minimum standards. Although respiratory care is not specifically identified in the codes, examination and patient treatment rooms should have 6 air exchanges per hour, while isolation and gas sterilization areas should have 10 exchanges per hour. These standards are designed to protect the patient, but higher rates are more suitable in certain situations. For instance, the Occupational Safety and Health Administration (OSHA) specifies at least 12 air exchanges per hour (without negative pressure) for employee protection. This level, however, is more appropriate in the cardiopulmonary function laboratory where patients have yet to be tested and evaluated (American Institute of Architects Committee on Architecture for Health, 1993). Remembering details like these when planning the pulmonary-rehabilitation space ensures compliance with structural codes and makes the area safer and more comfortable.

Finally, as long as schedules do not conflict, two or more departments, offices, or functions may be able to share an accessible area. Physicians share office space, which is an efficient and cost-effective allocation of resources. Like physicians, hospitals and medical-office centers offering pulmonary rehabilitation share space. When space is an issue, practitioners can use one room for class meetings and exercise activities. These options allow time for programs to develop and become established and for administrators to plan the programs' growth and expansion.

EQUIPMENT AND SUPPLIES

According to Frost & Sullivan, an international market and research firm, revenues from rehabilitation equipment in 1996 exceeded $600 million and will climb to over $950 million by 2002. This market growth is the result of four key factors: (1) the pressure to keep health-care costs down, (2) the growing interest in preventive medicine, (3) an increasing emphasis in sports medicine to prevent and treat injuries, and (4) an aging population that will continue to increase over the next 20 years. Respiratory-care departments will continue to become increasingly involved in the rehabilitation-equipment market through cardiopulmonary-rehabilitation programs (Inside Industry, 1996). Equipment acquisition can be expensive for any program. Oximeters, spirometers, treadmills, exercise cycles, and related equipment cost, but they are necessary to any pulmonary-rehabilitation program.

Recommended Equipment for Patient Monitoring.   The equipment needed and used in a pulmonary-rehabilitation program depends on the program or facility's operating budget, available space, patient numbers, and the program's focus and extent. Patient assessment and evaluation during and after physical exercise is imperative. Most patient monitoring is accomplished through pulse oximetry, simple spirometry, and blood-pressure readings. For this type of monitoring, any standard pulse oximeter with finger and ear probes, basic spirometer, and sphygmomanometer with stethoscope suffices. The numbers of oximeters, spirometers, and blood-pressure cuffs depend on the number of patients scheduled for any one session. Minimum requirements are one oximeter, one spirometer, and one blood-pressure cuff.

Programs may opt to monitor patients using transcutaneous CO_2 and O_2 determinations or with a combination of end-tidal CO_2 (capnographic) and pulse oximetry measurements. Noninvasive CO_2 assessment provides valuable data about the patient's overall condition and ventilatory status, especially during conditioning exercises. A number of transcutaneous monitors (Figure 4–2) and end-tidal/pulse oximeters (Figure 4–3) are available. This instrumentation increases a program's operating expenses, furnishes vital patient information, and adds a dimension to patient monitoring. Financially, CO_2 monitoring is a potential source of revenue from supplementary billing codes.

Peak flowmeters can be used instead of spirometers to assess airway obstruction. Peak flowmeters are a less informative but also much less expensive and less time-consuming

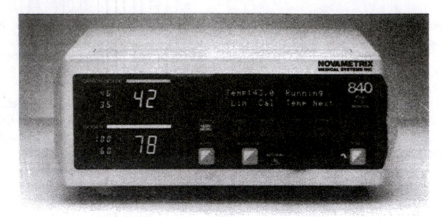

Figure 4–2 *A transcutaneous O_2/CO_2 monitor (Novametrix Model 840) for monitoring a patient's oxygenation and ventilatory status during pulmonary rehabilitation*

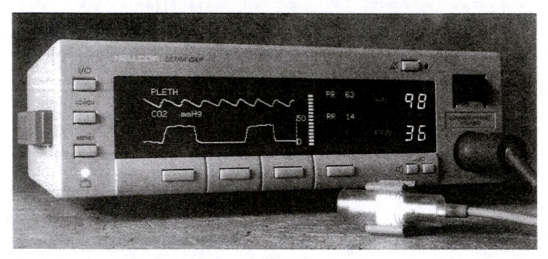

Figure 4–3 *A combined pulse oximeter and end-tidal CO_2 monitor (Nellcor Ultra Cap N-6000) may be used to monitor a patient's oxygenation and ventilatory status during pulmonary rehabilitation*

option for patient evaluation and monitoring. Each patient in the program should be given a peak flowmeter and instructed in its proper use. There is a wide variety of peak flowmeters on the market (Figure 4–4). Peak flowmeters should meet current standards for accuracy while also being durable and affordable. The three-zone system on many peak flowmeters allows patients to assess their conditions and identify any impending problems, which is an added benefit. In this system, green signifies above-normal readings, yellow denotes acceptable but cautionary readings, and red indicates below-acceptable levels.

Finally, in an effort to reduce the risk associated with adverse cardiovascular responses during exercise, some hospital-based programs are using electrocardiographic monitor-

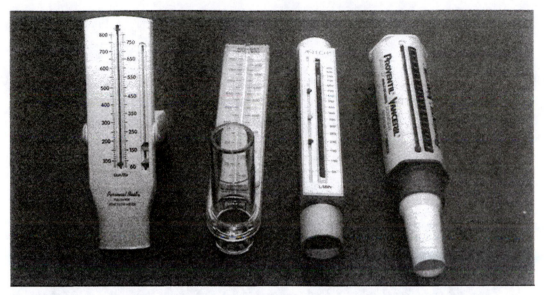

Figure 4–4 *Four peak flowmeters used to ascertain airway patency are the (from left to right): Personal Best, Assess, Astech, and Mini-Wright. (Photo courtesy of Bruce Wyka.)*

ing through telemetry to monitor patients. Programs that emphasize a patient's cardiovascular status (e.g., cardiac rehabilitation) use cardiac telemetry. However, because pulmonary patients are limited physically by dyspnea, cardiac telemetry may not be necessary, especially when a CPX test has already been performed to establish a patient's cardiac and pulmonary baselines. Any decision to use cardiac monitoring in pulmonary rehabilitation should be made only after carefully analyzing need and potential benefit.

Recommended Equipment for Physical Reconditioning.   Patients must incorporate and use a combination of aerobic or isotonic and isokinetic exercise in their pulmonary-rehabilition programs to enhance the strength and stamina of the upper and lower body. The equipment for achieving this conditioning should be varied and durable yet affordable. Programs ranging from four to ten patients should include combinations of any of the following exercise devices or appliances:

- Standard exercycles or bicycle ergometers (at least one for every two patients) with adjustable seats, tension control, and speedometers/odometers. (Figure 4–5). Some cycles come with pulse-monitoring systems.
- An automated treadmill with a timer and speed and elevation controls. (Figure 4–6). Each program should have at least one treadmill for every two patients.
- One to two rowing machines with timers and counters (Figure 4–7).
- One to two low-impact stepping units or stair simulators with timers and counters (Figure 4–8).
- Two to four arm ergometers with work tables (Figure 4–9).
- One to two wall-pulley units with adjustable weights (Figure 4–10).

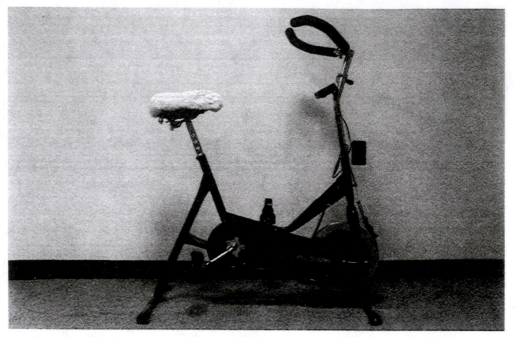

Figure 4–5 *A standard exercycle for lower-extremity conditioning with an adjustable seat, tension control, odometer, and speedometer. (Photo courtsey of Bruce Wyka.)*

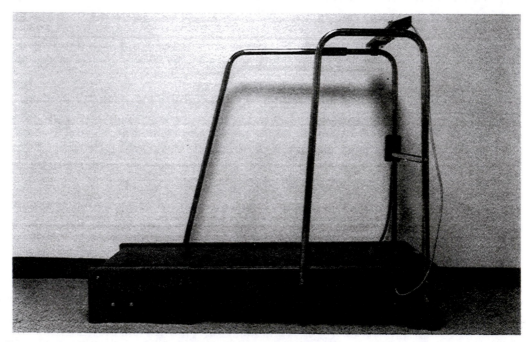

Figure 4–6 *Automated treadmill with elevation, speed, and timer controls. (Photo courtsey of Bruce Wyka.)*

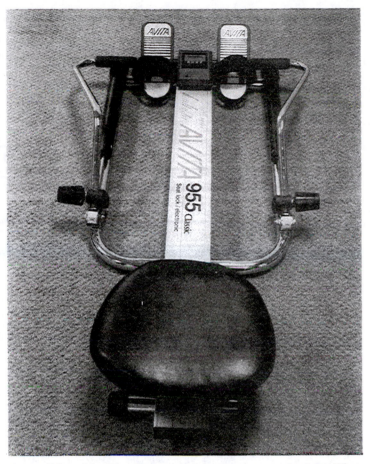

Figure 4–7 *Rowing machine with adjustable tension, a stroke counter, and a timer. (Photo courtesy of Bruce Wyka.)*

- At least four sets of free hand weights ranging from 1 pound to 10 pounds (0.5 kilogram to 4.5 kilogram).
- Two to four floor mats for floor exercises.
- An oxygen concentrator and/or portable oxygen cylinders with regulators, carts, and/or carrying packs. The number depends on class size and patient need.
- At least one compressor/nebulizer unit.

When space and cost are considerations, a floor pedal exerciser like the Pedlar® manufactured by Battle Creek (Figure 4–11) is a more inexpensive option than exercycles. The Pedlar® is simple and inexpensive and allows patients to pedal easily and safely from any chair. It comes with a tension control, but it does not have a speedometer or an odometer. The Pedlar® can also be used as an arm ergometer if placed on a desk or a table. While a floor-pedal unit can be used as an alternative to cycling at pulmonary-rehabilitation facilities, any standard exercycle with an adjustable seat, an odometer, a speedometer, and tension

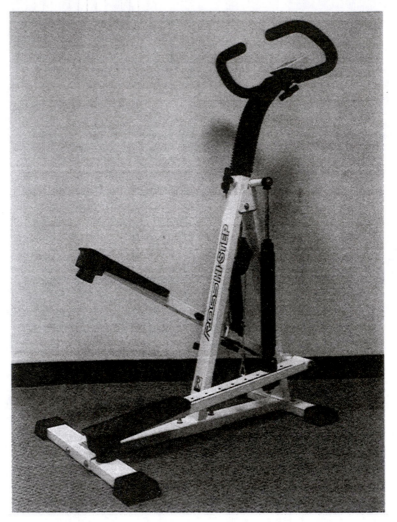

Figure 4–8 *Low-impact stepper or stair simulator with adjustable tension, step counters, and timers. (Photo courtesy of Bruce Wyka.)*

control is much more practical and useful because it provides better patient-performance data. Floor-pedal units are more appropriate for patient purchase and home use.

Other equipment, like NordicTrack® walking and skiing units, Lifecycles®, and universal-type gyms, may be too difficult or complicated for patients to use in pulmonary rehabilitation. The total-body workouts resulting from this equipment require simultaneous arm and leg motion, which excessively stresses most pulmonary patients. The affected muscle groups increase the oxygen demand to a level patients find insupportable. As a result, dyspnea and fatigue limit the patients' exercise sessions, and little or no physical conditioning occurs.

Many manufacturers currently market a wide variety of exercise apparatuses. Battle Creek Equipment, Burdick, Monark, Quinton Instrument, and Precor USA are among the

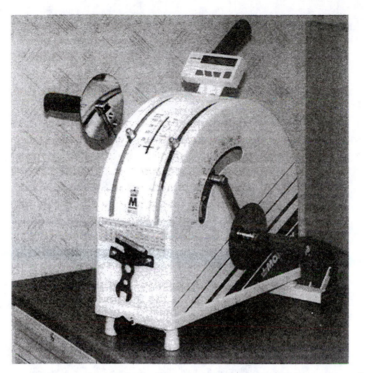

Figure 4–9 *Arm ergometer for upper-body conditioning with tension control, counter, and timer*

more popular exercise and rehabilitation-equipment suppliers. The many buyers' guides the professional and trade journals publish periodically provide detailed listings of these manufacturers and the products they supply. These guides also offer valuable information about the exercise equipment available for program or patient home use.

In addition to exercise apparatuses, other room accessories may include:

- a television
- a videocassette recorder (VCR)
- an audiotape player/radio
- a wall screen
- a flipchart or chalkboard
- a 35-mm slide projector
- an overhead projector
- wall charts of cardiopulmonary anatomy and breathing techniques
- motivational posters
- file cabinets
- wall clocks
- comfortable chairs
- a work table
- a water cooler
- refrigerator

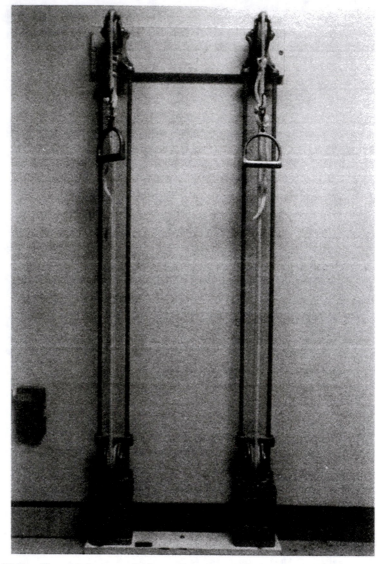

Figure 4–10 *Wall-pulley unit for upper-body conditioning. (Photo courtesy of Bruce Wyka.)*

Unused equipment and accessories are best stored in closets adjacent the classroom or exercise area. In the beginning, only essential equipment should be purchased. The program can incur additional expenditures as needs dictate.

Recommended Supplies.   Supplies vary from program to program, but they should include items like:

- a bag-valve-mask unit
- nasal cannulas and oxygen masks

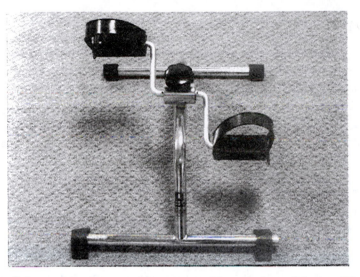

Figure 4–11 *Pedlar® floor pedal exerciser used for upper- and lower-body conditioning. (Photo courtesy of Bruce Wyka.)*

- nebulizer sets
- bronchodilator medications (in unit-dose and metered-dose forms)
- incentive spirometers
- inspiratory resistance breathing devices
- mouthpieces
- simple refreshments like cookies and juices
- batteries
- tissues
- cups
- patient booklets and handouts
- writing pads
- pens and related items

Like unused equipment and room accessories, supplies can be stored conveniently in closets or supply rooms close to where the rehabilitation sessions are held.

PERSONNEL

Any credentialed or licensed RCP with training and experience in pulmonary rehabilitation should be able to design, organize, and conduct individual and/or group sessions. Medical input and involvement is not only helpful but essential, especially if insurance reimbursement is an issue. Pulmonologists with expertise in pulmonary rehabilitation are best suited for these programs. Experience in performing and interpreting CPX test results is extremely advantageous.

Besides an RCP and a physician, other personnel who may be involved in implementing pulmonary rehabilitation include a nurse with rehabilitation experience, a physical therapist, an occupational therapist, a dietitian, a pharmacist, a clinical psychologist, and an office manager. The specific functions and responsibilities of this interdisciplinary team are listed in Table 4–3. All members of the team must be familiar with the goals and objectives of the program and should thoroughly understand pulmonary disorders (Kane, 1993).

While a variety of allied-health professionals adds significantly to the depth and quality of the overall pulmonary-rehabilitation program, there are drawbacks to having too

TABLE 4–3 Health-care practitioners or providers on the pulmonary-rehabilitation team and their specialty areas and specific functions and responsibilities

Practitioner	Area(s) of Specialty	Function/Responsibility
RCP	Respiratory care, patient assessment, breathing and rehabilitation techniques, chest physiotherapy, smoking cessation, pharmacology, physical reconditioning	Design, organize, conduct, and assess program outcomes. With training and experience, present most program topics.
Physician	Interpret exercise studies and prescribe treatment plans; evaluate and assess patient outcomes	Provide medical input; direct program; present program topics; assist with program design, implementation, and assessment.
RN	Patient assessment, breathing and rehabilitation techniques, chest physiotherapy, smoking cessation, physical reconditioning	With training and experience, design, organize, conduct, and assess program outcomes. Present most program topics.
Physical therapist	Breathing and rehabilitation techniques, chest physiotherapy, physical reconditioning	Assist with program planning and implementation, present topics related to ADL and physical reconditioning.
Occupational therapist	Rehabilitation techniques related to ADL and vocational counseling	Present topics related to ADL and vocational counseling.
Registered dietitian	Nutrition and weight control, specific diets	Present topics specific to nutrition and weight control.
Pharmacist	General and cardiopulmonary pharmacology	Present topics related to prescription and over-the-counter drug use and delivery.
Clinical psychologist	Group support, personal counseling, stress management, relaxation techniques, smoking cessation	Present psychological and behaviorally related topics, assist with smoking cessation, provide personal counseling.
Office manager	Organize and maintain office operations	Organize office, maintain patient files, handle office communication and patient billing, order supplies and equipment.

many professionals involved. Scheduling and expense are two main difficulties. At times, it may be extremely challenging to schedule specific individuals at specific times for specific presentations or functions. Other difficulties with a varied professional team include content, presentation, and workable time frames. Two-hour group sessions usually involve short presentations on special topics like medications, nutrition, stress management, smoking cessation, and other lifestyle aspects. Health professionals must gear their presentations to their audiences while allowing sufficient time for patient interaction, physician assessment, and conditioning exercises. If practitioners can agree to present within an allotted time frame, at an appropriate level, and for reasonable fees, the program will benefit from their involvement. If they cannot agree to these terms, fewer practitioners should be involved or just one or two rehabilitation specialists should conduct the sessions.

An RCP who is well-versed in cardiopulmonary pathophysiology, pharmacology, nutrition, exercise techniques, nicotine intervention, stress management, and basic respiratory home care should be able to implement a well-designed pulmonary-rehabilitation program. This individual should also be able to function as the program's director or coordinator, as well as be an active member of the interdisciplinary team (Connors, 1987). Tantamount to professional knowledge are good verbal and written communication skills, the ability to handle patients and the public effectively, and an adeptness at assessing outcomes. The number of specialists required to round out the team again depends on program size and scheduling. Most often, one specialist, one physician, and one office manager suffice. When possible, a secondary rehabilitation specialist to cover the primary practitioner's absences should be added to enhance the continuity of the sessions and the overall program.

PROGRAM CONTENT

An effective pulmonary-rehabilitation session can follow any format. A typical group session should be approximately 2 hours long, while individual sessions should range from ½ to 1 hour. The basic pulmonary-rehabilitation session format follows an outline that includes:

- review of patient activities since the last session;
- patient education (topic presentation with questions and discussion);
- exercise session;
- physician assessment (pre- or post-exercise); and
- establish objectives and activity plan for next session.

Patient Activities.   Patients will be instructed to maintain daily records or logs of their exercise routines and daily physical activities. These logs must be reviewed each session to ensure the patients are completing their assigned exercise prescriptions. Regularly inspecting patients' activities helps to ensure that individual objectives and performance goals are being met and that program outcomes are more favorable. Without regular checks, patients may become complacent or negligent. Patient records should be reviewed at the beginning of each session, either individually or within the group. Practitioners should try not to embarrass any patient but to reinforce the importance of performing daily exercise routines. Figures 4–12 and 4–13 are two sample daily patient log forms for documenting home-based activities. The exercises and routines follow any patient education session.

Patient Education.   Pulmonary rehabilitation is multidisciplinary in that it covers topics deemed important to each patient's condition and needs. Even individual patient sessions can follow topic outlines like that for groups. Some content areas covered include the concept and goals of pulmonary rehabilitation; cardiopulmonary anatomy, physiology, and pathology; breathing techniques; stress management; medications; nutrition; chest physiotherapy, and ADL. Normally, 30 to 60 minutes can be devoted to the patient-education portion of any rehabilitation class session. Table 4–4 lists topics that can be covered during the patient-education portion of pulmonary rehabilitation.

To facilitate learning, a number of relatively inexpensive patient booklets and learning guides are available. The American Lung Association offers *Help Yourself to Better Breathing,* which covers a wide variety of topics and issues deemed important to patients with chronic lung disease. A similar booklet is *COPD and You . . . A Patient Education Manual* by Judy Tietsort, RN, RRT. It is published by Allied Health Publications of National City, California, which also publishes *Better Breathers Club Panic Control Workbook* by Kim Golemb, RRT. Golemb's booklet specifically reviews key breathing techniques and procedures and

Name:					Week of:		
Date	Time	Pk Flow	Inhaled Medications	HR	Activity/ Exercise	How Am I Feeling?	Signs of Improvement
SUN							
MON							
TUES							
WED							
THURS							
FRI							
SAT							
Recognize negative thoughts. They only drag you down. It takes equal energy to think positive thoughts. So limit yourself to positive thoughts. You'll feel better about yourself. It will be easier to reach your goals. SMILE! FOCUS ON PURSED-LIP BELLY BREATHING! YOUR WORLD IS FRIENDLY!							

Figure 4–12 *Daily log form for recording patient status and home-based physical activities. (Courtesy of the Comprehensive Outpatient Rehabilitation Facility at St. Barnabas Medical Center, Livingston, New Jersey.)*

PATIENT ACTIVITY LOG

Patient Name _____

Week Number _____

Target H.R. _____

Day	PFLEX®	12 Minute Walk	Exercycle	Other	Assessment
	Setting _____ Minutes _____	Distance _____ No. of Stops _____ Pre-H.R. _____ Post-H.R. _____	Distance _____ Minutes _____ Pre-H.R. _____ Post-H.R. _____		
	Setting _____ Minutes _____	Distance _____ No. of Stops _____ Pre-H.R. _____ Post-H.R. _____	Distance _____ Minutes _____ Pre-H.R. _____ Post-H.R. _____		
	Setting _____ Minutes _____	Distance _____ No. of Stops _____ Pre-H.R. _____ Post-H.R. _____	Distance _____ Minutes _____ Pre-H.R. _____ Post-H.R. _____		
	Setting _____ Minutes _____	Distance _____ No. of Stops _____ Pre-H.R. _____ Post-H.R. _____	Distance _____ Minutes _____ Pre-H.R. _____ Post-H.R. _____		
	Setting _____ Minutes _____	Distance _____ No. of Stops _____ Pre-H.R. _____ Post-H.R. _____	Distance _____ Minutes _____ Pre-H.R. _____ Post-H.R. _____		
	Setting _____ Minutes _____	Distance _____ No. of Stops _____ Pre-H.R. _____ Post-H.R. _____	Distance _____ Minutes _____ Pre-H.R. _____ Post-H.R. _____		
	Setting _____ Minutes _____	Distance _____ No. of Stops _____ Pre-H.R. _____ Post-H.R. _____	Distance _____ Minutes _____ Pre-H.R. _____ Post-H.R. _____		

Questions or comments:

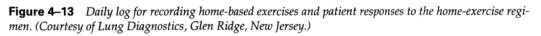

Figure 4–13 *Daily log for recording home-based exercises and patient responses to the home-exercise regimen. (Courtesy of Lung Diagnostics, Glen Ridge, New Jersey.)*

TABLE 4–4 A complete list of possible topics in a pulmonary-rehabilitation program and corresponding key issues for consideration and discussion

---

Presentation Topic	Key Issues for Consideration
Cardiopulmonary anatomy and physiology	Structure of the heart and lungs and how they work to supply the body with oxygen and remove carbon dioxide
Cardiopulmonary pathophysiology	Major differences between obstructive and restrictive lung diseases and specific examples; explanation of how chronic lung disease causes cardiac dysfunction
Breathing techniques and breathing retraining	Diaphragmatic and pursed-lip breathing techniques, inspiratory resistance breathing, basal expansion exercises, and sustained maximal inhalation through incentive spirometry (for patients with restrictive lung disease)
Stress management and relaxation	Ways to cope with stress, proper breathing techniques, avoidance of panic breathing, and relaxation methods
Physical reconditioning	Ways to exercise properly to promote agility, strength, and endurance using aerobic and isokinetic techniques and calisthenics
Pharmacology	Major cardiopulmonary medications and their effects on the body; proper use of metered-dose and dry-powder inhalers
Respiratory home care	Use of oxygen in the home and other forms of respiratory care, including small-volume nebulization and patient-monitoring systems
Chest physiotherapy	Postural drainage positions and techniques for percussion, vibration, coughing, and bronchial hygiene, including the use of the Flutter® device
Nutrition and diet	Key elements of good nutrition and weight control with focus on ways to avoid dyspnea after eating, the right food groups to eat, and trouble foods to avoid
ADL	Vocational counseling focusing on activities that enhance life and promote a more active, productive lifestyle

---

provides numerous helpful hints on saving energy, addressing panic situations, and approaching the ADL. All three publications are illustrated and written clearly and concisely. Additional patient materials are also available from other medical or professional organizations, health-care companies, and certain rehabilitation centers and programs. Practitioners should choose a few well-written and descriptive booklets and pamphlets to complement the topics they cover based on patient need, their relationship to the stated objectives, and overall cost to the facility. These materials will serve as the "course text" for the program. A patient manual or log should also be distributed and used by each patient as both a program syllabus and a record of daily exercise activities. Figure 4–14 shows two patient booklets and a daily log used in a pulmonary-rehabilitation program.

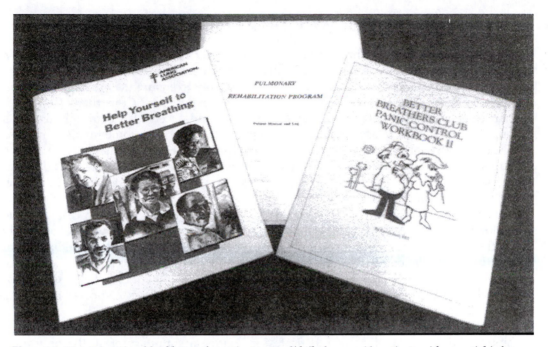

Figure 4–14 *Educational booklets and a patient manual/daily log provide patients with essential information about rehabilitating their conditions as well as a means of recording their daily exercise activities. (Photo courtesy of Bruce Wyka.)*

Every new program should begin with an orientation to the concept and goals of pulmonary rehabilitation. As with the CPX test, patients, and their witnesses, should read, date, and sign consent forms during the initial session. The form should specify the types and frequency of exercise required for each patient, possible complications, the extent of supervision and monitoring and by whom, and the anticipated duration of the program. Consent forms should be clear and concise with the intent to inform and protect the patient and the program from problems.

Nicotine intervention, while not an integral part of pulmonary rehabilitation because most enrolled patients no longer smoke, should be available to patients who are still addicted to nicotine. Methods of smoking cessation include using the nicotine patch or nasal spray while attending individual or group counseling sessions, "cold turkey," gradual weaning, and hypnotism. Patients should enroll in and complete nicotine intervention programs before they enroll in pulmonary rehabilitation.

Each education session of the pulmonary-rehabilitation program should begin with a welcoming remark followed by a brief "open mike" session, which gives patients the opportunity to comment on their progress and to voice their concerns. The formal presentation and patient questions and discussion can then follow. To increase the impact of any presentation, presenters should use audiovisuals, charts, demonstrations, and handout materials. Lectures should be focused and augment or explain material in any patient booklets used in the program. Presentations should be articulate, intelligible, and as simple as possible. Practitioners do not need to impress patients with medical knowledge and terminology.

Because many chronic pulmonary patients are elderly and may have hearing difficulty, practitioners should speak slowly and loudly. Practitioners should also maintain eye contact with group members and ask questions occasionally to ensure the group is following the presentation. Presentation skills develop with experience. Constructive criticism enhances a presenter's style and should be given and received accordingly. Patients should be encouraged to ask questions of the presenters and to become involved in class discussions. Patient participation enables a group to establish an identity and fosters group support and a greater degree of participation by all members of the class. Health-care practitioners with nonthreatening attitudes promote an atmosphere of healing, health, and patient progress in the program.

Practitioners must establish the patients' belief in the rehabilitation process, and the practitioner and the patients must establish trust. Patients will be more willing to comply with the rigors of their programs if they perceive tangible benefits and the dedication of the entire rehabilitation team. At the start of a program, some patients may be skeptical of rehabilitation, and they may require some assurance that it will work for them. Rehabilitation specialists must gain their patients' confidence if the program is to succeed in helping the patients manage their pulmonary impairments more effectively.

The final session of any pulmonary-rehabilitation program should be a graduation ceremony with presentations of certificates or honors, a summary of all the program's concepts and techniques, plans for continuing the rehabilitative process, a program evaluation, and an assessment of patient outcomes. A small party helps to accent the positive nature of the rehabilitation experience.

Patient Exercises.   To physically recondition patients and increase their exercise tolerances: (1) overall oxygen use must be improved, (2) essential muscle groups must be strengthened, and (3) the cardiovascular response to exercise must be enhanced. To achieve these three initiatives, patient exercises must be varied, focused, and performed during each class session and regularly at home. In addition, the three principles of exercise training, which are **specificity of training, overload,** and **reversibility,** must be followed (Faulkner, 1968). Specificity of training is founded on observations that programs can be designed to achieve specific goals and objectives and that exercising muscles is only beneficial to the targeted group. In other words, specific muscles or groups of muscles must be targeted to achieve beneficial results (Celli, 1994). The principle of overload contends that muscles must be forced or pushed beyond a certain level of activity to produce a training effect. The principle of reversibility or detraining effect implies that the benefits of exercise are transient and persist only as long as exercise is continued. Patients who stop exercising quickly lose any exercise-induced changes or benefits (Faulkner, 1968). All exercise incorporates these three key principles.

Breath-Retraining Techniques   The exercises used in pulmonary rehabilitation can be grouped into two major categories: breathing retraining and physical reconditioning. The first category includes breathing-retraining techniques and related exercises for both chronic obstructive and restrictive lung patients. Methods like pursed-lip diaphragmatic breathing, inspiratory or flow-resistive breathing, threshold loading, and sustained maximum inspiration (SMI) (incentive spirometry) can produce profound benefits by helping patients to control their breathing, improve their **ventilatory muscle endurance and strength**, and reduce the work of breathing and dyspnea.

Pursed-lip diaphragmatic breathing is considered the cornerstone of breathing retraining for COPD patients in pulmonary rehabilitation. Pursed-lip breathing, or PLB, comes naturally to many patients. By adjusting the size of the orifice their lips create, patients can vary the degree to which they retard expiration. This slows the patients' respiratory rates, reduces the work of breathing, creates a back pressure that prevents the smaller airways from collapsing, lessens the probability of air trapping and promotes more effective ventilation. Diaphragmatic or abdominal breathing, in contrast, is more difficult to master. Patients must practice this technique daily, first in a recumbent position with weights or resistance over the abdomen, then while sitting, standing, and walking. The time spent on diaphragmatic breathing depends on each patient's schedule and available time. Practice time can range from 15 to 30 minutes a day and, in most instances, can be performed with other types of breathing exercises or techniques. It may take some patients 6 to 8 weeks to breathe diaphragmatically, but the results are worth the effort. Diaphragmatic breathing decreases a patient's reliance on accessory muscle breathing, which in return reduces a patient's work of breathing while promoting a greater tidal volume and more effective ventilation.

Incentive spirometry using any currently available disposable device can be used to some degree in COPD, but this form of therapy is far more beneficial in treating restrictive lung disease by requiring patients to voluntarily perform hyperinflation maneuvers to increase lung capacity. Patients with sarcoidosis, pulmonary fibrosis, or any occupational lung disease should be considered candidates for this type of breathing exercise. Breathing retraining using sustained maximal inspiration with an incentive spirometer should be performed for up to 15 minutes, three to four times a day regularly to be effective.

On the other hand, respiratory dysfunction associated with COPD can be effectively improved with inspiratory muscle training (IMT) using either inspiratory or flow-resistive breathing or threshold loading. Inspiratory or flow-resistive breathing is accomplished with a device like the PFlex® (HealthScan Products Inc., Cedar Grove, NJ 07009) (Figure 4–15). The PFlex® uses decreasing hole sizes numbered from 1 to 6 to set the inspiratory training load as long as rate, tidal volume, and inspiratory time remain constant. Training starts at hole 1 for up to 30 minutes a day. When training at this level is easily tolerated, patients proceed to hole 2 and so on until they reach their highest inspiratory resistance levels.

Threshold loading is achieved with the Threshold® IMT device (HealthScan Products Inc., Cedar Grove, NJ 07009) (Figure 4–16). This apparatus uses a spring-loaded valve mechanism to provide a consistent inspiratory pressure training load, independent of inspiratory flowrate. Breathing pattern is not as critical as with inspiratory resistive breathing (Celli, 1994). The manufacturer recommends that the training load be set at approximately 30 percent of the patient's maximal inspiratory pressure (PI_{PImax}) and that training sessions increase gradually from 10–15 minutes a day to 20–30 minutes a day.

The results of using breathing techniques and retraining in pulmonary rehabilitation have been favorable. In one study, COPD patients who received breathing retraining with physical-reconditioning exercises performed better than a group receiving breathing

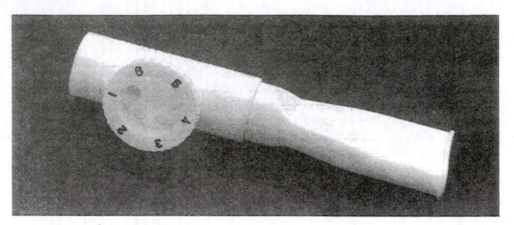

Figure 4–15 *PFlex® device for inspiratory resistive breathing exercises. (Courtesy of HealthScan Products Inc., Cedar Grove, New Jersey 07009.)*

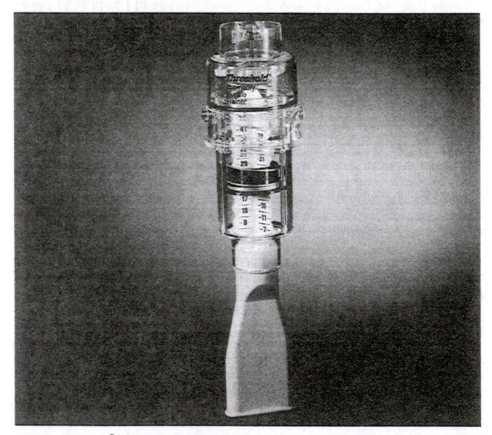

Figure 4–16 *Threshold® IMT device for inspiratory resistive breathing exercises. (Courtesy of HealthScan Products Inc., Cedar Grove, New Jersey 07009.)*

retraining only and a group performing no exercises. The group receiving breath retraining and physical reconditioning showed significant increases in ventilatory muscle endurance and exercise tolerance (Weiner, Azgad, & Ganam, 1992a). A companion study by the same investigators demonstrated that asthmatics who received IMT in the form of flow-resistive breathing displayed increased ventilatory muscle strength and endurance plus reduced asthmatic symptoms, emergency room visits, hospitalizations, days lost from school or work, and lower medication use (Weiner, Azgad, & Ganam, 1992b). Table 4–5 examines some of the major breathing-retraining techniques used in pulmonary-rehabilitation programs.

Techniques not mentioned or described in Table 4–5 include ventilatory isocapnic hyperpnea, biofeedback, yoga, and use of the Flutter® mucus-clearing device. With ventilatory isocapnic hyperpnea, patients sustain high levels of ventilation for approximately 15 minutes two to three times a day using a breathing circuit with fixed carbon dioxide and oxygen concentrations. Several studies report conflicting results of the benefits of this training method. In one study with no control group, COPD patients demonstrated both greater ventilatory capacities and exercise endurance in terms of arm and leg performance (Belman & Mittman, 1980). In two other controlled studies involving COPD patients, only the patients' ventilatory capacities increased. The patients showed no demonstrable improvement in exercise tolerance over the control group (Ries & Moser, 1986; Levine, Weiser, & Gillen, 1986). Biofeedback has been employed on mechanically ventilated patients during weaning using electromyographic signals to induce relaxation and greater tidal volumes. Results have been encouraging in terms of reducing ventilator days in the patient group treated with biofeedback (Holliday & Hyers, 1990). Yoga incorporates a philosophical approach in which patients learn to control their ventilatory patterns and responses. The exact mechanism is not yet fully understood, but COPD patients trained in yoga have demonstrated greater abilities to control dyspnea and to tolerate physical exercise better (Tandon, 1978).

While not exactly a breathing retraining method, the Flutter® device distributed by Nellcor Puritan Bennett is effective in removing mucus from the airways of patients with cystic fibrosis, chronic bronchitis, and bronchiectasis. The Flutter® is a small, handheld, pipelike device that is made of hard plastic and contains a small stainless-steel ball. As the patient exhales into the unit, the steel ball moves upward and downward, producing oscillations in expiratory pressure and airflow. These oscillations create a "fluttering" sensation and vibrations in the airway. The frequency of these oscillations ranges between 6 and 20 Hz, corresponding to the range of human pulmonary resonance frequencies. In principle, the Flutter® device can vibrate the airways, intermittently increase endobronchial pressure, and accelerate expiratory airflow. The upward movement of mucus, and its expectoration, is thereby facilitated (EdenTec®, 1996). This therapeutic modality actually falls under chest physiotherapy and bronchial hygiene, but because it involves a breathing maneuver, it has been covered here.

Finally, while it seems logical that increases in strength and endurance following ventilatory muscle training should enhance respiratory muscle function, it appears unlikely that this type of training has any impact on overall physical exercise performance. However, breathing retraining is essential when it comes to a patient's ability to cope with increased ventilatory loads resulting from any acute disease exacerbations (Celli, 1994).

TABLE 4–5 **Descriptions of the basic breathing techniques and exercises reviewed and practiced during pulmonary rehabilitation**

Technique/Exercise	Focus or Rationale	Application(s)
Pursed-lip breathing	To slow rate of breathing while creating back pressure to maintain airway patency, thus preventing airway collapse and air trapping. Pursed lips or cupped hands can be used to retard expiratory airflow.	Used during walking or any type of physical activity, especially stair climbing, bending, and lifting. Most effective in patients with COPD and during panic breathing.
Diaphragmatic breathing (abdominal breathing)	Abdominal muscles promote diaphragmatic excursions, resulting in more effective ventilation and reduced use of accessory muscles.	Constant use is advised to ensure adequate level of ventilation. Helpful in panic breathing. Most effective in COPD patients.
Segmental breathing	Promotes and maintains chest-wall mobility by having patients breathe against hand pressure applied over localized areas of the chest wall.	Useful after thoracic and abdominal surgery and in neurologic and musculo-skeletal conditions, asthma, and COPD.
Inspiratory resistance (flow resistance)	A flow-resistive device uses inspiratory load to strengthen ventilatory muscles. Promotes ventilatory muscle endurance.	Improves ventilatory muscle endurance in patients with COPD.
Threshold loading	A threshold-loading device uses inspiratory pressure as prescribed load to strengthen ventilatory muscles. Promotes ventilatory muscle endurance.	Improves ventilatory muscle endurance in patients with COPD.
Incentive spirometry	Inspiratory capacity maneuver with breath hold at the end of inspiration (sustained maximum inspiration) promotes lung expansion.	Improves overall ventilatory efficiency and effectiveness in patients with restrictive lung disease or conditions.
Glossopharyngeal breathing (frog breathing)	Use of glossopharyngeal muscles promotes capture and swallowing of air, resulting in some increase in vital capacity.	Ventilator-dependent or spinal-cord-injury patients who are able to leave ventilatory support for brief periods.

Physical-Reconditioning Techniques The second category of exercises involves physical-reconditioning techniques and exercises of four basic types: aerobic or isotonic conditioning, isokinetic exercises, isometric exercises, and calisthenics. Exercises that employ low resistance or tension with movement or repetition over a long duration overload enzymes of the tricarboxylic acid cycle and the electron transport system, causing increased endurance and stamina. This is aerobic or isotonic conditioning. Cycling without tension is an excellent way to achieve this type of conditioning. Conversely, exercises that incorporate resistance or tension with movement or repetition over a short duration are isokinetic and increase muscle tone and strength. Cycling with tension is one example of an isokinetic activity. Isometric exercises employ tension with muscle contraction, but without joint or limb movement. Pressing two hands together with periods of rest produces an isometric effect and increases muscle tone and strength. Patients can do isometrics any time and any place, even while sitting, without any special equipment or preparation. Lastly, calisthenics, which embody stretching and bending exercises, enable patients to develop flexibility and graceful movement (Celli, 1994). Table 4–6 looks at these physical-conditioning exercises in terms of their focuses and specific examples.

The time allotted group or individual physical-reconditioning exercises should range between 15 to 45 minutes depending on patient ability, available equipment, and group size. Exercise times should begin slowly at the onset of the program and gradually increase in duration and intensity as the program progresses. Music with a lively beat to which patients can exercise is recommended, as is a television to help pass time during longer exercise routines. Patients can view education tapes while exercising. Music and television are useful as long as they are not distracting.

Patients should be encouraged to reach their target HRs during each exercise activity. There appears to be a threshold of exercise activity to induce the training effects that benefit the muscles and cardiovascular system. This threshold or target, as determined during the CPX test, represents the HR at 50 to 70 percent of the $\dot{V}O_{2max}$ (Bellman & Wasserman,

TABLE 4–6 Descriptions of the four fundamental types of exercises for physical reconditioning conducted during pulmonary rehabilitation

Type of Exercise	Focus of Exercise	Specific Examples
Aerobic or isotonic conditioning (movement without resistance or tension)	To increase stamina and endurance, improve cardio-vascular status, and increase maximum oxygen consumption ($\dot{V}O_{2max}$)	Walking Cycling without tension Running in place Swimming Dancing
Isokinetic techniques (movement with resistance or tension)	To increase muscle strength and tone	Cycling with tension Walking with weights Weight lifting
Isometric exercises (resistance or tension without movement)	To increase muscle strength and tone	Pressing hands together Pushing on floor with feet Pushing against a wall or another immovable object
Calisthenics (the art of developing body strength and gracefulness)	To increase flexibility and agility	Modified and alternating toe touching Lateral bending and stretching Arm and leg lifts Controlled body movements (e.g., t'ai chi)

1982). Many programs have since found 65 to 75 percent of the $\dot{V}O_{2max}$ to be a safe and effective target because it is two thirds to three fourths a patient's maximum capability. When the target HR is achieved, cardiovascular fitness and overall conditioning occurs. However, patients must be cautioned not to exceed their targets by more than 10 percent because they begin to approach their maximum HRs.

To ensure safety, patients should be monitored before, during, and after exercise with pulse oximetry. Practitioners should perform blood pressure and peak expiratory flow rates or basic spirometry before and after an exercise session. They should document the patients' levels of activity or performance and monitor parameters in each patient's rehabilitation record. While the design of the rehabilitation record may vary from program to program, its content probably will not. Practitioners can ensure consistency by documenting what was done, for how long it was done, and what each patient observed and had as a monitored response. Figure 4–17 is an example of a patient attendance and exercise record. This form may be modified to include a rating of perceived exertion (RPE), which is a scale that indicates perceived intensity of various workloads during endurance evaluation and to monitor exercise intensity as part of the exercise prescription (Watchie, 1995).

Patients are instructed to perform their exercises at home between sessions or group meetings. The types of physical activities patients can perform at home depend on each patient's financial resources, available space, and ability to use equipment properly and safely. Realistically, most patients can perform breathing exercises, walking activities, and basic calisthenics at home, because these activities require little or no equipment. Cycling using a standard exercycle or a floor pedal unit like the Pedlar®, which can also be used as an arm ergometer on the table, is also possible for most rehabilitation patients. Most cycles used in the home are inexpensive, and patients can arrange to have them delivered and assembled. At home patients are usually required to perform 3 to 5 minutes of warm-up calisthenics, 15 to 30 minutes of breathing exercises using an inspiratory resistive device or incentive spirometer, a 6- or 12-minute walk, and cycling with gradual increases in duration and tension daily.

Walking is recognized as a safe and effective physical-conditioning technique that requires only a measured indoor area, or outdoors, if weather conditions allow. A treadmill can also be used, but it requires space and is an additional expense. The 12-minute walk, a standard in many rehabilitation programs, is a finite activity most chronic pulmonary patients should be able to perform. Because their physical activity is limited by dyspnea, it would be unrealistic to require chronic pulmonary patients to walk for up to an hour or for 2 to 3 miles like cardiac patients. Depending on patient condition and ability, a 6-minute walk may be prescribed instead. Pulmonary patients can walk for 6 or 12 minutes daily, noting the total distance in any unit of measurement and the number of stops, if any. As patients improve physically and develop greater levels of endurance and exercise tolerance, they will make fewer stops and note they have walked farther faster.

Patients who have stationary exercycles or floor pedal units are prescribed daily cycling. This cycling usually begins at a minimal level with no tension or resistance and increases gradually each week to a maximum 30 minutes a day with tension by the end of the program. If patients cannot cycle, additional walking or other physical activities, including swimming and aquatic exercises, can be recommended. Swimming, however, requires regular access to a pool. The duration of each exercise, as noted in the exercise

PULMONARY REHABILITATION EXERCISE FORM

Patient Name _____ I.D. _____ Physician _____

Target Heart Rate _____ Insurance _____ Therapist _____

DATE	PRE-	STEPPER	TREADMILL	ROWING	PULLEYS	BIKE	POST-
SpO$_2$ ____		____	____	____	____	____	____
Pulse ____		____	____	____	____	____	____
B/P ____							____

ACTIVITIES
PERFORMED: ____ min ____ min ____ min ____ min ____ min

____ steps ____ miles ____ strokes ____ reps ____ miles

____ tension ____ speed ____ tension ____ weight ____ tension

TOTAL TIME: ____

OTHER ACTIVITIES: ____ speed

DATE	PRE-	STEPPER	TREADMILL	ROWING	PULLEYS	BIKE	POST-
SpO$_2$ ____		____	____	____	____	____	____
Pulse ____		____	____	____	____	____	____
B/P ____							____

ACTIVITIES
PERFORMED: ____ min ____ min ____ min ____ min ____ min

____ steps ____ miles ____ strokes ____ reps ____ miles

____ tension ____ speed ____ tension ____ weight ____ tension

TOTAL TIME: ____

OTHER ACTIVITIES: ____ speed

Figure 4–17 *A patient exercise record to document patient activities and progress during pulmonary rehabilitation at a pulmonary-rehabilitation facility. (Courtesy of Lung Diagnostics, Glen Ridge, New Jersey.)*

prescription, can be adjusted based on patient objectives and overall condition. The level of performance for each activity, and the patient's physiologic responses in terms of HR, respiratory rate, and peak flow, should be documented in the daily log or record. Patients must be aware of their target HRs and how to modify their intensity levels once they reach their targets. Therefore, patients should be instructed how to determine their pulse rates correctly.

Patients should exercise no more than 5 days each week, including group and home exercise sessions. Two nonconsecutive days of rest each week allow muscles to repair and provide each patient with a respite from his or her daily physical routine. Patients should also be advised to premedicate with aerosolized bronchodilators (as prescribed); to ensure adequate intake of fluids, electrolytes, and vitamins; and to stop exercising if they experience angina, constant cough, extreme dyspnea, or excessive diaphoresis. Exercise should also be discouraged when patients experience fever, vertigo, or headache. Patients should document any untoward reactions to physical activity in the daily record and report it to the attending physician.

Patients who carry out their prescribed exercise routines regularly will begin to note some overall improvement after a few weeks. As they progress in their programs, patients will tolerate greater levels of exercise intensity and duration. A patient progress report like the one in Figure 4–18 should be completed periodically to document the patient's performance and improvement. These reports should be placed in each patient's rehabilitation record and sent to the referring physician.

To avoid losing conditioning or physical benefit, patients should be encouraged to continue their exercise regimens unless required to stop for medical reasons. The reversibility or detraining effect has been observed in patients who stop their physical-reconditioning routines. Patients who stop their routines can lose positive results in a matter of a few weeks. To regain what was lost takes patients almost 2 months of gradual increases in exercise duration and progressive resistance (Celli, 1994).

Often, simple motivation determines a patient's level of involvement and participation in pulmonary rehabilitation and its outcomes. The following case studies depict two patients involved in pulmonary rehabilitation. The first is highly motivated and takes an active role in group sessions and home activities. The second is an unmotivated patient who is skeptical of pulmonary rehabilitation and its benefits.

CASE STUDY

The Motivated Patient

L.M. is a 70-year-old black male diagnosed with severe chronic obstructive airways disease. His resting SpO_2 was 94 percent, but it decreased to 90 percent during walking activities and other forms of physical exertion. L.M.'s CPX evaluation demonstrated that dyspnea resulting from his pulmonary disease was limiting his physical activity. A target HR for L.M. of 120 to 130 BPM was derived from the study and deemed safe and effective. Concerned about his deteriorating respiratory condition and encouraged by his physician, L.M. willingly agreed to participate in a closed-format pulmonary-rehabilitation program for 12 weeks.

PULMONARY REHABILITATION
COMPREHENSIVE OP REHABILITATION CENTER
SAINT BARNABAS MEDICAL CENTER
(201)533-8990

PROGRESS REPORT

PATIENT NAME _____

ID # _____ AGE _____

REFERRING PHYSICIAN _____

DIAGNOSIS _____

INHALED MEDICATIONS_____

TRAINING COMPLETED:

__Lung Function	__Medications	__Panic Control	__Travel Enjoyment
__COPD	__Therapeutics	__Relaxation	__Sexual Counseling
__Breathing Exercises	__Activities of Daily Living	__Care & Use of Equip	__Smoking Cessation
__Bronchial Hygiene	__Nutrition	__Infection Control	__Home Exercise Program

EXERCISE PROGRESS:

Target SOB:_____ Telemetry Y/N Oxygen Y/N __LPM Target HR ____

Compliance: Excellent____ Good____ Fair____ Poor____

Abnormal Exercise Response: Chest Discomfort____ Leg Cramping____ Excessive SOB____

None____ Other_____

Pre 6 min walk: ____Total feet ____ MPH ____ Lo SpO2 ____ Hi HR ____/____ Hi SOB/Effort RA / O2 ____LPM

➢ **INITIAL WORKLOAD ACTIVITY SESSION** _____ **DATE** _____

MODE:	TIME	WORKLOAD		SPO2	O2	HR	SOB/EFFORT
ARM ERGOMETER	____MIN	____WATTS		____%	____L	____	____/____
BICYCLE ERGOMETER	____MIN	____WATTS	____RPM	____%	____L	____	____/____
ARM WEIGHTS		____KGS	____SETS OF 10	____%	____L	____	____/____
TREADMILL	____MIN	____MPH	____%ELEV	____%	____L	____	____/____
PULLEYS	____MIN	____KGS		____%	____L	____	____/____

TOTAL EXERCISE TIME ____ **MINUTES** WEIGHT _____

➢ **SESSION** _____ **DATE:** _____

MODE:	TIME	WORKLOAD		SPO2	O2	HR	SOB/EFFORT
ARM ERGOMETER	____MIN	____WATTS		____%	____L	____	____/____
BICYCLE ERGOMETER	____MIN	____WATTS	____RPM	____%	____L	____	____/____
ARM WEIGHTS		____KGS	____SETS OF 10	____%	____L	____	____/____
TREADMILL	____MIN	____MPH	____%ELEV	____%	____L	____	____/____
PULLEYS	____MIN	____KGS		____%	____L	____	____/____

TOTAL EXERCISE TIME ____ **MINUTES** WEIGHT _____

COMMENTS:_____

_____

Signature _____ Date _____

➢ **SESSION** _____ **DATE:** _____

MODE:	TIME	WORKLOAD		SPO2	O2	HR	SOB/EFFORT
ARM ERGOMETER	____MIN	____WATTS		____%	____L	____	____/____
BICYCLE ERGOMETER	____MIN	____WATTS	____RPM	____%	____L	____	____/____
ARM WEIGHTS		____KGS	____SETS OF 10	____%	____L	____	____/____
TREADMILL	____MIN	____MPH	____%ELEV	____%	____L	____	____/____
PULLEYS	____MIN	____KGS		____%	____L	____	____/____

TOTAL EXERCISE TIME ____ **MINUTES** WEIGHT _____

Post 6 min walk: ____Total feet ____ MPH ____ Lo SpO2 ____ Hi HR ____/____ Hi SOB/Effort RA / O2 ____LPM

COMMENTS:_____

_____

_____

Signature _____ Date _____

THANK YOU FOR YOUR REFERRAL,

PULMONARY REHAB RESPIRATORY THERAPIST

cc HOME EXERCISE PROGRAM
prprgrpt

Figure 4–18 *A patient progress report for periodically documenting patient performance and response to pulmonary rehabilitation. (Courtesy of the Comprehensive Outpatient Rehabilitation Facility at St. Barnabas Medical Center, Livingston, New Jersey.)*

During this time, L.M. actively participated in group sessions and exercises. He mastered diaphragmatic breathing, learned to use his inhaled medications more effectively, and discovered ways to cope with anxiety and panic. At home, L.M. reported that daily he performed inspiratory resistive breathing for 30 to 45 minutes using a PFlex® device. In addition, he reported a daily 12-minute walk, noting distance and number of stops, and cycling, which he gradually increased to 25 minutes a day with varying degrees of resistance. L.M. also did calisthenics and stretching exercises for about 5 minutes a day, but not routinely. L.M. performed most exercises four to five times a week.

As the weeks passed, L.M. demonstrated a lower resting pulse rate and blood pressure. During physical exercises that included walking, stair climbing, and cycling, L.M. achieved and maintained his target HR while exhibiting a lesser degree of desaturation as evidenced by SpO_2 monitoring. At the end of each exercise session, L.M.'s HR returned to its resting level in shorter periods. Subjectively, L.M. said he experienced less dyspnea, felt he had a greater exercise tolerance, and found himself participating in more physical activities at home and in the community.

1. What factors indicate L.M. performed the home-based physical activities and exercises he was assigned?
2. What indicator was used to verify L.M.'s improved recovery at the end of each exercise session?
3. What accounted for L.M.'s motivation?

CASE STUDY

The Unmotivated Patient

C.R. is a sixty-six-year-old white female diagnosed with emphysema and chronic asthma. Her resting PaO_2 on room air was 56 torr, and her physician prescribed home oxygen for nocturnal and ambulatory use. Perceiving the oxygen as a nuisance and feeling self-conscious, C.R. refused to use it regularly. Results from C.R.'s CPX test revealed a poorly conditioned individual in whom hypoxemia and dyspnea were limiting physical activity. Based on this study, C.R.'s target HR was determined to be 98 BPM. Skeptical of pulmonary rehabilitation, C.R. reluctantly agreed to participate in an open-ended pulmonary-rehabilitation program.

C.R. occasionally missed sessions and did not actively participate in any discussions unless encouraged to do so. She implied she was too busy at home or too tired and reported doing only minimal walking and cycling activities. She did not enjoy inspiratory resistive breathing exercises. When C.R. did attend group meetings, her HR, blood pressure, and oxygen saturation showed no overall improvement. During exercise, she was unable to achieve and maintain her target HR, and she complained of fatigue and dyspnea even though supplemental oxygen was in use. At the end of exercise sessions, C.R.'s HR took excessive periods to return to resting level. She reported no subjective improvements in her respiratory condition and wondered when the program would conclude.

1. What factors indicate C.R. was showing no progress or improvement due to pulmonary rehabilitation?
2. Why was C.R. so unmotivated? What could be done to motivate her?
3. Why might a closed-format rehabilitation program be better suited to C.R. than an open-ended one?

Physician Involvement.   Physician participation in pulmonary rehabilitation allows for accurate and ongoing patient assessment, and it is imperative for reimbursement. A physician can be scheduled for patient evaluation every time a session is held, but Medicare and other insurance payors will question the validity of such frequent assessments, especially if sessions are conducted two or three times a week. It is more acceptable for physicians to see patients once or twice a week. At each evaluation physicians should assess each patient's vital signs, oxygenation, breath sounds, other physical findings, level of activity, progress in the program, and potential problem areas. Physicians can write notes directly into the patient's rehabilitation record at the time of the evaluation or dictate them for later transcription. This type of timely medical follow-up enables physicians to closely monitor each patient in terms of overall improvement, difficulties with the exercise regimen, or the development of adverse responses to the rehabilitative effort. Physicians may also modify specific rehabilitation goals and objectives, including adding portable oxygen for ambulation/exercise or changing pharmaceutical prescriptions, during scheduled patient sessions.

Determining Performance Objectives and Activity Plans.   Time should be set aside at the end of each session to identify specific performance objectives and activity plans for each patient. Because patients may forget what their physicians have outlined or prescribed for them, these objectives and plans should be written by the patient or the program facilitator. Performance goals and related activities usually include breathing exercises and techniques like diaphragmatic breathing with inspiratory resistance or threshold loading, cycling, walking for 12 minutes, and performing arm exercises and/or designated calisthenics. Measuring HRs and peak expiratory flowrates before and after exercise helps patients monitor their activity sessions and assess their overall progress. Patients should enter their activities and related responses in their daily logs or records. These log or daily record sheets should be collected regularly and placed in each patient's rehabilitation record. Programs that have only weekly classes may need to document patient therapy and activity more regularly.

PROGRAM SCHEDULING

Pulmonary-rehabilitation programs may have weekly, biweekly, or thrice weekly sessions. Program length depends on whether the program is open ended or closed format. Most investigators agree that a minimum 4 weeks is required to achieve meaningful patient-related results. Most pulmonary-rehabilitation programs average 8 to 12 weeks, but some run for 1 year (Celli, 1994).

The schedules of pulmonary-rehabilitation programs depend on staff and patient availability, room availability, program expectations, and financial resources. According to Medicare, patients in pulmonary rehabilitation should require at least two to three exercise sessions per week to make the program beneficial. When sessions are only conducted weekly, it becomes imperative that patients fulfill their exercise requirements at home and document their activities in their daily records. The perception is that weekly therapy sessions indicate a patient's condition is not that serious and that rehabilitative measures are not necessary. Therapy sessions conducted two or three times a week indicate a more serious condition and the corresponding need for physical reconditioning and therapy.

PROGRAM MARKETING

A pulmonary-rehabilitation program may be successfully advertised and marketed in several ways. The purpose of any marketing campaign is to create or raise awareness of a program. There are three primary target groups when advertising pulmonary rehabilitation: chronic lung patients, physicians, and the general public. Secondary target populations include health-care practitioners and social-service or health organizations like the American Lung Association.

Once target audiences have been identified, a clear, concise message must be developed and delivered through various media. The message is usually in booklet or brochure form, but it may be an audio- or videotape. Such prepared messages describe components of the pulmonary-rehabilitation program and its special features and methods of referral. This program message may be communicated through the mail, in person to groups or individuals, through print media in local or professional newspapers, over the radio, on television, or over computer networks. In hospitals, public-relations departments can play a pivotal role in developing and implementing a marketing campaign.

Physicians remain an important target group in the marketing process for pulmonary rehabilitation. If they are unfamiliar with pulmonary rehabilitation, they must learn the benefits of breathing retraining and physical reconditioning. The RCP or the physician involved with the pulmonary-rehabilitation program are the team members who should meet with referring physicians to promote rehabilitation's value. Such meetings can be done individually or, when possible, to physician groups at seminars or open-house events. The rehabilitation team member must pay special attention to possible referral sources to allay any concerns they may have regarding patient loss via referral to a rehabilitation program. While some physicians are concerned with patient loss, regular communication, including patient progress reports, can help put many of their concerns to rest.

Advertising can be very expensive. If appreciable patient numbers result from advertising efforts, then marketing costs will be covered. If patient numbers are minimal, however, then some difficult marketing decisions must be made. Printing expenses, and expenses for mail and radio or television advertising, can be very expensive. In contrast, a well-written newspaper article or news reporting on the radio or television can promote a rehabilitation program effectively at little or no expense, as can presentations to patient, public, or professional groups. Usually, a well-defined marketing budget with a smart combination of flyers, some media advertising, news coverage, and personal presentations will make the targeted groups aware of the program.

PROGRAM IMPLEMENTATION

Pulmonary-rehabilitation programs are implemented when all the essential pieces and elements come together and a patient population has been identified and evaluated properly. All policies and procedures pertaining to the implementation of the program, including forms for documenting patient evaluation, patient assessment, patient activities, and equipment maintenance, should be included in a program policy-and-procedure manual. This manual will be invaluable during accreditation surveys or state-licensing inspections. Specifically, this manual should address and describe all aspects of the pulmonary-rehabilitation program, including policies or procedures that pertain to:

- the definition, description, and overview of the program and its related services;
- patient referrals;
- requirements of and diagnostic procedures for patient testing and evaluation;
- patient selection and rejection criteria;
- program design, scheduling, and implementation;
- equipment use and maintenance;
- personnel qualifications and responsibilities, including physician involvement;
- patient education and physical activities;
- monitoring and assessment of patient progress;
- patient discontinuation and discharge; and
- outcomes measurement and assessment.

This manual is the responsibility of the pulmonary-rehabilitation program and the medical directors. It should be revised and updated routinely to reflect the current status of the program.

Patient Performance Goals. A preprogram assessment and evaluation enables the rehabilitation specialist and physician to accurately identify specific performance objectives and rehabilitation goals for each patient in the program. Patient-specific performance goals and objectives must consider the extent or degree of each patient's disease or disorder, any underlying conditions, the patient's overall level of physical conditioning, the patient's special medical and social needs, and any other concern that may impact patient performance and progress. These goals and objectives should be short term and long term. Short-term goals include things that can be addressed during the program. They should focus on mastering breathing techniques, reducing levels of dyspnea, increasing physical conditioning and exercise tolerance, improving the ability to self-medicate, employing energy-conservation methods for self-care and routine chores, gaining self-confidence, and, if appropriate, stopping smoking. Long-term goals are somewhat higher targets. They should focus on an increased sense of well-being, fewer manifestations of illness (e.g., fewer emergency room visits or hospitalizations), an increased life expectancy, possible weight control, and an increased ability to carry out daily routines, especially those outside the home.

Specific goals and objectives address the need for breathing retraining; the type and level of prescribed physical activities; the need for oxygen, medications, or special monitoring during exercise; and any special patient needs. Performance goals should identify the targets each patient should attain in terms of work level, duration of activity, HR, oxygen saturation, dyspnea level, and other measurable outcomes. Patients must achieve and maintain their target HRs during exercise to help ensure that cardiovascular and physical conditioning are taking place. Patients complete and are discharged from open-ended programs when they achieve specific performance goals and rehabilitation objectives. Closed-format programs determine patient performance levels after designated periods.

Patient Treatment Plans.   **Patient-treatment** or **care plans** are essential if the full benefits of pulmonary rehabilitation are to be realized. All pertinent patient data, with input from various members of the rehabilitation team, will ensure the rehabilitation effort will be effective. The major purposes of a patient-treatment or care plan are to:

- improve communication among the various members of the rehabilitation or health-care team;
- enhance each patient's continuity of care;
- improve the quality of each patient's respiratory care;
- outline specific actions for relieving acute symptoms;
- formulate short- and long-term patient goals and objectives in the treatment and management of the pulmonary disorder;
- establish criteria for evaluating the effectiveness of pulmonary rehabilitation and monitoring each patient's progress and the progress of the pulmonary disorder; and
- identify the education and self-care needed to allow the patient and his or her family to participate fully in the implementation of the treatment plan (May, 1991).

According to Medicare, this plan of treatment must meet several requirements. Any therapy should be provided according to an ongoing, written plan and should include the following elements:

- patient diagnosis;
- specific statements of long- and short-term goals;
- a reasonable estimate of when the goals will be reached (estimated duration of treatment); and
- an exercise prescription that includes specific modalities and/or procedures to be used in treatment and the frequency of treatment (number of activities performed daily and/or weekly).

The physician determines the frequency and duration of the services by taking into account the accepted norms of medical practice and a reasonable expectation of improvement in each patient's condition. The treatment plan is individualized and established and periodically reviewed by a physician in consultation with staff members who are participating in the program (Xact Medicare Services, 1995). Treatment or patient care plans may have various designs. The cover sheet for one such plan is shown in Figure 4–19.

To achieve specific patient goals, an individualized treatment or care plan must be tailored to each patient in the program. This aids in monitoring patient progress and confirming when goals and objectives are met. A patient-treatment plan helps to identify the patient education topics that must be covered, the breathing-retraining techniques and exercises that are best suited to the patient, and the physical exercises that should be

PATIENT THERAPEUTIC OBJECTIVES AND TREATMENT PLAN

Patient _____   Patient I.D. _____

Diagnosis _____   Target Heart Rate _____

Physician _____   Date _____

Specific patient therapeutic objectives are as follows (check all that apply):

__ complete breathing retraining program
__ perform activities with less dyspnea and panic breathing
__ enhance activities of daily living (ADL)
__ improve or promote cough and expectoration
__ promote proper use of aerosolized medications with deeper deposition
__ promote upper extremity conditioning
__ promote lower extremity conditioning
__ improve exercise endurance and tolerance
__ improve arterial oxygenation
__ other: _____

Specific therapeutic regimen/treatment plan to achieve patient objectives (check all that apply):

__ diaphragmatic with pursed-lip breathing   __ twelve minute walk
__ inspiratory resistance breathing   __ daily calisthenic routine
__ cycling with increasing intensity   __ aerosol therapy instruction
__ chest physiotherapy procedures   __ other: _____

Proposed duration for prescribed regimen and treatment plan:

__ single session   __ twelve week session
__ single session with follow-up   __ other: _____

Type and frequency of patient assessment and follow-up (check all that apply):

__ by physician on a __ weekly basis or __ biweekly basis
__ by therapist on a __ weekly basis or __ biweekly basis
__ other: _____

Outcomes assessment. Patient will be evaluated regarding achievement of stated therapeutic objectives on the basis of (check all that apply):

__ patient performance criteria   __ pulmonary function test
__ post cardiopulmonary exercise test   __ other: _____

Figure 1 19 *A patient-treatment plan for pulmonary rehabilitation, which includes a list of therapeutic objectives and treatment regimens. This form must be completed by a physician with input from the rehabilitation team. (Courtesy of Lung Diagnostics, Glen Ridge, New Jersey.)*

promoted in an exercise prescription. A key component of any patient-treatment plan is the exercise prescription. It must be completed for each patient before rehabilitation starts by the physician overseeing the medical aspects of the program. Integral to an exercise prescription are the following elements:

- mode (the type of physical activity the patient performed, like walking, stair climbing, or cycling);
- duration (depends on a patient's fitness level. Very deconditioned patients should start with short intervals of exercise, with brief rest periods as needed. As the patients' conditioning increases, they should increase the duration of exercise 1 to 2 minutes a day, with a goal of performing 20 to 30 minutes of continuous exercise daily);
- frequency (if continuous exercise is less than 15 minutes a day, frequency should be two to three times a day. However, if continuous exercise is greater than 20 minutes a day, frequency should be once a day, 3 to 7 days a week); and
- intensity (depends on a patient's fitness level, health status, and program goals. Exercise intensity is usually based on the results of a patient's CPX test and is increased gradually according to a patient's tolerance).

Intensity may be determined based on a patient's target HR, as discussed previously, or on METs. To prescribe exercise for a patient based on METs, the desired range of energy expenditure is determined (usually 60 to 85 percent of maximal functional capacity), the range is expressed in terms of METs, and activities known to require this energy expenditure are prescribed. Another method of determining the intensity of exercise training uses the 15-point category RPE scale (ranges from 6 to 20) or the 10-point category-ratio RPE scale. These two scales are based on endurance evaluation and can be used to predict the percent of an individual's maximum HR during exercise. Healthy individuals can exercise within the 12-to-16 range on the 15-point scale (which is approximately 60 to 85 percent of maximum HR). This corresponds to a score of 4 to 6 on the 10-point scale. Chronic respiratory patients, limited by their dyspnea, physical conditions, and health statuses, will exercise with much lower scores within much lower ranges. It is important to note that most chronic respiratory patients in pulmonary rehabilitation find lower-intensity, longer-duration exercise more beneficial than higher-intensity exercise (Watchie, 1995). Figure 4–20 suggests an exercise-prescription format.

Patients should be encouraged to follow energy-saving techniques that include any or all of the following:

- establish a daily routine that is paced and has appropriate rest periods;
- sit whenever possible;
- eliminate unnecessary tasks;
- avoid strenuous arm activities;
- increase levels of activity gradually;
- organize the work area;
- use assistive devices when appropriate (e.g., shower chair or long-handled tools);
- adjust work heights; and
- avoid sustained positions.

PATIENT EXERCISE PRESCRIPTION

Patient name _____   Patient I.D. _____

Diagnosis _____   Target Heart Rate _____

Patient to perform the following physical activities, as prescribed, on the following basis:

_____ daily   _____ every other day   or   _____ times per week

_____ Oxygen to be used at _____ LPM during prescribed physical activities.

All physical activities performed must be recorded in each patient's daily log.

PHYSICAL ACTIVITY	INITIAL	INCREASE WEEKLY
Cycling (exercycle)	Distance _____ miles or Duration _____ minutes Tension _____	Distance _____ miles or Duration _____ minutes Tension _____
Twelve Minute Walk	Note distance and number of stops during this activity.	Note distance and number of stops during this activity. Increase walking speed on a weekly basis.
Arm Ergometry	Duration _____ minutes Tension _____	Duration _____ minutes Tension _____
Inspiratory Resistance Device: _____	Level or Setting _____ Duration _____ minutes	Increase level of setting _____ weekly _____ biweekly _____ as tolerated Duration _____ minutes
Stair Climbing	Number of Stairs _____ Duration _____ minutes	Number of Stairs _____ Duration _____ minutes
Other Activities (identify)		

PRESCRIBING PHYSICIAN _____   DATE _____

Figure 4–20   *The exercise prescription is a key part of a patient-treatment plan*

These suggestions help patients to perform more tasks with less discomfort and greater confidence (Watchie, 1995).

Patients must be allowed to engage in physical activities that they feel comfortable with and that will not aggravate any underlying conditions like arthritis or orthopedic injuries. Most patients will do well as the duration and intensity of physical exercise are increased gradually over the program. In essence, the patients develop a tolerance to exercise and dyspnea that allows them to perform higher levels of physical activity with greater levels of confidence. This growth tends to be slow, but it results in greater levels of patient performance and overall satisfaction with the program.

Patient Documentation. Program personnel and patients in the pulmonary-rehabilitation program must both maintain and keep records. These records document the patient's activity, response to therapy, and progress in the program. All patient records should be filed in the program office for medical-legal reasons, for use in any program-accrediting endeavor, and for insurance purposes, including any audit of program and patient activities.

Miscellaneous Considerations. Any practitioner involved with pulmonary rehabilitation should consider a few miscellaneous points or areas. These include the need to follow up or continue patient conditioning beyond that provided by the initial program and other patient-related activities that can enhance the rehabilitation effort. Maintenance activity, however, is suspect, and its validity will be questioned by payors like Medicare.

To avoid the detraining effect, all patients who have completed conditioning programs should be advised to continue their breathing retraining and exercise regimens at home on their own. Programs may decide to have patients complete regular check-ups, follow-ups, or reunions to ensure patients comply with this recommendation. Periodic pulmonary function testing, including CPX evaluations, should be scheduled to evaluate patient condition and overall progress.

Programs may also decide to form "better breathing" clubs to help continue the goals and focus of pulmonary rehabilitation. These clubs meet regularly to provide a social outlet while reinforcing program concepts. Guest speakers can be scheduled to present a variety of health-related topics and other group-related activities can be planned, including holiday parties, picnics, outings, weekend trips, and even cruise vacations. Rehabilitation groups can also become politically active by contacting their local, state, and federal representatives regarding any proposed changes in health-care benefits or programs. Activities like these contribute significantly to a patient's quality of life. Patients not only breathe and feel better, they are better able to cope with the devastating nature of their disease.

NATIONAL PULMONARY REHABILITATION SURVEY

In 1987, the AARC and the AACVPR conducted an inaugural joint survey to compile a national directory of pulmonary-rehabilitation programs and to identify and characterize the key components of these programs. Responses were received from 150 programs in 37 states spread evenly across the United States. The results revealed a fascinating, first-time look at pulmonary rehabilitation and its scope nationwide. Results from this survey are summarized as follows:

- programs enroll an average of six patients per class;
- class sessions run an average of 2.2 hours per day for an average of 2.6 days per week;
- programs run for an average of 8.3 weeks with a mean length of 47.5 hours;
- individual format is used by 28 percent of the responding programs, group format by 30 percent of the programs, and a combination of individual and group formats by the remainder;
- hospitals are the major site of pulmonary rehabilitation;
- of the responding programs, 97 percent are set up to serve outpatients, while 49 percent of the programs work with inpatients as well;
- of the responding programs, 23 percent accept COPD patients only, while most accept patients with other respiratory disorders;
- for 97 percent of the responding programs, patients come from within a 50-mile radius;
- nearly all (99 percent) the patient referrals come from physicians, while hospitals, clinics, HMOs, the American Lung Association, and industry comprise other referral sources;
- preprogram admission requirements include spirometry in 89 percent of the programs responding, chest radiographs in 70 percent of the programs, and exercise testing in 65 percent;
- postprogram assessment is achieved with exercise testing in 34 percent of the programs, while spirometry is performed in 29 percent of the programs;
- the health specialists most frequently represented on pulmonary-rehabilitation teams are physicians (88 percent), dietitians (85 percent), registered respiratory therapists (RRTs) (76 percent), and registered nurses (65 percent); and
- equipment used most includes pulse oximeters (97 percent), stationary bicycles (95 percent), treadmills (87 percent) and free weights (78 percent).

Other findings of the survey related to program content in terms of lectures, smoking cessation, exercise sessions, patient charges, and reimbursement which, the survey reported, is pulmonary rehabilitation's greatest challenge. The survey information was also useful in developing a national listing of pulmonary-rehabilitation programs. When reported in 1988, the list contained 265 programs, including the 150 that participated in the survey (Bickford & Hodgkin, 1988). However, twice as many programs may exist. Neil R. McIntyre, Jr., medical director of respiratory care services at Duke University Medical Center in North Carolina, believes there are approximately 500 centers throughout the United States offering some type of pulmonary rehabilitation ("Pulmonary Rehab Programs Are Cost Effective," 1989). Continuing to collect data like that acquired in the joint survey is essential to determining the true extent of pulmonary rehabilitation and should help to engender a more effective reimbursement mechanism.

─────────────── # SUMMARY ───────────────

A well-designed, well-organized, and well-implemented pulmonary-rehabilitation program has numerous components, all of which are essential to the program's overall success. Principal elements of any pulmonary-rehabilitation program include facility location, room space, operating budget, exercise and monitoring equipment, personnel, program format and focus, scheduling, and content. Because these elements vary and are available to different extents, pulmonary-rehabilitation programs can differ in focus, style, and delivery from center to center. Other issues revolving around program focus and structure include individual patient objectives, patient-treatment plans, and training specificity. The results and outcomes of pulmonary rehabilitation, discussed in Chapter 5, are a consequence of how well a program is designed and delivered. Program resources like equipment and staff are relatively easy to secure. While directing and motivating patients is more difficult, it is equally important to the overall development and success of the program.

Review Questions

1. What are five key components of a pulmonary-rehabilitation program?
2. What are the differences between an open-ended and a closed-format pulmonary-rehabilitation program? Which is more effective? Why?
3. What space and equipment needs are essential for a pulmonary-rehabilitation program?
4. What key health-care professionals should be involved in planning and conducting a pulmonary-rehabilitation program? What are the areas of expertise of each?
5. How can ventilatory muscle endurance be achieved during pulmonary rehabilitation?
6. What are the three principles of exercise training? Why are they important?
7. What are the key elements of a pulmonary-rehabilitation patient-treatment plan?

References

American Institute of Architects Committee on Architecture for Health. (1993). *Guidelines for construction and equipment of hospital and medical facilities (1992–93)*. Washington, D.C.: The American Institute of Architects Press.

Bellman, M.J., & Mittman, C. (1980). Ventilatory muscle training improves exercise capacity in chronic obstructive pulmonary disease patients. *American Review of Respiratory Disease, 121*(2), 273–280.

Bellman, M.J., & Wasserman, K. (1982). Exercise training and testing in patients with chronic obstructive pulmonary disease. (Monograph). *Basics of RD*. The American Thoracic Society.

Bickford, L.S., & Hodgkin, J.E. (1988, November). National pulmonary rehabilitation survey. *Respiratory Care, 33*(11), 1030–1043.

Burton, G.G., Gee, G.N., & Hodgkin, J.E. (1977). *Respiratory care—A guide to clinical practice*. Philadelphia, PA: J.B. Lippincott.

Celli, B.R. (1994, May). Physical reconditioning of patients with respiratory disease: Legs, arms, and breathing retraining. *Respiratory Care, 39*(5), 482–483, 488–491.

Connors, G.L. with A.L. Goldman (ed.). (1987, Spring). Role of the respiratory therapist. *Problems in Pulmonary Disease, 3*(1), 7.

EdenTec®. (1996). Flutter® mucus clearance device—Instructions for use for healthcare professionals. Eden Prairie, MN: EdenTec®—A Nellcor Company.

Faulkner, J.A. (1968). New perspectives in training for maximum performance. *JAMA, 205,* 741.

Holliday, J.E., & Hyers, T.M. (1990). The reduction of weaning time from mechanical ventilation using tidal volume and relaxation biofeedback. *American Review of Respiratory Disease, 141*(5) (Part 1), 1214–1220.

Inside Industry. (1996, May 20). Rehab equipment market to climb. *Advance for Respiratory Care Practitioners, 9*(10), 16.

Kane, C.S. (1993 February/March). An interdisciplinary approach to pulmonary rehabilitation. *RT— The Journal for Respiratory Care Practitioners, 6*(2), 16–24.

Levine, S., Weiser, P., & Gillen, J. (1986). Evaluation of a ventilatory muscle endurance training program in the rehabilitation of patients with chronic obstructive pulmonary disease. *American Review of Respiratory Disease, 133*(3), 400–406.

May, D.F. (1991). *Rehabilitation and continuity of care in pulmonary disease.* St. Louis, MO: Mosby-Year Book, Inc.

McMahon, P. (1988, November). The hospital-based pulmonary rehabilitation home care program. *AARCTimes, 12*(11), 50–51.

Pulmonary rehabilitation programs are cost effective. (1989, September 11). *Advance for Respiratory Therapists, 2*(37), 9.

Ries, A.L., & Moser, K.M. (1986). Comparison of isocapnic hyperventilation and walking exercise training at home in pulmonary rehabilitation. *Chest, 90*(2), 285–289.

Tandon, M. (1978). Adjunct treatment with yoga in chronic severe airways obstruction. *Thorax, 33*(4), 514–517.

Watchie, J. (1995). *Cardiopulmonary physical therapy: A clinical manual.* Philadelphia, PA: W.B. Saunders Company.

Weiner, P., Azgad, Y., & Ganam, R. (1992a). Inspiratory muscle training, combined with general exercise reconditioning in patients with COPD. *Chest, 102*(5), 1351–1356.

Weiner, P., Azgad, Y., & Ganam, R. (1992b). Inspiratory muscle training in patients with bronchial asthma. *Chest, 102*(5), 1357–1361.

Xact Medicare Services. (1995, April). *Medicare medical policy bulletins* (Bulletin No. Y-1C, Rev. 006, Chapter 7, pp. 7-53–7-54).

Suggested Readings

American College of Sports Medicine. (1995). *ACSM's guidelines for exercise testing and prescription* (5th ed.). Baltimore, MD: Williams & Wilkins.

American Lung Association. (1995). *Help yourself to better breathing.* New York, NY: American Lung Association.

Beckman, R. (1995, February/March). Rehabilitation of the ventilator-dependent patient. *RT—The Journal for Respiratory Care Practitioners 8*(2), 71–74.

Casaburi, R. (1992, February/March). Pulmonary rehabilitation: Improving exercise tolerance. *RT— The Journal for Respiratory Care Practitioners 5*(2), 15–22.

Chaff, L.F. (1994). *Safety guide for health care institutions* (5th ed.). A joint publication of the American Hospital Association and the National Safety Council. Chicago, IL: American Hospital Publishing, Inc.

Golemb, K. (1993). *Better breathers club panic control workbook.* (2nd ed.). National City, CA: Allied Health Publications.

Hodgkin, J.E., Connors, G.L., & Bell, C.W. *Pulmonary rehabilitation—Guidelines to success* (2nd ed.). Philadelphia, PA: J.B. Lippincott Company. 32–49.

Larson, J.L., Kim, M.J., Sharp, J.T., & Larson, D.A. (1988). Inspiratory muscle training with a pressure threshold breathing device in patients with chronic obstructive pulmonary disease. *American Review of Respiratory Disease, 138,* 689.

Make, B. (1991, April). COPD: Management and rehabilitation. *American Family Physicians, 43*(4), 1315–1324.

Morris, K.V., & Hodgkin, J.E. (1996). *Pulmonary rehabilitation administration and patient education manual.* Gaithersburg, MD: Aspen Publishers, Inc.

Scanlan, C. (Ed.). *Egan's fundamentals of respiratory care* (6th ed.). St. Louis, MO: Mosby-Year Book, Inc.

Tietsort, J. (1995). *COPD and you . . . A patient education manual.* National City, CA: Allied Health Publications.

CHAPTER FIVE

MEASURING AND ASSESSING THE OUTCOMES OF PULMONARY REHABILITATION

KEY TERMS

comprehensive
pulmonary rehabilitation
functional status

management by
objectives (MBO)

outcomes assessment
patient attrition

OBJECTIVES

Upon completing this chapter, the reader will be able to:

- List at least five patient expectations of pulmonary rehabilitation.
- Identify three accepted benefits of pulmonary rehabilitation.
- Identify three possible benefits of pulmonary rehabilitation.
- Identify three unlikely or debated benefits of pulmonary rehabilitation.
- Describe at least three ways in which pulmonary-rehabilitation outcomes may be ascertained and documented.
- List five reasons for attrition in pulmonary-rehabilitation programs and, explain how these problems could be addressed effectively.

INTRODUCTION

 Programs throughout the United States, in collaboration with research facilities, continue to document the beneficial effects of pulmonary rehabilitation. Patients appear to benefit objectively and subjectively from well-designed and well-implemented pulmonary-rehabilitation programs. These benefits must be reported properly to justify the program's continued existence and the need for reimbursing this important and vital therapy.

 This chapter examines patient expectations, the objective and subjective benefits of pulmonary rehabilitation, and the ways to measure and document the results of patient outcomes. Each step or component of pulmonary rehabilitation is as important as the next. While program design, organization, and implementation are crucial, no one can argue against the equally important function of measuring and assessing program and patient outcomes. Outcomes assessment must start at the beginning of the pulmonary-rehabilitation program. Practitioners must have clear ideas of what they want their patients to achieve or accomplish at the onset. A clear definition of each patient's goals and objectives at the onset enables practitioners to measure outcomes more objectively and completely.

THE PROCESS OF OUTCOMES ASSESSMENT

Outcomes assessment is an important facet of pulmonary rehabilitation that can be accomplished in various ways. Regardless of the method, outcomes assessment is essential to patient, provider, and reimbursement. With Medicare and other third-party payor reimbursement tightening, it is becoming increasingly more important to demonstrate to the medical and payor communities that pulmonary rehabilitation works. To verify these benefits and the overall value of pulmonary rehabilitation, practitioners must perform outcomes assessment continually by documenting progress and reporting results using appropriate measurement tools.

Outcomes assessment should be an ongoing process that looks at subjective and objective program results. Outcomes assessment offers insight into how a program may be improved or modified to operate more efficiently and effectively. In their simplest form, subjective patient surveys can tell whether a pulmonary-rehabilitation program was beneficial or not. However, objective measurements tend to be more reliable indicators of patient outcomes and patient benefits.

Patients often relate a number of subjective benefits they derive from the education, breathing retraining, and physical reconditioning of rehabilitation. Practitioners involved in pulmonary rehabilitation must be more objective. Outcomes assessment is a process that should start with identifying and addressing patient expectations and conclude with responses to the following:

1. In which way(s) did the patient progress?
2. In what aspects of pulmonary rehabilitation was the patient's participation most critical?
3. Which patient population seemed to derive the greatest benefit?

Improving the quality of pulmonary rehabilitation depends on how effectively patient expectations are met and how completely these three questions are answered (Peske, 1995).

PATIENT EXPECTATIONS

Patient expectations of pulmonary rehabilitation are tied closely to the goals and objectives established for each patient entering the program. While goals and objectives tend to be objective, patient expectations are subjective. It is important that practitioners address patients' expectations of what pulmonary rehabilitation can and cannot do at the beginning of the program during orientation. Coupling program expectations with specific patient goals and objectives personalizes the program for each patient while creating realistic targets. Patient expectations may include any of the following:

- feeling better overall;
- breathing properly and with less discomfort;
- performing physical activities with less shortness of breath;
- doing more and being more active;
- taking better care of oneself;
- relying less on oxygen or medications;
- experiencing fewer hospitalizations; and
- seeing one's physician less frequently.

Some of these expectations are subjective, while others are more objective and measurable. Expectations are often related to a patient's needs and condition. Properly identifying patient expectations in the beginning allows RCPs and other health-care providers to tailor class sessions and presentations to meet those needs. In most cases, a well-designed pulmonary-rehabilitation program covers nearly every topic and area for which patients need information, direction, and/or assistance.

A straightforward way of determining whether patient expectations were met is to use a questionnaire at the program's conclusion. The questionnaire simply should ask what the patients expected, were those expectations met, and why. The only difficulty with the questionnaire method lies in the patient's ability to read, write, and express him- or herself intelligently. Other ways to determine whether patient expectations were met include checklists and patient interviews, both of which also have shortcomings. Patients may simply check boxes on a checklist, or they may be less than truthful in an interview. Some interviewers may inadvertently coach patients to give certain responses and even suggest answers.

IDENTIFYING THE BENEFITS OF PULMONARY REHABILITATION

The benefits of pulmonary rehabilitation may be classified as those that are accepted, those that are possible, and those that are unlikely or debatable. Controversy continues regarding the benefits of pulmonary rehabilitation. As research in this area continues, and reconditioning methods and techniques continue to be refined, the real benefits and outcomes of pulmonary rehabilitation should become more apparent. It is now becoming more evident that patients who finish **comprehensive pulmonary rehabilitation** programs tend to have fewer infections and hospitalizations, experience less dyspnea, and lead more active and productive lives than those who do not. In addition to breathing retraining and physical reconditioning, comprehensive pulmonary rehabilitation programs cover all facets of care for the respiratory patient, including stress management, medication use, nutrition, personal hygiene, and ADL.

Accepted Benefits of Pulmonary Rehabilitation. The COPD patients who complete pulmonary-rehabilitation programs demonstrate three major and accepted benefits, all of which account for the fewer respiratory symptoms and lesser degrees of dyspnea the patients claim to experience. The first accepted benefit of pulmonary rehabilitation is increased endurance and exercise tolerance. The second involves an increase in $\dot{V}O_{2max}$. The third is an increase in physical performance as evidenced by increased anaerobic threshold and decreased ventilation, oxygen consumption, and HR (Hughes & Davison, 1983). The postrehabilitation CPX test is useful in illustrating and confirming these accepted benefits, but only when performed as part of the program admission criteria. Comparing the pre- and postprogram CPX studies indicates any degree of improvement in terms of exercise tolerance, $\dot{V}O_{2max}$, and physical performance.

Possible Benefits of Pulmonary Rehabilitation. A number of possible or probable benefits of pulmonary rehabilitation have been demonstrated through program evaluations and assessments. Subjectively, patients may experience increased senses of well-being, less anxiety and depression, and better qualities of life. Objectively, patients may have increased hypoxic drives and increased left ventricular function. Most of these benefits are observed in patients without obstructive airways disease (Hughes & Davison, 1983). Possible benefits tend to be less objective than accepted benefits and do not require pre- and post-CPX testing. In addition to ABG analysis, cardiac output determinations and other hemodynamic parameters are necessary to demonstrate the authenticity of some possible benefits.

Unlikely Benefits of Pulmonary Rehabilitation. A number of pulmonary-rehabilitation benefits remain unlikely, debated, or unknown. Some of these questionable benefits include improved survival or longevity, improved pulmonary-function tests, improved ABGs, changes in muscle oxygen extraction, changes in step desaturation, and episodes of apnea (Hughes & Davison, 1983). If these benefits were more demonstrable, pulmonary rehabilitation would be more widely offered and accepted. Table 5–1 lists all the accepted,

TABLE 5–1   A comprehensive listing of the accepted, possible, and unlikely benefits of pulmonary rehabilitation

Accepted Benefits	Possible Benefits	Unlikely Benefits
Increased exercise tolerance and endurance	Increased sense of well-being with less anxiety and depression	Increased longevity and survival
Increased $\dot{V}O_{2max}$	Better quality of life	Improvement in PFT
Increased physical performance (with increased anaerobic threshold and decreased ventilation, oxygen consumption, and HR)	A more active lifestyle with an enhanced ability to carry out ADL	Improvement in ABG
	Increased mucociliary clearance	Lowered pulmonary artery pressure
	Fewer infections and hospitalizations	Improved blood chemistry, including blood lipids
	Increased hypoxic drive	Change in muscle oxygen extraction
	Increased left ventricular function	Change in step oxygen desaturation and apnea

rehabilitation would be more widely offered and accepted. Table 5–1 lists all the accepted, possible, and unlikely benefits of pulmonary rehabilitation.

METHODS OF MEASURING AND ASSESSING OUTCOMES

The CPX test is not only essential to identifying and admitting patients into pulmonary rehabilitation, it is equally important in measuring and assessing patient outcomes and overall improvement. As noted earlier in this chapter, the accepted benefits of pulmonary rehabilitation and physical reconditioning are determined based on the positive changes observed between pre- and postexercise studies, particularly in the areas of work performance and $\dot{V}O_{2max}$. Figure 5–1 is a form used to compare patient performance during CPX testing before and after pulmonary rehabilitation. Tools like these help to identify changes in patients' conditions and physical abilities. Most postrehabilitation CPX testing is done at the program's conclusion and should be repeated once every 3 years thereafter. More frequent testing may be warranted by a patient's condition.

In most instances, postrehabilitation CPX testing parameters that change or increase by 15 percent or more suggest significant improvement. Parameters that deserve special attention or consideration because they indicate specific changes and/or improvement in patient condition include:

- test duration;
- highest workload or capacity (in watts);
- $\dot{V}O_{2max}$;
- time patient reached anaerobic threshold;
- METs achieved;
- oxygen saturation at maximum;
- maximum ventilation;
- maximum HR;
- maximum blood pressure;
- ECG;
- reason(s) for terminating the test.

While patients who have improved physically because of pulmonary rehabilitation show positive changes in these parameters, others who have improved physically may exhibit negative changes. These negative changes are usually cardiovascular and manifest as cardiac arrhythmias or blood pressure elevations. Pulmonary patients who are physically limited by dyspnea may terminate their initial CPX tests based on their impaired ventilatory statuses and abilities before any cardiovascular abnormality can be detected. In these cases, the patients' pulmonary defects are able to mask the presence of cardiac defects because the study was short. However, once pulmonary rehabilitation is completed, these patients are usually able to increase their test durations and work capacities, thereby allowing any cardiovascular problem to manifest itself. When this occurs, patients should be referred to a cardiologist for follow-up. The following case study examines five patients who, based on CPX testing, completed a pulmonary-rehabilitation program. Key

RETROSPECTIVE STUDY ON REHAB PATIENT PERFORMANCE

Patient _____ Sex _____ DOB _____

Physician _____ Diagnosis _____

Dates of Initial Rehab Program Attendance _____

Type(s) of Physical Activity Performed _____

PRE-REHAB TEST		Date _____
Workload Achieved =		
METS Achieved =		Resting: Heart Rate = _____
Maximum Heart Rate =		Blood Pressure = _____
Maximum Blood Pressure =		O_2 Saturation = _____
O_2 Saturation at Max =		Reason Test Stopped:
O_2 Consumption at Max =		
Ventilation at Max =		Duration = _____

PRE-REHAB TEST I	% Change	Date _____
Workload Achieved =		
METS Achieved =		Resting: Heart Rate = _____
Maximum Heart Rate =		Blood Pressure = _____
Maximum Blood Pressure =		O_2 Saturation = _____
O_2 Saturation at Max =		Reason Test Stopped:
O_2 Consumption at Max =		
Ventilation at Max =		Duration = _____

POST-REHAB TEST II	% Change	Date _____
Workload Achieved =		
METS Achieved =		Resting: Heart Rate = _____
Maximum Heart Rate =		Blood Pressure = _____
Maximum Blood Pressure =		O_2 Saturation = _____
O_2 Saturation at Max =		Reason Test Stopped:
O_2 Consumption at Max =		
Ventilation at Max =		Duration = _____

Figure 5–1 *A comparison of pre- and postrehabilitation performance as measured by CPX testing can be documented using a form such as this. It also allows for another study to be performed to document any further changes in a patient's condition. (Courtesy of Lung Diagnostics, Glen Ridge, N.J.)*

testing parameters were used to demonstrate the patients' responses to rehabilitation and physical reconditioning.

CASE STUDY

Results of Pulmonary Rehabilitation Based on CPX Testing

Five patients completed a 12-week, closed-format pulmonary-rehabilitation program. Sessions, approximately 2 hours each, were conducted weekly. At home, each patient kept a daily log of exercise activities that included cycling on a stationary bicycle, 12-minute walks, calisthenics, and breathing retraining using inspiratory resistance and diaphragmatic breathing with pursed lips. At the facility, the patients cycled, walked, and used arm ergometry for upper extremity conditioning. All patients were monitored accordingly. Physician follow-up was biweekly. The pulmonary rehabilitation was comprehensive, and patients received instruction in breathing techniques, stress management and relaxation, exercise routines, medication delivery, respiratory home-care equipment and therapy, nutrition, secretion clearance, personal hygiene, and ADL. At the conclusion of the program, these patients completed evaluation surveys and postrehabilitation CPX testing. Results of this testing were as follows:

Patient	Age	Sex	Test Duration	Workload at Max	SpO_2 AT MAX	$\dot{V}O_{2max}$	METs
R.A.	68	F	4:25/6:30	65/90	94%/95%	805/1110	3.5/4.8
P.C.	74	M	5:15/7:45	75/120	93%/94%	775/1080	3.2/4.5
K.C.	61	F	3:30/5:10	55/80	91%/93%	638/902	2.9/4.1
C.M.	58	F	6:10/7:50	95/120	95%/95%	1200/1425	4.8/5.7
K.W.	73	M	4:00/5:30	70/95	91%/94%	529/1058	2.3/4.6

In the preceding data, duration is expressed in minutes:seconds, workload at maximum is expressed in watts, and results as prerehabilitation/postrehabilitation.

1. Of the five patients who completed pulmonary rehabilitation, which demonstrated the greatest degree of improvement? On what basis is this determination made?
2. Based on these data, which patient was in the "best" condition upon entering the program? On what basis is this determination made?
3. What additional information would have been helpful in assessing the outcomes of this program?

Patients may also be evaluated after pulmonary rehabilitation using standard pulmonary-function testing, ABG analysis, chest radiographs, blood chemistries, and dyspnea indices. Improvement in any of these functions is not always evident, and it appears unlikely in most cases. Nevertheless, results do relate to each patient's overall condition. This type of information may prove invaluable to any retrospective studies and should therefore remain part of the medical record.

Another effective way to measure patient outcomes resulting from pulmonary rehabilitation is the process known as **management by objectives (MBO).** First used in the late 1960s and early 1970s, MBO is an effective way to monitor and follow a patient's activity and improvement within the rehabilitation program. The benefits of MBO are clear. It provides the health-care provider with structure and a means of assessing patient performance and progress; it provides patients with a clear understanding of what is expected of them (Olsson, 1968; Tosi & Tosi, 1973). By establishing distinct, concise, and measurable rehabilitation goals and objectives for each patient, health-care practitioners are in a better position to supervise each patient's activities and to redirect patients when and if necessary. Following are key elements to an effective MBO process in any pulmonary-rehabilitation program:

- mutual goal setting by patients and health-care providers in the program;
- patient and practitioner commitment to this approach;
- frequent performance reviews; and
- the freedom to develop alternative methods for achieving stated objectives.

The MBO process may be used in closed-format rehabilitation programs, but it is essential for open-ended programs in which patients complete their rehabilitation regimens only when they attain specific personal goals and objectives. There are pitfalls to the MBO process, like lack of patient and practitioner commitment, poor implementation, poor coaching, little assistance, lack of follow-up, overemphasized evaluation, and a process that is too mechanical. However, MBO can be viable if these pitfalls are recognized and avoided. The MBO process enables practitioners to measure patient outcomes effectively and to identify deficiencies or problem areas, thereby justifying the need for continued rehabilitation and physical reconditioning.

Finally, evaluation forms that identify patient comments and compare physical activities at the beginning and end of the program provide information that is useful in appraising patient performance and progress. A section of the evaluation form should allow patients to indicate their performance levels at the start of the program and at its conclusion. In general, most patients start cycling at 10 minutes per day with no tension. A 6- or 12-minute walk remains at 6 or 12 minutes for the duration of the program, but patients walk faster, for greater distances, and with fewer stops as they acquire greater endurance and exercise tolerance. Arm ergometry may start at 5 minutes per day with no tension or resistance. Inspiratory resistance breathing usually begins at the lowest level for 15 to 20 minutes a day. Depending on the program's length, cycling will increase to 25 to 30 minutes per day with varying amounts of tension. Arm ergometry will increase to well over 10 minutes a day with significant resistance, and most patients will achieve very high levels of inspiratory resistance for at least 30 minutes a day using any currently available training device. Other physical activities a patient completes, like stair climbing, should also be included. An example of a program evaluation form used to document this type of patient activity is found in Figure 5–2. Patient-rehabilitation records and daily log sheets should be used to verify this information as it appears on the evaluation form. Daily log sheets should be collected at the end of the program and placed in each patient's pulmonary-rehabilitation record.

PHYSICAL ACTIVITY	AT START OF PROGRAM	AT END OF PROGRAM
Cycling (exercycle)	Distance _____ miles or km Duration _____ minutes Tension _____	Distance _____ miles or km Duration _____ minutes Tension _____
Twelve Minute Walk	Distance _____ Number of Stops _____	Distance _____ Number of Stops _____
Arm Ergometry	Duration _____ minutes Tension _____	Duration _____ minutes Tension _____
Inspiratory Resistance Device: _____	Level or Setting _____ Duration _____ minutes	Level or Setting _____ Duration _____ minutes
Stair Climbing	Number of Stairs _____ Duration _____ minutes	Number of Stairs _____ Duration _____ minutes

Patient name _____ Date of Evaluation _____

Figure 5–2 *A section of a patient evaluation form that compares patient performance at the beginning and end of a pulmonary-rehabilitation program. (Courtesy of Lung Diagnostics, Glen Ridge, N.J.)*

Some patients may require assistance in completing these forms. However, practitioners should not volunteer information, coach patients in their responses, or unwittingly suggest answers or responses. Information obtained from these evaluations should be tabulated, analyzed, and used to modify or revise the program.

An important part of any evaluation process is to ascertain the degree of patient satisfaction. Particular areas include room comfort, scheduling, time allotted for sessions, competency and skills of the health-care providers conducting sessions, available equipment, and scope of the program. Many MCOs are interested in patient comments and may require patient satisfaction survey data when a rehabilitation facility applies for acceptance into any health-care provider networks.

PATIENT ATTENDANCE AND ATTRITION

Even though the benefits of pulmonary rehabilitation are tangible, patients either miss sessions or do not complete programs in which they enroll. Attendance and **patient attrition** continue to be issues that program and medical directors must address. Causes for patient absence and attrition are numerous. Some are easily identified. Some are not so obvious and require inquiry. Remember that patients who stop attending sessions do not complete evaluation forms or questionnaires at the end of the program. It is important that program personnel contact these patients to ascertain their exact reason(s) for withdrawing from the program. If patients cannot provide this information, the referring physician may be able to explain why the patients left.

Attrition in pulmonary-rehabilitation programs seems to be associated with the degree to which patients' psychosocial needs are met. Other reasons for absence and attrition include illness; inclement or adverse weather conditions like humidity, wind, and temperature; problems with program personnel or other patients in the group; transportation and parking problems; personal emergencies; vacation; dissatisfaction with routine; and lack of interest or loss of enthusiasm.

Obviously, some of these reasons cannot be controlled by the patient or the program, but others can. Practitioners involved with the program should monitor patient enthusiasm and motivation as well as performance. Identifying patient dissatisfaction or lack of interest early allows practitioners to make changes that may reduce program attrition. Practitioners must allow for illness, holidays, vacations, and personal emergencies. Makeup sessions can be offered at the program's discretion, which enables patients to continue in the program despite interruptions. Finally, programs should ensure there is adequate parking and assist in making arrangements for transportation with local agencies or between patients.

PROGRAM RESULTS AND FINDINGS

Pulmonary-rehabilitation programs throughout the United States have been collecting and analyzing data on patient outcomes and benefits. There has been particular interest in the effects of comprehensive pulmonary-rehabilitation programs versus those of programs offering education alone on the physiological and psychosocial outcomes of patients with COPD. Findings strongly suggest that comprehensive pulmonary rehabilitation results in significantly greater exercise tolerance and exercise endurance, lesser degrees of muscle fatigue and dyspnea, and enhanced self-efficacy in activities like walking. Differences in survival and duration of hospital stays were noted but were not significant. Other areas, like pulmonary function, psychological depression, and overall quality of life, did not differ between the two groups (Ries et al., 1995).

Other studies have reported encouraging results regarding the benefits of pulmonary rehabilitation in COPD patients. For instance, follow-up studies conducted since 1985 at Duke University Medical Center have demonstrated that almost two thirds of patients who complete pulmonary-rehabilitation programs continue to progress or at least remain stable. These findings are based on CPX studies that show significant increases in $\dot{V}O_{2max}$. However, no significant changes in pulmonary functions have been recorded. Improvement in patient condition is clearly the result of increased exercise tolerance and endurance on the basis of $\dot{V}O_{2max}$ increases. Other studies conducted at Duke University clearly document that pulmonary rehabilitation reduces the number of hospital days per year for patients with chronic lung disease (Scott, 1989).

Findings from another study concluded that pulmonary rehabilitation can produce the following results in chronic lung patients:

- improved walking capacity and overall **functional status** unassociated with changes in airflow or oxygen saturation; and
- functional benefits measurable with indices of functional status, namely the MDI, the MRCI, and the Modified Pneumoconiosis Research Unit Score (MPRUS).

Of the three indices, the MDI appears to be the most sensitive for ascertaining functional improvement in patients with chronic lung disease. *Functional status,* defined as the impact of a patient's dyspnea on the performance of daily activities, has emerged as another important indicator of clinical response to rehabilitation. It appears that both exercise tolerance and functional status are clearly enhanced in patients with lung disease after physical reconditioning. These conclusions corroborate those of other investigations that suggest pulmonary rehabilitation is in fact beneficial (Holden et all, 1990).

One study involving forty-four subjects with chronic obstructive disease demonstrated that pulmonary-rehabilitation programs can in a cost-effective manner significantly improve exercise capacity with sustained benefits. The program in the study was 6 weeks long and had a continuing home component. The cost of the basic program was approximately $800 per patient. Findings using CPX testing revealed a 73 percent (± 16 percent) improvement in aerobic capacity in these patients, and a 250 percent (± 78 percent) improvement in physical exercise endurance. There was no change in spirometry, degree of exercise desaturation, maximum HR or ventilation, and little improvement in oxygen consumption and O_2 pulse, which implies that most of the reconditioning was related to increased muscle efficiency. Follow-up testing in twenty-four of the forty-four patients showed that 89 percent (± 7 percent) of the peak exercise performance was maintained up to 1 year after completing the formal 6-week program. This was attributed to the rehabilitation efforts continued at home after the program was completed (Holle et al., 1988).

Other centers and programs continue to report similar findings and results. Patients demonstrate improvement in exercise tolerance but little or no change in spirometric values and oxygen saturation. While patients who have completed pulmonary rehabilitation appear to have improved general health, future studies must be more comprehensive when dealing with the other aspects of physical health that include social functioning, role functioning, and mental health. In addition, therapeutic modalities will have to be studied individually to monitor and assess their relative benefits. With this information, pulmonary rehabilitation can then be prescribed individually using the most appropriate components, be based on the needs and goals of each patient, and employ techniques more extensively to benefit greater numbers of patients (Make, 1990).

SUMMARY

Determining and assessing outcomes of pulmonary rehabilitation is a labor-intensive process that is critical to establishing credibility for pulmonary rehabilitation and helping to justify its continued existence. Meeting patient expectations and objectives, comparing before and after activity levels, and surveying degrees of patient satisfaction are several ways of ensuring program quality and overall success. More importantly, evaluating outcomes through objective measures like CPX testing and other laboratory tests may be more reliable and more useful than simple subjective analysis. Increased physical conditioning and improved cardiopulmonary status usually indicate patients have benefitted from pulmonary rehabilitation. However, neither of these is advantageous unless the patients experience greater freedom and less dyspnea while performing daily activities, have greater levels of self-confidence, and perceive that they are better.

The obstacles keeping patients from attending and completing their pulmonary rehabilitation must also be addressed effectively. While some reasons for nonattendance and attrition, like transportation, dissatisfaction, and loss of enthusiasm, can be managed, others, like weather conditions and patient illness, cannot. Attendance is critical to the success or failure of any pulmonary-rehabilitation effort.

Review Questions

1. List five patient expectations of pulmonary rehabilitation, and explain how programs can help meet these expectations.
2. Identify three accepted benefits of pulmonary rehabilitation, and describe how they are measured or determined. Do the same for three possible benefits and three unlikely or debated benefits.
3. Discuss the importance of CPX testing in determining results and outcomes associated with pulmonary rehabilitation.
4. What are five reasons for patient attrition in pulmonary rehabilitation?
5. How can patient attendance and attrition issues can be handled effectively?

References

Holden, D.A., Stelmach, K.D., Curtis, P.S., Beck, G.J., & Stoller, J.K. (1990, April). The impact of a rehabilitation program on functional status of patients with chronic lung disease. *Respiratory Care, 35*(4), 332–338.

Holle, R.H., Williams, D.V., Vandree, J.C., Starks, G.L., & Schoene, R.B. (1988, December). Increased muscle efficiency and sustained benefits in an outpatient community hospital-based pulmonary-rehabilitation program. *Chest, 94*(6), 1161–1168.

Hughes, R.L., & Davison, R. (1983, February). Limitations of exercise reconditioning in COLD. *Chest, 83*(2), 242.

Make, B. (1990, April). Pulmonary rehabilitation—What are the outcomes? *Respiratory Care, 35*(4), 329–331.

Olsson, D.E. (1968). *Management by objectives*. Palo Alto, CA: Pacific Books.

Peske, G.W. (1995, February/March). The power of outcomes research. *RT—The Journal for Respiratory Care Practitioners 8*(2), 18–19.

Ries, A.L., Kaplan, R.M., Limberg, T.M., & Prewitt, L.M. (1995). Effects of pulmonary rehabilitation on physiologic and psychosocial outcomes in patients with chronic obstructive pulmonary disease. *Annals of Internal Medicine, 122,* 823–832.

Scott, F. (1989, September 11). The bottom line: Does it help patients? *Advance for Respiratory Care Practitioners, 2*(37), 14–15.

Tosi, C., & Tosi, H. (1973). *Management by objectives*. New York, NY: MacMillan Press.

Suggested Readings

Artunian, J. (1995, February/March). Designing a yardstick for rehabilitation. *RT—The Journal for Respiratory Care Practitioners 8*(2), 27–28.

Bickford, L.S., & Hodgkin, J.E. (1988, November). National pulmonary rehabilitation survey. *Respiratory Care, 33*(11), 1030–1043.

Couser, J.I. (1996, February/March). Focus on the elderly—Pulmonary rehabilitation's benefits among COPD patients are not age-specific. *RT—The Journal for Respiratory Care Practitioners, 9*(2), 59–66.

Hodgkin, J.E., Connors, G.L., & Bell, C.W. (1993). *Pulmonary rehabilitation—Guidelines to success* (2nd ed.). Philadelphia, PA: J.B. Lippincott Company.

Marsh, P., & Hilling, L. (1992, June). Pulmonary patients speak out about life-quality issues. *AARCTimes, 16*(6), 31–33.

Morris, K.V. (1992, June). Evaluating the effects of pulmonary rehabilitation. *AARCTimes, 16*(6), 29–30.

Ries, A.L., Kaplan, R.M., & Blumberg, E. (1991). Use of factor analysis to consolidate multiple outcome measures in chronic obstructive pulmonary disease. *Journal of Clinical Epidemiology, 44*(6), 497–503.

CHAPTER SIX

REIMBURSEMENT FOR PULMONARY REHABILITATION

KEY TERMS

current procedural terminology (CPT) coding
HCFA common procedure coding system (HCPCS)

International Classification of Diseases, 9th Revision or *ICD-9-CM*

insurance co-payment
Medicare—Part A
Medicare—Part B
third-party reimbursement

OBJECTIVES

Upon completing this chapter, the reader will be able to:

- Identify at least five factors that affect the cost of a pulmonary-rehabilitation program.
- Identify at least three legitimate ways to obtain reimbursement for pulmonary rehabilitation from third party payors.
- Discuss the importance of patient diagnosis when it comes to patient billing and the role of the *International Classification of Diseases, 9th Revision* (*ICD-9-CM*).
- Define *CPT coding* and describe its role and importance to billing for pulmonary rehabilitation.
- Define HCFA common procedure coding system (*HCPCS*) and describe its role and importance to billing for pulmonary rehabilitation.
- Compare and contrast insurance reimbursement for pulmonary rehabilitation as it is paid for by commercial carriers, Medicare, and Medicaid.
- Explain some of the reasons pulmonary rehabilitation is not recognized and reimbursed universally.

INTRODUCTION

It is difficult to argue against the importance of finances to any pulmonary-rehabilitation program. Without a "healthy bottom line," pulmonary-rehabilitation programs struggle financially and have difficulty staying viable. As with any facet of health care, a sound fiscal basis is an essential component to the continued existence and operation of any pulmonary-rehabilitation program. Without institutional and outside funding or insurance reimbursement, pulmonary-rehabilitation programs would not be able to afford space, equipment, supplies, or personnel. With proper budgeting, resource use, and funding, most programs can become self-supporting. However, much depends on the climate of insurance reimbursement. Like the weather, insurance payment for services provided under pulmonary rehabilitation changes constantly, especially when Medicare is involved in the process. This chapter looks at the issue of finances, including the current and projected reimbursement for pulmonary rehabilitation from Medicare, Medicaid, and commercial/private insurance companies.

FACTORS AFFECTING PROGRAM AND PATIENT COSTS

A number of factors relate directly to the costs of a pulmonary-rehabilitation program. These factors include things like personnel, location and space expenses, utilities, equipment and supplies, marketing and advertising, equipment maintenance and repair, and incidental or miscellaneous items. While these factors vary from program to program, commonly the largest budget item is personnel, which includes salary and benefits. Exercise and monitoring equipment is usually second, with location and space expenses occupying third. Marketing and promotional costs can be very expensive if not monitored and regulated closely. However, these tend to be higher at the onset of a program and decrease as the program establishes itself and physicians begin to refer patients for pulmonary rehabilitation routinely.

Most program costs can be kept down by budgeting effectively and using all program resources efficiently. While it might be desirable to involve a number of specialists from different health-care disciplines to conduct a comprehensive pulmonary-rehabilitation program, it might be too expensive. If primary program personnel have knowledge and skills in various subject areas like pharmacology, nutrition, and stress management, those personnel should be used accordingly as long as the quality of the program is not jeopardized. Sharing space, equipment, and supplies are other ways programs can control and reduce expenditures and become more cost-effective.

PATIENT CHARGES

Patient charges often reflect the costs of conducting pulmonary rehabilitation. These charges are established on a cost-per-patient basis. By examining these figures, the cost-effectiveness and overall efficiency of a program may be determined. These figures can also be used to compare similar programs based on productivity, financial viability, and operational stability. Individual sessions are less cost-effective than group sessions simply because they have lower patient numbers. In terms of billing, patients are charged for rehabilitation services rendered. These services often relate to some form of patient monitoring like serial pulse oximetry or end-tidal CO_2 determinations. Other charges may include spirometry, peak flowrate measurements, exercise therapy sessions, aerosol therapy instruction, ADL, chest physiotherapy, and physician assessment. These charges and corresponding codes are discussed in greater detail later in this chapter. In an effort to control costs or increase revenue further, some programs also charge patients directly for supply items like educational booklets, incentive spirometers, peak flowmeters, and inspiratory resistance devices.

Programs that depend solely on pulmonary-rehabilitation services for reimbursement often find it difficult to stay financially solvent or to realize profits. Additional revenues from PFT, ABG analysis, and CPX evaluations are needed to make pulmonary rehabilitation profitable. While profit motive alone should not justify the existence of a pulmonary-rehabilitation program, it is essential if the program is going to remain viable and be able to meet the needs of its patients.

As discussed in Chapter 4, in 1987 the AARC and the AACVPR conducted a joint survey to compile a national directory of pulmonary-rehabilitation programs and to examine in detail the key components of these programs. The survey reported that 40 programs (27 percent) bill for their programs with one comprehensive charge, while 110 programs (73 percent) bill for individual services. It also reported that 102 programs (68 percent) reported charges for outpatient programs. Inpatient programs become part of a patient's hospital stay and are covered by prospective payment or the DRG system. Depending on format and duration, outpatient program charges ranged from $35 to $4,000 for the entire program; the average charge was $1,232. The survey also reported that outpatient programs run an average 8.3 weeks with a mean length of 47.5 hours. One reason for the wide variation in outpatient program charges may be that some programs included charges for patient testing (e.g., PFT, CPX evaluation, ABG, and blood chemistry) while others did not (Bickford & Hodgkin, 1988).

Patients can only be charged for sessions they attend. Fees should be structured so as not to discourage a patient from attending sessions. Many pulmonary-rehabilitation patients are on fixed incomes and may choose not to attend sessions if they consider the fees excessive. Medicare providers and other insurance carriers may cap payments for any rehabilitative services a patient receives, including those for pulmonary rehabilitation. Any capped payments must be considered when planning program schedules and fees. The charge per session depends on the level of patient education, monitoring, and therapy. Current nationwide charges range from $60 to over $200 per session. Assuming health insurance pays 80 percent of these charges, patients are responsible for the remaining 20 percent, or approximately $12 to $40 per session. Grants or scholarships from health-related companies or health organizations like the American Lung Association may be available to help patients who must participate in pulmonary rehabilitation.

BILLING PRACTICES AND CODING SYSTEMS

Although programs are billing and receiving Medicare and other third-party reimbursement for pulmonary rehabilitation, which procedures or services can be charged and billed remains controversial. According to Medicare, physical therapy exercises are covered when performed with the expectation of restoring the patient's level of function that has been lost or reduced by injury or illness. However, therapy performed repetitively to maintain a level of function is not eligible for reimbursement. Maintenance or follow-up program activities involve therapeutic procedures that sustain a patient's current level of function and prevent any regression, as in the detraining effect. Maintenance usually begins when the therapeutic goals and objectives of the patient treatment plan have been met or when no further functional progress is apparent or expected to occur. Medicare does not reimburse providers for this type of activity (Xact Medicare Services, 1995).

To obtain reimbursement for pulmonary rehabilitation, a specific patient treatment plan (see Chapter 4) must be devised and implemented. A physician involved with the case should authorize the plan and exercise prescription with a signature. These services should be provided two to three times a week for 6 to 8 weeks for a total of 12 to 18 therapeutic sessions. Most patients requiring rehabilitation are expected to show some degree of improvement over this period. Providing services less than twice a week implies that a patient is not seriously ill or is not in dire need of therapy or rehabilitation. Periodic assessment of patient progress by a physician is also recommended (Xact Medicare Services, 1995).

Although currently there is no blanket code for pulmonary rehabilitation, it is a recognized therapeutic service. Therefore, there are several legitimate ways to obtain reimbursement from Medicare and other third-party payors for pulmonary rehabilitation. Some suggestions for obtaining payment include charging sessions as:

- physical therapy exercises for patients with COPD (because physical therapy is being billed, the services of a licensed physical therapist may be required);
- office visits with therapeutic exercises; or
- physician office visits (intermediate).

This billing would be in addition to patient monitoring procedures like end-tidal CO_2 measurements, spirometry, and serial pulse oximetry determinations, which may be considered other reimbursable rehabilitation services. However, providers should be cautioned to become thoroughly familiar with and observe all current Medicare policy pertaining to any reimbursement for pulmonary-rehabilitation service components.

Billing for any delivered pulmonary diagnostic, therapeutic, or rehabilitative services must meet certain requirements, including a patient diagnosis coded according to the fourth edition of the *International Classification of Diseases, 9th revision, Clinical Modification* or *ICD-9-CM*. The ICD-9-CM is recommended for use in all clinical settings, but it is required for reporting diseases and diagnoses to the federal government, in particular to the U.S. Public Health Service and HCFA.

Patient billing revolves around a system of approved procedural coding from HCFA and the American Medical Association (AMA). In 1992, HCFA proposed a plan to promote cross-coding between the AMA's **current procedural terminology** or **CPT coding** and HCFA's **common procedure coding system (HCPCS).** However, there appears to be little need for cross-coding between the two systems, because CPT coding focuses mainly on procedures and services while HCPCS focuses mostly on equipment and supplies. To avoid confusion between the two systems, cross-referencing is used. For example, when a procedure or a service is assigned a CPT code, the HCPCS system deletes it but still refers the individual to the CPT system. The AARC, in response to concerns its members voiced, formed an ad hoc Committee on Procedural Coding in 1993 to review and study these coding systems and to make recommendations for:

- codes requiring clarification and/or redefinition;
- respiratory care services, equipment, and supplies needing codes; and
- methods that could be used in revising these systems to accurately reflect the services being provided.

The AARC is actively involved with both the AMA and HCFA regarding any proposed changes in procedure coding in an effort to obtain recognition for RCPs and the healthcare services they provide (Molle, 1993). The following section briefly describes the three major coding systems.

The *International Classification of Diseases, 9th Revision, Clinical Modification* or *ICD-9-CM*, which is updated annually, is published by the Public Health Service of the U.S. Department of Health and Human Services in recognition of its responsibility to circulate this classification throughout the country for morbidity or disease coding. The *International Classification of Diseases, 9th Revision* (*ICD-9*), published by the World Health Organization (WHO), is the foundation for the *ICD-9-CM*, which is now in its fourth edition. The concept of expanding the *International Classification of Diseases* or *ICD* for use in hospital indexing initially arose in response to the need for more efficient storage and retrieval of diagnostic data. Work on this project began in 1950 when the U.S. Public Health Service and the Veterans Administration (VA) examined the *ICD* for hospital indexing purposes. By 1966, the attention given hospital indexing was evident in the publication of the *ICD-8*. In 1968, the U.S. Public Health Service published the *Eighth Revision International Classification of Diseases, Adapted for Use in the United States* or *ICDA-8*, which served as the basis for coding diagnostic data for and official morbidity and mortality statistics in the United States.

The *ICD-9-CM* has three volumes. The first is a tabular list of diseases, the second is an alphabetic index, and the third is a disease classification. Specifically, these volumes contain the following information:

- Volume 1 has five appendices:
  Appendix A—Morphology of Neoplasms
  Appendix B—Glossary of Mental Disorders
  Appendix C—Classification of Drugs by the American Hospital Formulary Service
  Appendix D—Classification of Industrial Accidents According to Agency
  Appendix E—List of Three-Digit Categories
- Volume 2 has many diagnostic terms that do not appear in Volume 1 because Volume 2 includes most currently used diagnostic terms.
- Volume 3, *ICD-9-CM Procedure Classification*, has a tabular list and an alphabetic index of surgical and investigative and therapeutic procedures that are based on a modification of WHO's "Surgical Procedures." It also contains increased clinical detail over its predecessors, made possible by expanding the rubrics from three to four digits.

All three volumes represent extensive input from clinicians, nosologists, epidemiologists, and statisticians from the public and private sectors.

A basic disease or diagnostic code is a three-digit rubric that represents a specific disease classification. Subclassifications referring to a specific anatomic site or a variation of the disease in the body are coded with a fourth and/or fifth digit. For example, the general diagnostic code for asthma is *493*. Asthma is therefore coded *493.00*, while asthma with status asthmaticus is *493.01*. Extrinsic asthma is coded *493.0*, and intrinsic asthma is coded *493.1*. Procedure classifications, in contrast, use four-digit rubrics or code headings.

The *ICD-9-CM* is recommended for use in all clinical settings and is required when reporting to the U.S. Public Health Service or HCFA. A properly coded diagnosis is essential to obtain reimbursement, especially when billing Medicare for any diagnostic or therapeutic service. Coding must correctly and consistently follow these basic steps:

1. Always start with Volume 2, the Alphabetic Index, which is arranged by condition. Locate the main entry term and select the appropriate code, but be aware that some conditions have multiple entries under their synonyms.
2. Refer to Volume 1 and locate the selected code. Exclusion notes or other instructions may direct the researcher to use a different code from that selected in the Volume 2 index.
3. Read and follow the conventions specified and used in the Tabular Index of Volume 1 (Public Health Service [PHS], 1991).

The layout of this diagnostic coding procedure is illustrated in Figure 6–1 (Rowell, 1996).

COMMON PROCEDURAL TERMINOLOGY CODING

The *Physicians' Current Procedural Terminology* manual is published annually by the AMA with input from many individuals and organizations, including national medical specialty societies, state medical associations, professional health care organizations, health-insurance organizations and agencies, and HCFA. It lists descriptive terms and codes used in reporting medical services and procedures. This CPT coding and related terminology provides a uniform language that accurately depicts medical, surgical, and diagnostic procedures and services and therefore serves as an effective means for communicating reliably between physicians, patients, and third parties. The CPT coding relates specifically to procedures and services performed by physicians and health-care practitioners. Any patient charge must be designated properly with a CPT code that consists of a five-digit identifying code number and a descriptor for that specific procedure or service. For example, the code and descriptor for spirometry are as follows:

> 94010 Spirometry, including graphic record, total and timed vital capacity, expiratory flow rate measurement(s), and/or maximal voluntary ventilation (American Medical Association [AMA], 1995).

When a service or procedure has been altered by some circumstance but not changed in definition or code, a modifier, such as a GB modifier, should be employed. Modifiers are used when billing for procedures that are separate but necessary, as when performing multiple spirometries or flow volume loops before and after a CPX test to determine

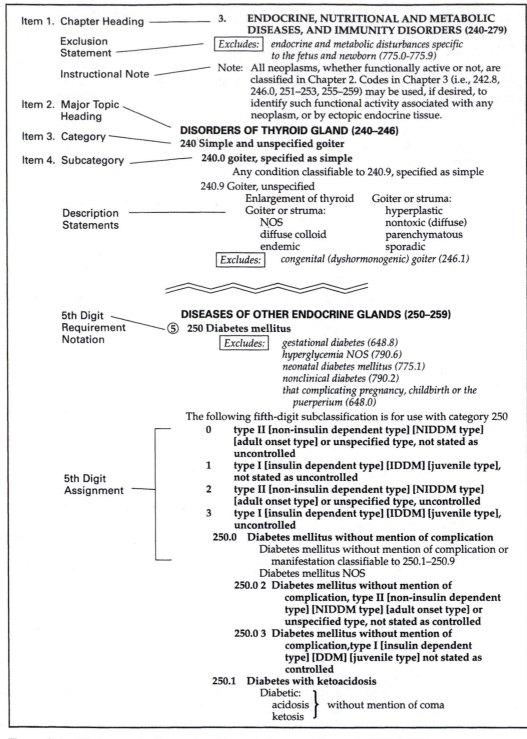

Figure 6–1 *The layout of a diagnostic coding procedure according to the ICD–9–CM*

the presence of exercise-induced asthma (EID). However, a considerable number of respiratory-care procedures or services have not been assigned CPT codes, including oxygen therapy, transcutaneous monitoring, and the use of metered dose inhalers (MDIs) to administer respiratory medications. One area of the CPT coding system that would significantly impact reimbursement for pulmonary rehabilitation involves the RCPs' ability to use the "evaluation and management services" codes, such as code *99361* for case management services—team conferences (for pulmonary-rehabilitation programs) and code *99411* for preventive medicine services—group counseling (for smoking-cessation programs as part of or in addition to pulmonary rehabilitation). A modifier for use with these codes has been recommended to indicate these services were performed by RCPs (Molle, 1993).

The *Physicians' Current Procedural Terminology* manual is available at the end of each year, but the codes it lists do not take effect until January 1 of the new year. Should any procedures be added or revised during the year, a newsletter is published and sent to all subscribers advising them of the changes. However, procedural coding usually changes annually as reflected in each year's manual. The AARC, through its ad hoc Committee on Procedural Coding, has been providing input to the AMA regarding modifications and/or deletions of CPT codes (Molle, 1994a).

Program administration and personnel, especially those in the billing office, must completely know CPT coding and any changes that are proposed and/or that have been adopted, because coding affects reimbursement policies and practices. What is reimbursable one year may not be the next. Like disease coding, CPT coding must be performed correctly and consistently.

HCFA COMMON PROCEDURE CODING SYSTEM

Each year HCFA publishes the *HCFA Common Procedure Coding System* manual, which outlines reimbursable items, including durable medical equipment (DME), oxygen and related respiratory equipment, and services like patient transportation (Health Care Financing Association [HCFA], 1995). The HCPCS coding is most frequently used by hospitals, physician offices, and home-care companies supplying DME, oxygen, and related forms of respiratory-care equipment (Molle, 1993). The AARC's ad hoc Committee on Procedural Coding has been working with the HCFA on proposed coding revisions, especially in the sections of the HCPCS coding system pertaining to supplies for oxygen and related respiratory equipment and DME. The AARC's active role in this process is deemed to be an important move by the respiratory-care profession into procedural coding (Molle, 1994b). However, other than portable oxygen for ambulation and some respiratory home-care modalities, the HCPCS applies little to pulmonary rehabilitation. The HCPCS codes are discussed further in Chapter 12.

Table 6–1 presents examples of coding associated with the *ICD-9-CM*, CPT, and HCPCS. Again, these codes are subject to change, and practitioners must remain aware of any revisions, modifications, or deletions by referring to any updates or newsletters that publicize proposed or enacted changes.

TABLE 6–1 Examples of coding with the *ICD-9-CM*, the CPT system, and the HCPCS for billing patients

System	Function	Sample Codes	Description of Code
ICD-9-CM	Classifies diseases and procedures	491	Chronic bronchitis
		491.2	Obstructive chronic bronchitis
		491.21	Obstructive chronic bronchitis with acute exacerbation
CPT	Covers procedures and services	94620	Pulmonary stress testing, simple or complex
		97110	Therapeutic procedure, one or more areas, each 15 minutes; therapeutic exercises to develop strength and endurance, range of motion and flexibility. (Note: Physician or therapist is required to have direct [one on one] patient contact.)
		97535	Self-care/home management training (e.g., ADL and compensatory training, meal preparation, safety procedures, and instructions in the use of adaptive equipment); direct, one-on-one contact by provider, each 15 minutes
HCPCS	Covers transportation services, medical or surgical supplies, and oxygen or related respiratory equipment	E0431	Portable gaseous oxygen system, rental; includes regulator, flowmeter, humidifier, cannula or mask, and tubing. (Note: Special coverage instructions apply.)

THIRD-PARTY REIMBURSEMENT

Third-party reimbursement refers to the situation in which an agency or an organization other than the patient pays for the medical care provided the patient. These agencies or organizations include private or commercial insurance, managed-care plans like HMOs, Medicare, Medicaid, VA benefits, and worker's compensation (Connors et al., 1992). Third-party reimbursement also refers to insurance payment for the delivered medical services. The major payors for pulmonary rehabilitation are Medicare, Medicaid, and private or commercial insurers, including managed-care plans. The national pulmonary-rehabilitation survey, conducted by the AARC and the AACVPR in 1987, reported that 51 percent of the pulmonary-rehabilitation patients were covered by combinations of private insurance and Medicare. Patients covered by Medicare alone accounted for 45 percent of the client pool, while HMOs covered only 9 percent (Bickford & Hodgkin, 1988). These statistics have changed since 1987 because of health-care reform and the consequent widespread enrollment in managed-care plans. Carriers have reimbursed providers for recognized components of pulmonary rehabilitation.

An **insurance co-payment,** which is based on a patient's health-insurance policy, is the patient's financial responsibility for any uncovered medical costs. Patients are usually responsible for any annual deductibles and unpaid balances. Table 6–2 identifies some procedures, and their CPT codes, programs have used for billing purposes. Personnel

TABLE 6–2 This is a partial listing of some of the procedures, with corresponding CPT codes, which have been used for patient billing of pulmonary rehabilitation

Procedure	Code
Complete PFT—Pre- and postpatient evaluation	
Flow volume loop	94375
Pre- and postbronchodilator spirometry	94070
Lung volume determination (He or N_2 washout method)	94240
Diffusing capacity (DL_{CO})	94720
Aerosol inhalation	94664
ABG analysis—Pre- and postpatient evaluation	
Arterial puncture	36600
Analysis of blood gas values	82803
CPX test—Pre- and postpatient evaluation	
Continuous electrocardiogram	93015
Pre- and postexercise spirometry	94070
Oxygen uptake and carbon dioxide output	94681
Pulmonary stress testing (complex)	94620
Therapeutic procedures during rehabilitation	
Oxygen saturation (multiple determinations)	94761
Carbon dioxide expired gas determination	94770
Peak expiratory flowrate determination	94160
Exercises to develop strength/endurance (each 15 minutes)*	97110
Therapeutic procedures in group (two or more)	97150
Self-care and training in ADL (each 15 minutes)*	97535
Aerosol instruction/demonstration	94664
Aerosol instruction/demonstration (subsequent)	94665
Chest wall manipulation (initial)	94667
Chest wall manipulation (subsequent)	94668
Physician assessment of patient (intermediate office visit)	99213

*Requires one-on-one patient contact.

should refer to the most current edition of the CPT coding manual or any communication regarding coding changes.

PRIVATE OR COMMERCIAL CARRIERS

Most private or commercial insurances have requirements similar to those of Medicare, namely patient diagnosis, treatment plan, and physician authorization. However, a predetermination and other related documentation may be necessary before a patient receives an authorization to begin care. A managed-care plan like an HMO also requires that a pulmonary-rehabilitation provider is a member of its network before any patient is admitted into a program.

MEDICARE

According to HCFA, claims for Medicare patients should be submitted to **Medicare—Part A** for any pulmonary-rehabilitation component performed during a hospital stay. Conversely, claims for rehabilitation components performed on an outpatient basis should be submitted to Medicare—Part B. In addition, the Medicare provision that authorizes the reimbursement for outpatient services provided by an RCP are found in the CORF regulations released in December 1982 (American Association for Respiratory Care [AARC], 1983). Chapter 2 discusses CORFs in detail and defines the roles and responsibilities of RCPs at this type of alternate site. For reimbursement, Medicare requires documentation by the attending physician of the patient's diagnosis; an individualized treatment plan with therapeutic objectives, an exercise prescription that specifies the type, amount, duration, and frequency of services; and a plan for periodic patient review and assessment. Because HCFA allows Medicare intermediaries to interpret HCFA policy regarding pulmonary rehabilitation, there is no consistency in Medicare reimbursement from state to state. Providers should become familiar with the policies of their Medicare intermediary (Connors et al., 1992).

Until there is a blanket code for pulmonary rehabilitation, programs are responsible for billing and justifying each component of a patient's care so payment will not be denied. Programs should not bill for any component that is not a medical necessity. For example, if a patient does not demonstrate arterial oxygen desaturation during exercise, the patient should not be billed for serial oxygen saturations via pulse oximetry. This does not imply the procedure should not be performed or that the patient should not be monitored. Instead, it simply means the procedure should not be billed because Medicare will not reimburse it.

MEDICAID

Medicaid is jointly funded by the federal and state governments. It currently provides health care to almost 39 million low-income Americans, including women, children, and those who are elderly, blind, and disabled. Medicaid appears to be the fastest-growing component of state budgets and the second largest state expense after education. As a result, there are a number of proposals to restructure Medicaid to give enrollees greater access to health care while reducing the growth in state spending for the program (Eicher, 1996).

There is a rehabilitation category under Medicaid, and payment for pulmonary reha-bilitation services does exist, but it varies greatly from state to state. These variations relate to the type and degree of state control and to the amount of reimbursement allotted pulmonary rehabilitation. Both inpatient and outpatient services have been defined, along with a competitive fee schedule resulting from contracts with rehabilitation services providers. However, some programs may be reluctant to accept Medicaid patients into pulmonary rehabilitation if they feel the established fees are too low.

PROBLEMS WITH INSURANCE REIMBURSEMENT

It is apparent that pulmonary-rehabilitation programs conducted for inpatients in a hospi-tal or for outpatients through a hospital or a CORF have fewer problems and experience little difficulty when it comes to insurance reimbursement. In these cases, Medicare covers correctly structured pulmonary outpatient rehabilitation programs. Furthermore, the *Medicare/Medicaid Coverage Manual*, published in 1988 by HCFA, defines the role of respi-ratory care in a hospital and describes outpatient hospital services, outpatient therapeutic services, and instructional and home-care patient-education programs. This manual also indicates that respiratory therapies can entail pulmonary-rehabilitation techniques that include: (1) exercise conditioning, (2) breathing retraining, and (3) patient education of the management of the patient's respiratory problems (Brown, 1988).

Other outpatient programs at non-CORF facilities, especially those offered at private, freestanding clinics or centers or physician offices, tend to encounter more obstacles and to have greater difficulty in receiving payment for services. Some insurance carriers, espe-cially Medicare intermediaries, have denied payment for pulmonary-rehabilitation services conducted at these outpatient facilities. This remains evident even though pul-monary rehabilitation is now viewed by the medical and health-care communities as an integral component of good, comprehensive patient care (Bunch, 1988).

REASONS FOR REIMBURSEMENT DIFFICULTIES

Initially, lack of professional licensure was an issue because many insurance carriers only reimbursed those medical procedures provided by licensed personnel. Since the 1980s, almost every state has passed some form of respiratory-care licensure or credentialling measure. However, there are several additional reasons why HCFA and other insurance carriers appear to be hesitant about clarifying coverage and reimbursement policies for outpatient pulmonary rehabilitation. These reasons include:

- lack of time and staff to process claims;
- outlining a standard pulmonary-rehabilitation program would increase reimburse-ment because more programs would exist (Brown, 1989);
- most carriers are trying to reduce health-care costs, not increase them;
- lack of proper documentation of patient activities, progress, and benefit; and
- traditional conviction that only physical therapists are trained and qualified to con-duct pulmonary-rehabilitation programs.

Programs may experience meaningful results from pulmonary rehabilitation and patients may perceive significant benefits, but if nothing has been documented, carriers will continue to deny payment to the facility or provider. Every program must be able to document patient assessment and evaluation; short- and long-term patient goals; the patient treatment plan, including exercise prescription; patient activity records (program and home); routine physician assessment of patient progress; and follow-up assessment and evaluation at the end of the program. This documentation demonstrates the focus a program places on each patient and also proves useful in the event of a patient audit or a denial of payment. In addition, this documentation may help to establish a clinical case by justifying the need for, and involvement of, an RCP in pulmonary rehabilitation instead of a physical therapist.

An interesting argument lies in the fact that Medicare recognizes pulmonary rehabilitation as a clinical modality because it reimburses physical therapists and nurses for delivering related clinical activities. It would be more cost-effective to simply recognize and reimburse RCPs for their role in pulmonary rehabilitation. The questions remain: Who better understands respiratory dysfunction and related physiology, and who is better able to implement and monitor the breathing retraining and physical reconditioning of patients with chronic pulmonary disease? The key to reimbursement may be found in the answers to these questions.

THE APPEALS PROCESS

If payment for pulmonary rehabilitation is denied, the facility or provider may appeal the action. The appeals process gives Medicare beneficiaries, providers, and suppliers the opportunity to exercise their rights to due process should they disagree with a claim determination. The appeals process involves the following steps:

- Review, the first step in the appeals process, involves experienced personnel conducting an independent review of the claim. The time limit for requesting a review is 6 months from the date of the Explanation of Medicare Benefits (EOMB). A decision is rendered within 45 days.
- Hearing is the second step in the process if the patient is not satisfied. Request for a hearing must be made within 6 months from the date of notification of the review decision. To be eligible for a hearing, the amount in question must be at least $100. In the hearing, an impartial hearing officer considers testimony regarding the claim and renders a decision.
- Administrative law judge is the third step in the appeals process. The hearing officer's decision is final and binding unless the amount in question is at least $500. The hearing officer's decision may be appealed to an administrative law judge within 60 days of receiving the hearing decision.
- Review by the appeals Council of the Office of Hearings and Appeals is the fourth step in the process if the party is dissatisfied with the administrative law judge's decision. Requests for review must be in writing and specify the issues of the case and the disagreement of the findings of fact and conclusions of law.
- The U.S. District Court is the fifth and final step in the appeals process. The party is entitled to a judicial review in the U.S. District Court if still dissatisfied with the

outcome of the case. The amount in question must be at least $1,000. There is no time limit on this reopening or reevaluation of the claim determination (DMERC Region A Service Office, 1996).

This appeals process is designed to ensure the rights of any party seeking restitution for claim denial. However, it is anticipated that with further clarification of the reimbursement picture and universal acceptance of pulmonary rehabilitation as a vital therapeutic modality, problems with insurance claims will decrease both in scope and number.

SUMMARY

Payment by insurance carriers for pulmonary rehabilitation remains controversial. Although pulmonary-rehabilitation programs can bill for pre- and postprogram patient testing and evaluation and for the components of physical reconditioning and patient monitoring, the billing issue will not be resolved until pulmonary rehabilitation becomes a fully accepted and recognized clinical modality with its own standard codes. Until then, RCPs must continue to work within the existing reimbursement environment. By properly identifying and using recognized diagnostic and therapeutic procedures, and related coding systems like the *ICD-9-CM* and CPT, programs should be able to bill and receive payment for services. This is essential for the existence and viability of the pulmonary-rehabilitation program and to patients with chronic pulmonary disease.

Review Questions

1. List five factors affecting the cost of pulmonary rehabilitation. Which is highest?
2. What are three legitimate ways programs can obtain reimbursement from third-party payors for pulmonary rehabilitation?
3. What is the *ICD-9-CM*, and what important role does it play in identifying and coding a patient's diagnosis for patient billing?
4. What does *CPT coding* mean? What role does it play in billing for pulmonary rehabilitation?
5. What is HCPCS, and how important is it to pulmonary-rehabilitation billing?
6. Compare and contrast insurance reimbursement for pulmonary rehabilitation as it is perceived and paid for by commercial carriers, Medicare, and Medicaid.
7. What are some reasons pulmonary rehabilitation is not recognized and reimbursed universally?

References

American Association for Respiratory Care. (1983, March). CORF regulations released. *AARCTimes,* 7(3), 40–52.

American Medical Association. (1995). *Physicians' current procedural terminology (CPT '96)* (4th ed.). Chicago, IL: American Medical Association (Department of Coding & Nomenclature).

Bickford, L.S., & Hodgkin, J.E. (1988, November). National pulmonary rehabilitation survey. *Respiratory Care, 33*(11), 1033–1034.

Brown, C. (1988, September). Washington overview. *AARCTimes 12*(9), 22.

Brown, C. (1989, April). Washington call to action. *The AARC Record, 10*(2), 11–12.

Bunch, D. (1988, March). Pulmonary rehabilitation: The next ten years. *AARCTimes 12*(3), 54.

Connors, G., Hilling, L., Morris, K.V., Hodgkin, J.E., & Duckett, D. (1992, June). Obtaining third-party reimbursement for pulmonary rehabilitation. *AARCTimes, 16*(6), 50–51.

DMERC Region A Service Office. (1996, March). Hearing and reviews. *DME Medicare News, 27,* 38–39.

Eicher, J. (1996, April). The nation's governors propose plan to restructure Medicaid. *AARCTimes 20*(4), 8.

Health Care Financing Administration. (1995, January). *HCFA common procedure coding system (HCPCS 1995).* U.S. Department of Health and Human Services.

Molle, C.J. (1993, September). More than Morse . . . Procedure coding for the respiratory cryptographer—Part I: CPT coding. *AARCTimes 17*(9), 72, 74.

Molle, C.J. (1993, October). More than Morse . . . Procedure coding for the respiratory cryptographer—Part II: HCPCS coding. *AARCTimes, 17*(10), 52–55.

Molle, C.J. (1994a, July). More than Morse . . . Procedure coding for the respiratory cryptographer—Part I: Update on CPT coding recommendations. *AARCTimes 18*(7), 36–38, 40–41, 43–44.

Molle, C.J. (1994b, October). More than Morse . . . Procedure coding for the respiratory cryptographer—Part II: Update on HCPCS coding recommendations. *AARCTimes 18*(10), 18–21, 23–26.

Public Health Service. (1991, October). *International classification of diseases, 9th revision, clinical modification, 1,* iii, xiii–xvi, xxiii, 419–420. U.S. Department of Health and Human Services Publication No. (PHS) 91-1260.

Rowell, J.C. (1996). *Understanding medical insurance—A step-by-step guide* (3rd ed.). Albany, NY: Delmar Publishers.

Xact Medicare Services. (1995, April). *Medicare medical policy bulletins.* Bulletin No. Y–1C, Revision 006, Chapter 7.

Suggested Readings

Aftias, D. (1993, September 20). California rehab program cuts health care costs. *Advance for Respiratory Care Practitioners 6*(33), 11.

Bunch, D. (1990, June). Obtaining reimbursement for your pulmonary-rehabilitation program. *AARCTimes, 14*(6), 38–40.

Bunch, D. (1991, July). A matter of interpretation: Pulmonary rehabilitation directors struggle with reimbursement. *AARCTimes, 15*(7), 48–49.

Cox, R. (1996, January 29). Low-cost pulmonary-rehabilitation program yields major savings for small hospital. *Advance for Respiratory Care Practitioners 9*(2), 18.

Hodgkin, J.E., Connors, G.L., & Bell, C.W. (1993). Reimbursement: A determinant of program survival (Chapter 30). *Pulmonary rehabilitation—Guidelines to success* (2nd ed.). Philadelphia, PA: J.B. Lippincott Company.

Scanlan, C. (Ed.) (1995). *Egan's fundamentals of respiratory care* (6th ed.). St. Louis, MO: Mosby-Year Book, Inc.

CHAPTER SEVEN

PAST AND CURRENT CONCEPTS OF RESPIRATORY HOME CARE

KEY TERMS

continuing care
continuum of care
durable medical
equipment (DME)

home health care
home medical equipment
(HME)

Joint Commission on
Accreditation of Healthcare
Organizations (JCAHO)
respiratory home care

OBJECTIVES

Upon completing this chapter, the reader will be able to:

- Define *home health care* and explain its current importance as an alternate site for patient care.
- Define *respiratory home care.*
- Identify five historical factors or developments that increased respiratory home care's application and acceptance.
- Explain how home care, and respiratory home care in particular, has become an integral component of continuing or seamless patient care.
- Identify at least five specific goals and/or objectives of respiratory home care.
- Briefly explain the reimbursement issues facing respiratory home care today.
- List and define the four standards outlined in the AARC's position statement on respiratory home care.
- Identify and discuss the major ethical issues of respiratory home care.

INTRODUCTION

The home is the most extensive and challenging alternate-care-site opportunity for RCPs. More patients are being cared for and more procedures are being performed in the home than ever before. Health care has its roots in the home. Because hospitals were not accessible, people relied on common home remedies, and any available physician made house calls. However, as patient care grew more demanding, complex, and involved, it could no longer be delivered safely and effectively in the home. With the advent of surgery and more complex diagnostic and therapeutic procedures, health care shifted to hospitals and other types of medical facilities that arose to meet this level of care.

Society today, and health care in particular, has appeared to come full circle. The trend now is back to home health care. The question is no longer what can be done in the home, but what cannot be done. While home oxygen therapy is still the backbone modality, airway management, mechanical ventilation, nasal continuous positive airway pressure (nasal CPAP), spirometry, ABG analysis, and other forms of patient monitoring are now routinely performed at home.

Home health care, with its respiratory specialty, is a major component of subacute care. As health care continues to shift from the hospital to more cost-effective alternate-care sites, professional and employment opportunities will abound for the RCP and other related health-care providers. The future is full of opportunities for those ready and able to take advantage of them. **Respiratory home care** is one of those opportunities. This chapter takes a closer look at its history and evolution.

BASIC DEFINITIONS

Any area of specialization seems to develop its own unique terminology. Home care is no exception. Several key home care terms are defined and discussed here as an orientation and a foundation.

HOME HEALTH CARE

Home health care is defined as "the provision of services and equipment to the patient in the home for the purposes of restoring and maintaining his or her maximal level of comfort, function, and health" (Council on Scientific Affairs, 1990). It encompasses medical and health-related services or care provided in the home and implies any procedure can be delivered, performed, and/or administered to a patient at home provided the patient is willing and capable of receiving the care or that adequate family and/or professional support for the patient exists (American Association for Respiratory Care [AARC], 1988). Since Medicare initiated DRGs or the prospective payment system in hospitals in October 1983, there has been an increased emphasis on, and shift to, patient care at alternate sites, especially the home (May, 1984). Coupled with recent health-care reform measures, including managed care, this interest and growth in home care should not only have been predicted but expected.

The primary goal of home care is to provide quality health care to patients in their homes, thereby reducing the patients' dependence on hospitals for this care. Home care is best provided when:

- the care is in the patient's best interests;
- the patient is willing, cooperative, and/or capable of receiving or performing the prescribed care or procedure; and
- adequate family and/or professional support exists for the patient.

CONTINUING CARE

Home health care is an important component of the **continuing care** or **continuum of care** setting that is prevalent in today's health-care climate. Continuing care denotes a constant delivery of patient care and related services, particularly when multiple facilities or sites are involved. It also implies seamless care, a concept that suggests patient care is uninterrupted and ongoing from acute to subacute to home-care settings. Seamless care was discussed in detail in Chapter 1.

RESPIRATORY HOME CARE

The AARC defines *respiratory home care* as "those specific forms of respiratory care provided in the patient's place of residence by personnel trained in respiratory therapy working under medical supervision" (AARC, 1979). Respiratory home care is an area of specialization that focuses on and meets a patient's respiratory care needs within the home. Diagnostic and therapeutic procedures that can be delivered to and administered at a patient's residence make seamless care possible. Patients are able to receive care and related services effectively and safely without interruption. More medical and therapeutic procedures are now available in the home-care arsenal for safe and effective delivery or administration. Psychologically, the patient is more receptive and adapts more readily to prescribed therapy. Economically, respiratory home care is cost-effective because it reduces health-care expenditures and, in many cases, eliminates or prevents the need for more costly hospitalization.

DURABLE AND HOME MEDICAL EQUIPMENT

Durable medical equipment (DME) and **home medical equipment (HME),** are synonyms. The original term, DME, generically implied any type of substantial or long-wearing equipment available for home use. HME is now used to describe this type of medical, therapeutic, or diagnostic equipment. In most cases, home-care services provided by RCPs are not reimbursed by Medicare or other insurance carriers. For the most part, only oxygen and other forms of respiratory home-care equipment are covered. In terms of reimbursement, equipment is approved by and paid for by the HCFA through Medicare based on monthly rentals or, in some cases, capped rentals. Depending on their terms of coverage, insurance carriers also pay for home oxygen and types of respiratory-care equipment.

HISTORICAL DEVELOPMENTS

Before 1970, very few chronic lung patients were treated and cared for adequately at home. Respiratory home care existed only in isolated cases involving selected therapeutic modalities (Wyka, 1984). The history and evolution of respiratory home care to its present status can be attributed to eight major factors. Each factor contributed significantly to the growth, acceptance, and application of respiratory care. These factors are:

1. equipment and technology advancements;
2. institution of a reimbursement mechanism through Medicare and Medicaid;

3. proliferation of HME companies and providers;
4. increased availability of skilled and credentialed RCPs;
5. passage of state licensure laws;
6. development of position statements and regulatory standards;
7. change in professional and societal attitudes; and
8. impact of health-care reform measures.

The following section examines key aspects of each factor and its impact on the growth of respiratory home care.

ADVANCES IN EQUIPMENT AND TECHNOLOGY

Respiratory home care began with oxygen therapy. The development of more efficient oxygen concentrators, liquid oxygen (LOX) systems, and oxygen-conserving devices has made home oxygen therapy practical and common. Other types of therapy, including intermittent positive pressure breathing (IPPB) and aerosol treatments, became feasible with the advent of electrically driven, easy-to-use devices like the Bennett AP-5$_R$ and Monaghan 515$_R$ and portable air compressors. Disposable IPPB circuits, as well as other supply items that could be reused with proper cleaning and disinfection, became available and made home treatments more user friendly.

The development of compact positive pressure ventilators has made home mechanical ventilation a reality for ventilator-dependent patients. Adjuncts like portable suction units and monitoring devices also helped make home ventilation more accessible and safer. Noninvasive ventilatory modes, including the rocking beds, iron lungs, and cuirass-type ventilators that were available in the 1930s and 1940s in a hospital or a specialty-care center, have also found home applications. Negative-pressure pneumosuits, nasal CPAP, and bilevel pressure devices are used in the home treatment of neuromuscular dysfunction, COPD, and sleep apnea.

Technology has made patient monitoring and diagnostic testing within the home more practical. Overnight oxygen saturation determinations, sleep studies, spirometry, and ABGs are all now routinely performed at home. Compact, computerized, and easy-to-use systems have made it possible to perform these types of procedures safely and accurately at home.

MEDICARE AND MEDICAID REIMBURSEMENT

The second major factor in respiratory home care was the inception of Medicare and Medicaid legislation in 1966. This legislation created a reimbursement mechanism, not for the services of RCPs (inhalation therapists at that time), but for home-care equipment. In the mid-1960s, respiratory care was a developing health-care discipline, with approximately 5,000 practitioners nationwide (AARC, 1988). As such, it was not recognized as a profession by Medicare and Medicaid and therefore omitted from reimbursement regulations.

The AARC has continually challenged Medicare to cover and reimburse the RCP in the home. In 1990, the AARC proposed a demonstration project to authenticate the cost-effectiveness of respiratory home care by RCPs (Giordano, 1990). On May 21, 1991, Senator Don Riegle introduced S1120, the Medicare Home Respiratory Care Act of 1991, to the U.S. Senate. This bill, drafted and supported by the AARC, would establish a respiratory home care demonstration project. Its counterpart in the House, HR1120, would add respiratory care as a Medicare nursing home facility benefit (Cathcart, 1991).

However, HR1120 required a cost analysis by the Congressional Budget Office (CBO). Because the measure appeared to require some type of funding, it had little chance of passing. In addition, there were changes in both houses of Congress. Health-care reform became a major issue, and attention focused on reducing Medicare spending. Consequently, neither respiratory-care measure passed (Brown, 1993). Other measures and projects to secure a reimbursement mechanism for RCPs have been undertaken. However, the result remains the same. The reimbursement issue is still being debated.

HOME MEDICAL EQUIPMENT PROVIDERS

The proliferation of HME companies and providers was another major factor affecting respiratory home care. Initially, HME providers were not involved in respiratory home care. No mechanism for sending therapists and compensating them for visits had been developed. However, this changed with the advent of payment for home oxygen and other related therapy beginning in 1967 under Medicare—Part B. Companies not only offered equipment on a rental basis, they were able to provide respiratory home care by an RCP. These RCPs were reimbursed for services based on equipment rental fees paid for by Medicare and other insurance carriers (Wyka, 1984).

SKILLED AND CREDENTIALED RCPS

In the early 1960s, most respiratory-care training was hospital based and on-the-job. It was not until the late 1960s and early 1970s that more colleges and universities began offering formal respiratory-care programs. The American Registry of Inhalation Therapists (ARIT) began examining and credentialing respiratory therapists in 1961, followed by the Technician Certification Board (TCB) of the then American Association for Inhalation Therapy (AAIT), which examined and credentialed technicians beginning in 1969. Currently, the National Board for Respiratory Care (NBRC) has assumed responsibility for credentialing RCPs. With a credentialing mechanism in place, programs increased throughout the country, which increased the number of graduates assuming patient care responsibilities both in the hospital and in the home. Respiratory home care continued to evolve as more RCPs looked to home care as a career option.

STATE LICENSURE LAWS

Although Arkansas is recognized as the first state with some form of legal credentialing, California is credited as the first state to enact a contemporary respiratory care practice act. Assembly Bill (AB) 1287 was signed into law by California Governor Jerry Brown on September 24, 1982 (Lopez, 1982). Since then, forty-two states, the District of Columbia (DC), and Puerto Rico have passed some form of licensure or legal credentialing for RCPs.

As of June 1996, thirty-four states, plus the District of Columbia (DC) and Puerto Rico, have enacted licensure laws. Eight states have certification laws. The remaining eight have passed no legislation to this effect (Eicher, 1996).

While credentialing pertains to peer recognition within a profession, licensure involves government control and recognition of a profession. Licensure or legal credentialing defines and validates a profession's scope of practice, enhances professional recognition, and creates opportunities for insurance reimbursement. Insurance carriers recognize and reimburse licensed professionals for services rendered. Ultimately, state licensing and legal credentialing of RCPs should positively affect the home care reimbursement issue. State licensing is discussed further in Chapter 11.

POSITION STATEMENTS AND REGULATORY STANDARDS

As respiratory home care developed, a number of position statements and standards aimed at directing or regulating respiratory home care were developed and distributed. In 1977, the ATS's Scientific Assembly on Clinical Problems and its Section on Nursing approved a position paper entitled, "Skills of the Health Team Involved in Out-of-Hospital Care for Patients with COPD." This statement identified the skills or competencies required of practitioners who provide services to ambulatory and homebound patients with COPD. The statement concluded that successful patient management depended on the cooperation of many disciplines, services, and support systems (American Thoracic Society [ATS], 1977).

In 1978, the AARC instituted specialty sections. Initially, this concept had limited success. However, the AARC was aware of its enormous potential and decided in 1986 to revitalize specialty sections, including the Continuing Care/Rehabilitation Section (Walters, 1986). In 1993, the AARC instituted a separate Home Care Section to foster interaction and information sharing among RCPs with interests in respiratory home care. The AARC's recognition of respiratory home care as a specialized clinical entity was responsible for forming and growing this specialty section.

The AARC took a major developmental step in 1979 when it published an official statement entitled, "Standards for Respiratory Therapy Home Care." This statement defined respiratory home care and identified goals for this care. It also recommended four standards:

Standard I   The need for therapy must be clearly established. There must be criteria and therapeutic objectives for program-entry requirements. A unified approach should exist between the physician and the therapist for the objectives and modalities of therapy.

Standard II   A medical record that includes the prescription must be established and maintained on all patients receiving any form of respiratory home care.

Standard III   Respiratory therapy equipment must be safe and appropriate. The patient must demonstrate its effective use, and the patient or family must demonstrate its proper maintenance, including sterilization or cleanliness standards.

Standard IV   There must be evidence that patients are receiving follow-up evaluations at least once per month, and more often if necessary, by some member of the home care team (AARC, 1979).

These standards were first distributed in 1979. Since then, home-care practice and perspective have changed significantly, necessitating standards updates to reflect the current scope and direction of respiratory home care.

Specific regulatory standards that have affected respiratory home care include the Six-Point Plan and the **Joint Commission on Accreditation of Healthcare Organizations (JCAHO)** standards for home-care companies. The Six-Point Plan contained HCFA's guidelines to Medicare carriers for calculating the new fee screens for HME reimbursed by Medicare (Segedy, 1989). This measure immediately impacted reimbursement for oxygen and other types of home-care equipment. This measure, and other aspects of home-care equipment reimbursement, are discussed in detail in Chapter 12.

Another profound development involved the accreditation of home-care companies. In 1986, the JCAHO initiated a 2-year project to study home care and to develop standards for home-care providers. These standards were first published in 1988 to assist home-care companies in providing quality patient care in the home. There were two levels of standards. General standards, which applied to all home-care providers, addressed home medical-equipment management. Specific standards, in contrast, were unique to certain types of home-care providers. Specific standards, like those that applied to respiratory home care, focused on the clinical aspects of care. Companies could be accredited on the first level of standards only or on both, depending on the extent of their home-care services. These home-care standards were revised in 1994 (Joint Commission on the Accreditation of Healthcare Organizations [JCAHO], 1994) and again in 1996 (JCAHO, 1996). Currently, JCAHO accreditation is voluntary, but it will assume a more important role in the managed-care environment, especially in provider networks and reimbursement practices by Medicare and other third-party payors. The JCAHO standards are discussed in greater detail in Chapter 11.

PROFESSIONAL AND SOCIETAL ATTITUDES

Before 1970, respiratory home care was viewed with some skepticism. Some doubted respiratory care could be delivered safely and effectively at home. Others were concerned about patients' abilities to perform and adhere to prescribed therapeutic routines involving oxygen and/or medication delivery. Still others believed that patient care could only be delivered safely and effectively in the hospital. However, technological advances, and a concern for rising health-care costs, have changed societal attitudes toward respiratory home care. Society now views the home as a place where patients can not only convalesce but be treated and managed practically and competently. The home now represents a safe and cost-effective environment in which patient care and related therapy can be delivered and performed increasingly.

There have been other advances related to society's increased awareness and acceptance of home care. In 1989, the National Center for Home Ventilation (NCHV) formed with sponsorship from the AARC and several leading physicians' groups. The NCHV is a nonprofit research group funded by ventilator manufacturers, national home health providers, and professional organizations. The NCHV is focusing on a number of key areas. First, it wants to ensure that the field of home ventilator care is moving in the right direction. Second, it wishes to improve the safety and efficacy of home ventilation and to address the fundamental problem areas of equipment, training, follow-up care, and the role of caregivers. Finally, it is taking an active role in collecting data to be used in the creation of a national home-care database (Bunch, 1991).

In 1991, the AARC joined twelve other organizations to form the Home Care Coalition. This coalition is a nonprofit entity representing consumers/patients, family caregivers, health-care providers, and equipment manufacturers serving patients in their homes. The Home Care Coalition was created to:

- preserve Medicare benefits for home-care equipment;
- support quality HME, supplies, and services; and
- improve patient access to these services.

The coalition also promotes the interests of all organization members and supports the AARC's ultimate goal of securing reimbursement for respiratory-care services provided in the home (RC Currents, 1992). The Coalition has continued to meet and work and in 1996 announced plans to publish a document entitled, "Home Care: It's the Answer." This publication will explain ways in which home-care providers, including RCPs, contribute to the quality of life and cost/benefit of caring for patients at home (AARC, 1996).

HEALTH-CARE REFORM

As Chapter 1 discussed, health-care reform, including managed care, has been a major force affecting health-care delivery and the change in focus from hospital-based care to care at alternate sites. This shift to alternate-site care is the industry's attempt to curtail increasing health-care costs while ensuring a safe and effective level of care. Hospital-based care has simply become too expensive. Hospital restructuring and downsizing have also contributed to the movement toward alternate sites, and the home in particular. Both society and the health-care industry now view home care as a practical alternative that delivers patient care and related services effectively and efficiently.

GOALS AND OBJECTIVES

The primary goal of respiratory home care is to provide and deliver quality respiratory care, including diagnostic and therapeutic services, to patients in their homes, thereby reducing the need for hospitalization. From this goal, several objectives can be derived. They are to:

- support and maintain life;
- promote a better quality of life;

- improve each patient's physical, emotional, and social well-being;
- promote patient and family self-sufficiency;
- ensure safe and cost-effective delivery of patient care within the home; and
- foster the continuum of patient care (Scanlan, 1995).

BASIS FOR CARE

The scientific basis of respiratory care has been well established. It appears that whatever can be performed in the hospital can now be modified or tailored for home-care application. However, several key needs must be considered when choosing home care. They include the need for:

- Periodic assessment of patient care delivery. In most instances, professional support is not routinely available. Adjustments in patient assessment must be instituted.
- Modified use of supplies and medications, because no central supply department or pharmacy will be available. Resources must be expended with an eye on conservation because availability will be different.
- Need for backup equipment, in some cases to ensure patient safety and continuity of care should power and/or equipment fail.
- Modifications in infection-control measures. Most equipment and related supplies used in the home must only be clean and routinely disinfected to prevent any possible iatrogenic infection. Sterilizing home-care equipment is difficult for patients and, in most cases, not even necessary.
- Patient and family education of equipment use and troubleshooting, therapy administration, and infection-control procedures. In addition to initial instruction, follow-up and reinforcement are often necessary to ensure compliance with prescribed home-care treatment.
- Established protocols for emergency procedures involving patients and equipment. Rapid-response networks involving physicians, health-care professionals, and/or equipment suppliers should be in place, especially with ventilator-dependent patients.

These key needs help to form the basis for respiratory home care. Safe and effective delivery of patient care depends on the extent to which these needs are addressed.

MODALITIES AND PROCEDURES

A number of respiratory procedures and therapeutic modalities can be delivered and performed in the home. These procedures can be classified as diagnostic, therapeutic, life support, and supportive (Table 7–1). These procedures and related equipment are discussed in detail in Chapters 9 and 10. It should be emphasized here that the primary focus in respiratory home care is the patient. While practitioners should attend to equipment and related care, their ultimate effect on patients' well-being should always be the primary concern.

TABLE 7–1   Respiratory home care therapeutic modalities and related procedures

Category	Specific Procedures
Diagnostic	ABG sampling and analysis*
	PFT, namely spirometry
	Assessment of pulmonary mechanics, including determining negative inspiratory force and minute volume
	Pulse oximetry, including overnight saturations*
	Sleep studies, specifically screening for sleep apnea syndromes
Therapeutic	Oxygen therapy
	Hyperbaric oxygen therapy
	Aerosol treaments (handheld, using small volume nebulizer)
	Continuous aerosol therapy
	IPPB therapy
	Nasal CPAP and bilevel pressure therapy
	Airway management, including suctioning and tracheostomy care
	Chest physiotherapy and bronchopulmonary hygiene
Life support	Mechanical ventilation (positive or negative pressure using invasive and noninvasive techniques)
	Apnea monitoring
Supportive	Pulmonary rehabilitation, including breathing retraining, physical reconditioning, and ADL
	Smoking cessation using nicotine-intervention techniques
	Infection-control measures
	Patient assessment

*HCFA prevents home-care companies and providers from performing this testing to qualify patients for home oxygen because it may be a conflict of interest.

ETHICAL STANDARDS AND BEHAVIOR

> "That into whatsoever house I shall enter, it shall be for the good of the sick, holding myself aloof from wrong, from corruption, and from the tempting of others to vice."

This quote is from the Oath of Hippocrates. While it is directed to physicians, other health-care providers, including RCPs, would do well to heed it. This wisdom from approximately 2,400 years ago holds true today. Ethics and ethical behavior have held, and will continue to hold, important and even expanded roles in health care, especially home health care. Broadly defined, *ethics* is acting according to the principles of right and wrong that govern a business or a profession. Ethics has frequently been associated with issues of patient rights, like do-not-resuscitate orders. The do-not-resuscitate matter is very involved and complicated, demanding thoughtful attention from any health-care provider (Biere & Brinton, 1994). Unfortunately, corruption, vice, and unscrupulous behavior in home health care exist. As a result, rules and standards have been established to guide practitioners in proper home care behavior and to discourage unscrupulous acts of discharge planning, referral practices, and patient interactions.

The AARC Code of Ethics applies to all respiratory-care practices, regardless of the environment in which they are delivered. To enhance this code and to address inquiries from a number of practitioners regarding ethical conduct in the home-care setting, the Standards Committee of the AARC published a position statement on "Ethical Performance of Respiratory Home Care." This statement defines *conflict of interest* both generally and specifically. In general, conflict of interest occurs when RCPs "engage in any activity which compromises the motive for the provision of any therapy procedures, the advice or counsel given patients and/or families, or in any manner profit from referral arrangements with home-care providers." Specifically, the AARC document defines *conflict of interest* as "any act of a respiratory-care practitioner during or outside the practitioner's principal employment for which the practitioner receives any form of consideration for:

a. the referral of patients to specific home-care providers;
b. the solicitation of others for specific home-care provider referrals;
c. recommendations for ordering specific therapy procedures and/or equipment;
d. recommendations for the continuation of unwarranted procedures and/or equipment;
e. the association of any practitioner with any home-care provider, when profit or revenue generation influences the selection, evaluation, or continuation of any home care procedure and/or equipment;
f. individuals who are either employed by or receive remuneration from both health-care institutions which may refer patients and by durable medical equipment suppliers who offer respiratory home care must openly disclose this relationship to both parties; and
g. institutionally based respiratory-care practitioners who have significant ownership interest in a durable medical equipment company which provides respiratory home care must openly disclose this relationship to the employing institution, Medicare—Part B carriers, and all others who may be involved in the referral process. Therapists must remove themselves from the process of patient referrals to that provider" (AARC Standards Committee, 1986).

The home-care standards of the JCAHO have also helped organizations and health-care providers to address ethical issues. Over 3,300 home-care organizations subscribe to and follow these standards. Some ethical dilemmas in the home are:

- maintaining confidentiality of patient records;
- providing various types of financial information to patients;
- patients who are possible victims of child or elder abuse;
- patients who refuse therapy;
- patients who do not comply with a physician's prescription;
- patients who do not fulfill their responsibilities regarding their care;
- patients can no longer take care of themselves;

- patients who live in environments that threaten their personal safety or that of the staff providing care; and
- patients whose continued care imposes financial burdens on either the provider or caregiver (Biere & Brinton, 1994).

Medicare, through HCFA, is concerned with other practices involving unethical, unscrupulous, and/or illegal behavior on the part of HME companies, RCPs, or other health-care providers. Some of these practices, which are blatantly unethical or can be misconstrued as unethical or illegal, involve:

- finders fees (payment by an HME provider to an RCP for patient referrals);
- hiring hospital RCPs (HME providers hire hospital-based RCPs in return for patient referrals);
- consultation services (is only unethical when fees are connected to patient referrals);
- patient inducements (free, noncovered equipment or services are offered to patients using a certain HME provider);
- home blood gases and oximetry (definite conflict of interest when performed by an HME provider to qualify a patient for home oxygen or when an HME company rents equipment to a hospital for use in a home-evaluation program and then refers its patients back to the hospital to be qualified for coverage. Lease or rental fees for blood gas analyzers or oximeters must be at fair market price);
- stock options (given in return for consultation services involving patient referrals);
- cash payments for clinical evaluations resulting in referrals to a particular HME provider; and
- free equipment offered to a hospital or physician office by an HME provider in return for patient referrals (Larson, 1986).

Practices like these can bring about rather harsh penalties, like those prescribed under the Medicare/Medicaid Anti-Fraud and Abuse Amendments of 1977 (PL 95–142). Practitioners found guilty of fraud or abuse can face fines of not more than $25,000, not more than 5 years in prison, or both (Scanlan, 1995). There is also the antikickback statute (42 U.S.C. 1395nn), which states that anyone who knowingly or willfully solicits, receives, offers, or pays any remuneration in return for Medicare business is guilty of a criminal offense carrying a similar penalty (Thornton, 1986). The following case study helps to illustrate a potential ethical dilemma in home care.

CASE STUDY

Respiratory Department Manager
Plans to Establish a Home-Care Company

C.K. is a licensed RCP and RRT with a bachelor's degree who manages a respiratory-care department in a 300-plus bed community hospital. Before this, she was a staff therapist who also made respiratory home care visits on a fee-for-service basis for a local HME company. C.K. enjoyed both the challenges and satisfaction of respiratory home care.

Because she understood the needs of homebound patients, C.K. seriously considered establishing her own respiratory home-care company. Other physicians, including C.K.'s medical director, encouraged her to pursue this undertaking and indicated they would refer patients to her. C.K. was thinking of establishing her new company while maintaining her role as department manager. She planned to continue both roles until her company became profitable. However, when she realized there may be a conflict of interest, C.K. decided to rethink her career plans.

1. Could C.K. legally and ethically serve both roles? If so, how?
2. What major conflicts of interest would C.K. face if she assumed both roles?
3. What would be the most appropriate path for C.K. to follow?

Joint ventures between hospitals, HME providers, and/or physicians are also questionable regarding legality and must be structured and implemented carefully to avoid possible areas of conflict. There is always concern when business mergers or alliances are formed involving patient referrals and insurance reimbursement. This is especially true when physicians are involved or included as owners (Thornton, 1986). Clearly, patient referrals and ethical behavior are of vital concern to all parties involved in home care, including HME providers, hospitals, physicians, and RCPs.

CURRENT NEEDS AND RECOMMENDATIONS

While respiratory home care has grown and progressed significantly in terms of its level and extent of patient care, supportive equipment, and overall acceptance, it still has a number of needs. Most of these needs pertain to education and training, equipment operation and maintenance, reimbursement, and research. Specifically, they include:

- enhancing professional education to identify the minimal skills needed to support homebound respiratory-care patients appropriately;
- introducing home care as part of the respiratory-care curriculum and allied-health program;
- granting patients and caregivers greater access to training involving equipment, related supplies, and patient-care modalities;
- allowing homebound respiratory-care patients greater access to the services of trained and credentialed RCPs by obtaining reimbursement from third-party payors for the services of RCPs in the home;
- enhancing the dependability of respiratory home-care equipment;
- increasing the traceability of home-care equipment defects and/or problems;
- establishing a clearinghouse for directing patients to appropriate home-care resources;
- regulating through the government HME providers and home health-care professionals via some form of legal credentialing;
- revising and updating the discharge-planning process to better meet the needs of home-care patients;
- addressing the unique environmental conditions of home-care patients; and
- continuing the research, demonstration, and information-gathering projects that substantiate the extent and cost-effectiveness of respiratory home care (AARC, 1988).

Not all the problems of respiratory home care can be solved by addressing these needs or meeting these recommendations. However, respiratory home care will continue to advance as a specialty area as practitioners take on more responsibilities, assume more active roles, and effect changes in home-care delivery and perception. The respiratory-care profession must increase its value to the health-care system and expand its scope of practice in ways that allow more comprehensive support of patients cared for outside the hospital. Ultimately, third-party payors will recognize this value and reimburse RCPs for their home-care services (Giordano, 1994).

SUMMARY

Respiratory home care is a key component of primary care, the continuum of care, and patient care at alternate sites, but it has not always been this way. Respiratory home care has experienced significant growth, development, and acceptance since 1970. Historical developments and events like those involving equipment and technology, personnel availability, home-care company proliferation, professional standards, professional/societal attitudes, and health-care reform have all helped to foster the manner in which respiratory home care is provided and viewed today. This chapter introduced some of the major issues and challenges facing respiratory home care. The following chapters will demonstrate how the profession is reacting and responding to these considerations.

Review Questions

1. What is meant by *home health care,* and what is its importance to alternate-site care?
2. Define *respiratory home care.*
3. List five historical factors or developments that increased the application and acceptance of respiratory home care.
4. How has home care, and respiratory home care in particular, become an integral component of seamless patient care?
5. List at least five specific goals and/or objectives of respiratory home care.
6. What are the reimbursement issues facing respiratory home care today?
7. What are the four standards outlined in the AARC's position statement on respiratory home care?
8. Identify and discuss two major ethical issues in respiratory home care.

References

American Association for Respiratory Care. (1979, November). Standards for respiratory therapy home care. An official statement by the AARC. *Respiratory Care, 24*(11), 1080–1082.

American Association for Respiratory Care. (1988). *Final report of the consensus meeting on home respiratory care equipment.* Dallas, TX: AARC, Food and Drug Administration and Health Resources and Services Administration.

American Association for Respiratory Care. (1996, July). AARC participates in home care project. *AARC Report,* 1.

American Association for Respiratory Care Standards Committee. (1986, August). Ethical performance of respiratory home care. Position statement for the AARC. *AARTimes, 10*(8), 21.

American Thoracic Society. (1977, Summer). Skills of the health team involved in out-of-hospital care for patients with COPD. Position paper approved by the ATS's Scientific Assembly on Clinical Problems and its Section on Nursing. *ATS News.*

Biere, D., & Brinton, K. (1994, April). Playing by the rules: JCAHO home-care standards offer insight into typical ethical issues. *HomeCare, 16*(4), 50.

Brown, C. (1993, January). Congress gears up for 1993. *AARCTimes, 17*(1), 6.

Bunch, D. (1991, March). Establishing a national database for home care. *AARCTimes, 15*(3), 62, 64.

Cathcart, M. (1991, June). AARC introduces home care bill. *AARCTimes, 15*(6), 44–48.

Council on Scientific Affairs. (1990, September). Home care in the 1990's. *Journal of the American Medical Association, 263*(9), 1241–1244.

Eicher, J. (1996, June). 1996 state licensure update. *AARCTimes, 20*(6), 10.

Giordano, S.P. (1990, May). Proposed demonstration project for Medicare reimbursement of respiratory care practitioners' services rendered in the home. *AARCTimes, 14*(5), 51–53, 59.

Giordano, S.P. (1994, April). Current and future role of respiratory care practitioners in home care. *Respiratory Care, 39*(4), 321–326.

Joint Commission on Accreditation of Healthcare Organizations. (1994). *1995 Accreditation manual for home care—Volume I.* Oakbrook Terrace, IL: Joint Commission on the Accreditation of Healthcare Organizations.

Joint Commission on Accreditation of Healthcare Organizations. (1996). *1997–98 Comprehensive accreditation manual for home care.* Oakbrook Terrace, IL: Joint Commission on the Accreditation of Healthcare Organizations.

Larson, K. (1986, August). DME referrals: What's legal and what's not. *AARTimes, 10*(8), 28–31.

Lopez, B. (1982, December). State credentialing: A reality in California. *AARTimes, 6*(12), 57–60.

May, F.L. (1984, July). The HCFA perspective on DRGs. *AARTimes, 8*(7), 28–30.

RC Currents. (1992, September). Home care coalition. *AARCTimes, 16*(9), 17.

Scanlan, C. (Ed.). (1995). *Egan's fundamentals of respiratory care* (6th ed.). St. Louis, MO: Mosby-Year Book, Inc.

Segedy, A. (1989, January). Six-point plan: Carriers, dealers say new HME rates too low. *HomeCare, 11*(1), 59–62.

Thornton, D.M. (1986, August). Medicare fraud and abuse: "Let's be careful out there." *AARTimes, 10*(8), 44–47.

Walters, S. (1986, July). Specialty sections cater to individual needs. *AARTimes, 10*(7), 21.

Wyka, K.A. (1984, October). A review of respiratory home care. *RX Home Care, 6*(10), 41–49.

Suggested Readings

Kim, H. (1996, January). Respiratory distress—As managed care and pending oxygen cuts loom, respiratory therapy providers prepare for the future. *HomeCare, 18*(1), 73–76, 120.

Oakland, K. (1994, April). Ethics in home care. *HomeCare, 16*(4), 46–48.

Saposnick, A. (1995, April). Opportunities abound for RCPs in home care. *AARCTimes, 19*(4), 66–70.

Smith, R. (1996, February/March). Home care's imminent golden age. *RT—The Journal for Respiratory Care Practitioners 9*(2), 35–38.

Waite, J.W., & Russo, D. (1995, October). Hospitals expand into the continuum of care: Setting up a true hospital-based home care division. *AARCTimes, 19*(10), 32–33, 49.

CHAPTER EIGHT

PATIENT SELECTION AND DISCHARGE PLANNING

KEY TERMS

caregiver
discharge plan
discharge planning

disease-management
program
high-technology
home care

homebound patient
organ specific or disease
specific
ventilator-assisted individual
(VAI)

OBJECTIVES

Upon completing this chapter, the reader will be able to:

- Describe three conditions or situations that qualify a patient as homebound.
- Specify three criteria that must be satisfied before a patient can be discharged to the home-care environment.
- Identify eight patient conditions that are appropriate for respiratory home care.
- Describe the discharge planning process as it pertains to respiratory home care.
- Identify six members of the discharge planning team who should be involved with the discharge planning process for the homebound respiratory patient.
- Identify five characteristics that make RCPs ideal care coordinators.
- Differentiate between care coordinator and case manager.

INTRODUCTION

A *patient* is someone who receives care or services or is represented by an appropriately authorized person. Depending on interpretation, *patient* may also mean client, customer, patient/family unit, consumer, or health-care consumer. A patient who is cared for at home is a **homebound patient.** The HCFA specifies that the homebound patient does not have to be bedridden to be considered confined to the home. Homebound patients should be unable to leave home. Leaving home requires significant effort on the part of the homebound patient. Patients are also considered homebound if they leave their homes infrequently or for short periods. Patients are not considered homebound if they can obtain health care outside the home as outpatients (Health Care Financing Administration [HCFA], 1991).

This chapter considers the homebound patient with regard to patient selection and **discharge planning** for respiratory home care. To be carried out properly and effectively, these two processes require RCPs to participate actively. Patients who no longer require acute or subacute levels of attention but still require continued treatment or therapy are candidates for outpatient or home care. This type of care is recommended when the:

- treatment or therapy cannot be provided or administered outside the hospital due to therapeutic complexity, safety, or staff and/or equipment availability;
- patient has transportation and is physically able to travel to the hospital; and
- treatment is short-term.

With today's technology and the availability of trained, qualified personnel, home care is preferred. It is financially more responsible and eliminates the need for patient travel. Meeting the needs of homebound chronic respiratory patients is a challenging task and one in which the RCP must be involved. Appropriate recommendations for respiratory home care help to ensure the care is a success, particularly from the patient's point of view. The process starts with patient selection and discharge planning and culminates with the safe and proper implementation of respiratory care in the home.

PATIENT SELECTION PROCESS

Any patient with a chronic respiratory condition can be cared for at home properly if certain conditions or situations exist, including:

- the patient is stable and no longer requires acute or subacute levels of care at a health-care facility;
- patients can care for themselves and can correctly and safely administer the prescribed treatment or therapy;
- for patients who cannot care for themselves, family members or **caregivers,** who may be lay or professional health-care providers, must be available to administer the prescribed care; and
- the home environment permits the safe and effective delivery of care, which is verified by an environmental safety check before discharge.

PATIENT SELECTION BASED ON PATIENT CONDITION

Patients receiving respiratory home care may be categorized based on their conditions or diseases or equipment/therapies. Patients are also classed based on age, specifically neonatal, pediatric, adolescent, adult, or geriatric. The following lists conditions or diseases that can be adequately managed at home.

Obstructive Pulmonary Diseases
- chronic obstructive pulmonary disease (COPD)
- pulmonary emphysema
- chronic bronchitis

- bronchial asthma
- bronchiectasis
- acute bronchitis
- bronchiolitis

Restrictive Pulmonary Diseases
- pulmonary fibrosis
- sarcoidosis
- cystic fibrosis
- pneumoconioses (occupational lung conditions)
- tuberculosis
- pneumonia, including pneumocystis carinii
- lung cancer
- neuromuscular paralysis and related anomalies, including myasthenia gravis, polio-myelitis, and amyotrophic lateral sclerosis (ALS)
- skeletal abnormalities involving the bony thorax, like kyphoscoliosis
- severe obesity

Cardiovascular Conditions
- congestive heart failure
- postmyocardial infarction

Atypical Conditions
- sleep apnea syndromes
- sudden infant death syndrome (SIDS)
- bronchopulmonary dysplasia (BPD)
- migraine headaches
- ulcerative conditions involving the skin

PATIENT SELECTION BASED ON THERAPY

Respiratory home-care patients may also be categorized based on therapy, including modalities like oxygen therapy, hyperbaric oxygen (HBO), aerosol therapy (intermittent or continuous), airway management (tracheobronchial toilet and/or tracheostomy care), chest physiotherapy, breathing retraining and physical reconditioning, IPPB, nasal CPAP and bilevel positive airway pressure, mechanical ventilation (invasive and noninvasive), and specialized cardiopulmonary monitoring.

Respiratory patients may receive one, two, or more of the therapeutic modalities identified here depending on their conditions, needs, and statuses. Chronic respiratory patients demonstrating hypoxemia with a PaO_2 of 55 torr or less or an oxygen saturation of 88 percent or less qualify for home oxygen therapy, one of the most common forms of respiratory home care. These patients, along with millions of asthmatics, may also benefit from handheld or small-volume nebulization powered by electrical or battery-powered air compressors. Patients with obstructive sleep apnea syndrome may require nasal CPAP, oxygen, and aerosol treatments. Ventilator-dependent patients may not only require mechanical ventilation but oxygen, aerosol therapy, chest physiotherapy, airway management, and specialized monitoring. HBO therapy has been used at home on patients with skin ulcers, while infants who are considered high risks for SIDS may be monitored at home with apnea detection systems. Conditions often dictate patient needs and treatment or therapy. The goal of discharge planning is to identify and meet these patient needs properly.

DISCHARGE PLANNING PROCESS

According to the CPG developed and promulgated by the AARC, discharge planning involves a multidisciplinary effort to successfully transfer the respiratory patient from a primary health-care facility to an alternate care site, like an SNF, an extended-care facility, or the home. Implementing the **discharge plan,** the central component of the discharge planning process, ensures both safety and efficacy of continuing care for the respiratory patient. This discharge plan, which embodies the discharge planning process, consists of:

- evaluating the patient for the appropriateness of discharge;
- determining the optimal site of care and required patient care resources; and
- verifying that financial resources are adequate.

Discharge planning is indicated for any respiratory care patient being considered for discharge or transfer to alternate sites, including the home, and should begin as early as possible (AARC, 1995a).

MEMBERS OF THE DISCHARGE-PLANNING TEAM

The first step in the discharge process is to select the discharge planning team members and assign their responsibilities. A coordinator should also be selected to orchestrate the activities of the team members. According to the AARC's CPG on discharge planning, the team member with expertise in respiratory care should be the coordinator (AARC, 1995a). Figure 8–1 identifies the key members of the discharge planning team, and Table 8–1 identifies all team members and their primary responsibilities and/or functions.

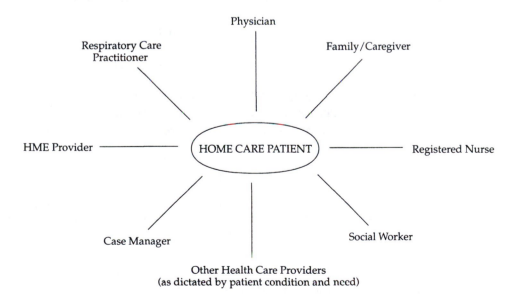

Figure 8–1 *The home-care patient is the focal point of the discharge planning team*

TABLE 8–1   **Members of the discharge planning team and their responsibilities
and/or functions**

Team Member	Responsibility or Function
Utilization review	Documents patient's in-hospital care and recommends discharge when appropriate.
Physician	Initiates discharge and prescribes home-care therapy.
Social worker	May include discharge planning or community health department. Usually functions as team coordinator. Organizes and coordinates all prescribed patient home care. Contacts all team members and outside resources and ensures patient can be discharged safely and properly.
Case manager	Acts as gatekeeper while ensuring continuity of patient care. Grants authorization for purchasing costly equipment or services and reviews outpatient and/or home-care procedures.
Registered nurse	Develops home-care plan, provides necessary follow-up, and evaluates patient status and response to prescribed home care. Can function as team coordinator.
Respiratory care practitioner	Recommends respiratory home care based on patient condition and need and may set up home-care equipment and therapy as required. Evaluates home-care environment and patient response to therapy. Can function as team coordinator.
HME Provider	Provides prescribed home-care equipment and supplies and possibly RCPs for equipment set up and scheduled follow-up. Handles all emergencies involving equipment.
Clinical psychologist	Evaluates patient's emotional status and provides counseling as necessary.
Physical therapist	Recommends and provides all forms of prescribed physical therapy.
Occupational therapist	Recommends and provides all forms of prescribed occupational therapy.
Dietitian or nutritionist	Evaluates patient's nutritional needs and prepares dietary plan. As necessary, arranges meal delivery.
Family/caregiver	Implements patient home care daily and notifies team members of any changes in patient status or condition.

In 1977, the ATS, through its Scientific Assembly on Clinical Problems, released a position paper identifying skills of the health-care team involved in out-of-hospital care for patients with chronic lung disease. This paper indicated that members of the team should be able to:

- examine the patient;
- provide continuous medical follow-up, observation, and evaluation;

- evaluate the patient's psychosocial response to illness;
- teach patients and families about patient care;
- perform and interpret spirometry and ABG analysis;
- recognize the need for and teach bronchial hygiene, exercise conditioning, and ADL;
- use and maintain respiratory therapy equipment;
- assist patients in identifying and using appropriate community resources;
- safely transfer an acutely ill patient to a hospital as required;
- determine vocational potential and provide job retraining and placement; and
- plan, coordinate, and evaluate care.

The paper went on to recommend that these skills and competencies be made available to each patient and that care be coordinated by one professional health practitioner. Practitioners should decide who will provide and who will coordinate care based on who on the health-care team has the greatest number of skills and abilities to provide the care (American Thoracic Society [ATS], 1977).

Much of what was proposed in 1977 applies today. Based on this ATS position paper, nurses, RCPs, physical therapists, social workers, and case managers all have, to a degree, the skills listed. However, the physician is the key health-care provider in patient care, both in the hospital and the home. The relationship between a physician and the patient/family is often the most important variable in determining the success or failure of the discharge and home-care plan. The physician is responsible for authorizing and supervising all medical care while also providing follow-up, reinforcement, and encouragement (May, 1991).

Other members of the discharge-planning team must work closely and communicate effectively with the physician to provide effective respiratory care at home. This teamwork:

- allows for consistency and continuity in the quality of respiratory care;
- ensures that proper and timely care is provided;
- enhances communication when patient condition changes;
- promotes ideas for improving overall patient care;
- confirms that all patient care modalities are consistent with other aspects of the overall care plan;
- ensures effective transmission of physician orders; and
- facilitates the coordination of various aspects of patient care, including timing treatments with other prescribed therapy, performing tests, providing social outlets, and scheduling family or leisure activities (May, 1991).

THE DISCHARGE PLAN

Members of the discharge planning team should develop and agree on a written discharge plan that clearly and concisely delineates:

- educational materials and training aids for the patient, family, and/or caregiver;
- assessment tools to evaluate the effectiveness of patient, family, and/or caregiver training;
- realistic estimate of the time needed to complete the training process and discharge the patient safely;

- the team members who will be assigned to the patient, family, and/or caregiver to gather information and implement the training program; and
- source of and limits to funds for implementing the discharge plan.

This plan must also determine that physical and financial support are adequate to implement discharge (AARC, 1995a). A plan like this is indispensable to patients who are going home with **high-technology home care,** which involves a complex level of services that include infusion therapy and mechanical ventilation. This care necessitates periodic patient visits and assessment, as well as education and training. High-tech respiratory home care involves ventilator-dependent or **ventilator-assisted individuals (VAI).**

Patients requiring more routine types of care, including home oxygen and aerosol therapy, require discharge planning and appropriate training and follow-up but at much lower intensities. Other components of the discharge plan may include the planned discharge date, therapeutic goals, therapeutic modalities, equipment and supply needs, education and training for patient, family and/or caregivers, selection of the HME provider, and other agencies and plans required for patient follow-up and routine assessment.

The care ventilator-dependent individuals or VAI require necessitates intensive education and training with clear demonstration of skill and ability on the part of family members and/or assigned caregivers, as well as documentation of these competencies before any patient discharge. The VAI is an excellent example of how the discharge plan should be developed and implemented. According to the AARC's CPG on long-term invasive mechanical ventilation in the home, the five goals of home mechanical ventilation are to:

1. Sustain and extend life.
2. Enhance the quality of life.
3. Reduce morbidity.
4. Improve or sustain physical and psychological function of all VAIs and enhance growth and development in pediatric VAIs.
5. Provide cost-effective care.

This CPG also mandates that an assessment of need focusing on four primary areas be conducted. These four primary areas are the determination that:

1. Indications are present and contraindications are absent.
2. The goals of mechanical ventilation in the home can be met.
3. No continued need exists for higher level of services.
4. Frequent changes in the plan of care will not be needed. However, when changes in the care plan are needed, implementation may take longer than in a health-care facility (AARC, 1995b).

Consequently, some of the factors that must be considered when discharging a VAI to the home include the:

- Selection of appropriate candidates for home ventilation. The most successful cases have involved patients who have neuromuscular or skeletal disorders with little or no disease progression. Inappropriate candidates appear to be those with rapid disease progression like ALS. Losing body functions and independence causes depression and feelings of hopelessness, which make successful home care difficult.

- Clinical and physiologic stability of the patient.
- Home environment must be safe, comfortable, and accessible.
- Availability of respiratory-care practitioners to provide necessary support and patient follow-up.
- Availability of nursing agencies and community resources for continuous or intermittent care.
- Availability of family and social support systems. Many patients who cannot provide their own care will need others to assume the care responsibility.
- Ability to educate and train the patient, family, and/or caregivers on aspects of mechanical ventilation, equipment operation and maintenance, airway management, and infection control. The individuals responsible for patient care must be able to understand and assimilate all the concepts of medical and physical care and equipment application.
- Ability to pay for services through adequate financial assets and insurance coverage, which results in fewer problems and worries regarding patient care. While financial considerations should never be a contributing factor in the delivery of patient care, the health-care industry is very sensitive about cost containment and reimbursement. As a result, financial issues can be an obstacle to discharging the ventilator-dependent patient. (Gilmartin, 1991)

Considering these factors during the discharge planning process increases the likelihood that the goals of home mechanical ventilation will be achieved. The outcome will be home care that meets each patient's needs and is more efficient and cost-effective overall. Unsuccessful care usually results from inadequate home-care resources, namely financial and personnel. Financial considerations pertain to personal assets and/or insurance coverage, while personnel issues relate to inadequate medical follow-up, inability of the VAI to care for self, lack of or inadequate numbers of caregivers, or inadequate respite care for caregivers (AARC, 1995b).

DISCHARGING THE HOMEBOUND RESPIRATORY PATIENT

Patient discharge requires the discharge planning team to work together, a coordinated care plan to be developed, and periodic assessments and evaluations of the patient to be conducted. The home-care patient benefits when these three principles are honored. With the physician, the RCP can play a major role in the home to help ensure the patient realizes benefits by becoming more involved in the coordination of patient care.

RCP ATTRIBUTES

The RCPs are vital members of the respiratory home care discharge planning team because they have a number of unique attributes. More than other health-care providers, RCPs know respiratory home-care equipment intimately and the situations in which it is used. The RCPs also have extensive experience with and knowledge about a wide variety of cardiopulmonary problems and are familiar with the policies, procedures, and personnel of most local HME providers (Sorbello, Fluck, & Wiezalis, 1988). The RCPs have always had the ability and skill to assess and evaluate patients with chronic cardiopulmonary disease and to make appropriate recommendations for equipment application and patient care. Therefore, RCPs involved in home care should have:

- extensive clinical and medical backgrounds;
- extensive knowledge of varied home-care equipment;
- the ability to troubleshoot equipment and to teach patients and caregivers to do the same;
- excellent organizational skills;
- superior communications skills and the ability to teach patients and caregivers the basics of respiratory home care;
- the motivation and ability to work independently;
- the ability to instill confidence in patients, family, and/or caregivers to perform procedures like CPR and tracheostomy care; and
- the ability to handle daily logistical challenges.

Because the home-care RCP may be the only health-care provider who visits the patient routinely, the RCP must accept a number of responsibilities that include:

- evaluating and selecting the home-care equipment that meets a patient's physiological, psychological and environmental needs most effectively;
- instructing the patient, the patient's family, and/or the caregivers on equipment use and maintenance;
- developing patient care plans;
- monitoring and assessing patient progress and the abilities of the patient, the patient's family, and/or caregivers to administer care; and
- communicating the patient's status and progress to other members of the home-care team.

By assuming these responsibilities, RCPs help to ensure that their home-care patients receive the additional respiratory care by reporting situations to the attending physician, the social service department, or the case manager. In this way, RCPs are dynamically involved in the coordination and total management of their patients' care (Saposnick, 1995). Finally, RCPs are taking more active roles in the continuum of patient care, including care at alternate sites. No other health-care practitioner is as well-versed in respiratory home care.

Role as Care Coordinator.   Unfortunately, the care coordinator, a key player in home-care delivery, has not been recognized for reimbursement. The characteristics identified here make it imperative to include RCPs on both the discharge planning and respiratory home-care teams and to reconsider them for third-party reimbursement for the home services they deliver. In addition, the role of RCPs within the home must be expanded beyond that of high-technology caregivers and task performers to those who are responsible for controlling utilization and care rendering. They must also become care coordinators for respiratory patients, which means they must coordinate all resources, equipment, and personnel in such a way as to balance cost and benefit properly. Care coordinators must be able to effectively administer all respiratory-care protocols. To achieve this, RCPs must continue to develop skills and assume responsibilities in the discharge-planning process and in the implementation of respiratory home care (Giordano, 1994).

Role as Case Manager.   Case management involves identifying and allocating resources for patient care. Some practitioners perceive care coordination and case management as the same. However, the two actually denote different levels of involvement with or responsibility for ensuring effective patient care. Care coordination can be very general or very focused. For RCPs, care coordination deals primarily with chronic pulmonary patients receiving respiratory care.

Case management, on the other hand, centers on the holistic needs of a patient. Although their focus is different, case managers must have the same skills as care coordinators. Case management is multidisciplinary, requiring the orchestration of various scopes of practice to effect competent delivery of care. When patients receive primarily respiratory care, case management can be **organ specific** or **disease specific.** Even primary respiratory home-care patients can develop myriad complications and other health-related problems involving various organ systems. Therefore, any RCP functioning as a case or a disease manager must be able to effectively address a wide variety of patient-related conditions, not just those affecting the respiratory system.

Case management is not a new concept to health care. Traditionally, public-health nurses and physicians who visited patients at home to guide them toward the most effective treatments and health practices were the first case managers. However, case management has evolved into something entirely different for strictly economic reasons. This evolution will continue as capitation of payments to acute and primary care facilities becomes normal and accepted practice. Currently, utilization review, utilization management, quality assurance (QA), continuous quality improvement (CQI), total quality management (TQM), intake and admissions, discharge planning, and social service are being encompassed under case management.

Of particular interest is the value CQI and TQM add to home-care planning and case management. Properly implemented programs can help improve patient care, empower staff, expand practitioner roles and functions, and help to reduce health-care costs. The foundation of effective programs involves a commitment to staff training. The CQI process should be employed routinely at all levels of an organization to improve performance. It should also enhance team building and employee participation. The CQI process can also bring about cost savings by eliminating waste in daily functions. Efforts involving CQI should focus on "doing the right things right" (Stewart, 1995).

The TQM process, on the other hand, involves applying principles, like the definition of *quality,* orientation of consumer, focus on work processes, preventive systems, and CQI, to a set of clinical or critical pathways. These pathways are flowcharts illustrating key events or decision points that lead, in most cases, to successful treatment and care of patients. Care maps are more intricate because they reflect a patient's response to an action or an intervention while identifying time frames in which actions should be taken. A **disease-management program** may be used to focus on a diagnosis or a condition. Both critical pathways and care maps can be used to organize the sequence of patient care, and both are useful for treating most patient conditions. Patient outcomes become the quality standards toward which all work processes and related activities should be directed. A TQM process is actualized when patient care is planned, provided, documented, and evaluated using critical pathways and care maps (Tierney, 1996).

Both CQI and TQM can be very helpful and useful in developing a patient-treatment plan and/or managing the administration of patient care. Besides their applications to case management, CQI and TQM can also be useful in meeting JCAHO accreditation standards, even though the Joint Commission does not require adoption of any one specific management style, school of thought, or tool (Joint Commission on Accreditation of Healthcare Organizations [JCAHO], 1996).

The current state of case management parallels the respiratory-care profession. Both are trying to respond to gaps in the delivery of health care in an efficient and cost-effective manner. Chapter 1 examined case management in detail and the roles the RCP can assume. Depending on the type of health-care facility and individual position, RCPs as case managers conduct predischarge visits to ensure a patient's home is safe and appropriate, provide information to develop or to adjust patient-care plans, advocate new or expanded services, promote systems changes to better meet the needs of a patient, assist in arranging clinic visits or hospitalizations, provide supportive counseling to patients and families, meet with service providers to plan improvements in service systems, and respond to family crises (Anguzza, 1991).

THE RESPIRATORY HOME CARE PLAN

Clinically speaking, the general respiratory care plan has five main components:

1. identification of problem areas and/or complaints
2. subjective findings
3. objective findings
4. patient assessment
5. patient care plan

Each component should be addressed completely when developing a plan of care (May, 1991). According to the AARC CPG on discharge planning, this care plan should also reflect the multidisciplinary nature of home care and should be consistent with recommended practices and guidelines for each patient's condition. The care plan should also address or delineate:

- integration of the patient into the community;
- appropriate patient self-care;
- roles and responsibilities of home-care team members for daily care management;
- the mechanism for securing and training additional caregivers;
- emergency and contingency plan for care;
- the use, maintenance, and troubleshooting of all prescribed equipment;
- monitoring and responding to changes in a patient's medical condition;
- administration of all medications;
- time frame for plan implementation;
- ongoing assessment of outcomes;
- method of assessing growth and development of pediatric patients;
- medical and respiratory care follow-up; and
- mechanism for communicating between all members of the health-care team.

This plan should always be developed and modified on the basis of a patient's condition, needs, and goals (AARC, 1995a).

ASSESSMENT OF OUTCOMES

The discharge and home-care plan should be assessed routinely by members of the respiratory home-care team. Desired outcomes should be based on the following criteria:

- no readmission to a hospital or alternate care site due to discharge or home-care plan failure;
- satisfactory performance of all treatments and modalities by caregivers as instructed;
- caregivers demonstrate the ability to assess the patient, troubleshoot, and solve problems as they arise;
- treatments meet the patient's needs and goals;
- equipment meets the patient's needs and goals;
- care site can provide the necessary patient services; and
- patient and family are satisfied.

Undesired outcomes necessitate further evaluation and possible modification or adjustment to the care plan (AARC, 1995).

Factors Affecting Home Care Outcomes. A number of factors can be used to predict the outcomes of respiratory home care, including:

- primary diagnosis;
- comorbidity;
- potential for aspiration;
- reason for respiratory home care;
- therapeutic modalities and frequency;
- age;
- physiology;
- nutrition;
- degree of dyspnea;
- functional capability;
- cognitive status;
- family support;
- insurance coverage and available financial resources;
- coping style; and
- ability to communicate.

The RCPs are obliged to weigh all factors when determining the appropriateness and effectiveness of prescribed respiratory home care (Gilmartin, 1994).

ADDITIONAL CONSIDERATIONS

A number of things must be considered before any patient is discharged into the home. Major components of the process, like identification of the discharge planning and respiratory home-care teams; development of the discharge and patient care plans, and training of patients, family, and/or caregivers, have been discussed thoroughly. There are, however, additional considerations.

The first consideration involves an inspection of the home living quarters and a corresponding environmental safety check before patient discharge. While this is more critical to home mechanical ventilation and VAI, patients receiving home oxygen and other forms of routine therapy should also have this service. Electrical systems and outlets to operate oxygen concentrators and compressors and heating and ventilation systems should be inspected and evaluated in any home where respiratory care is to be provided. This inspection may be conducted by any member of the discharge planning team, but it is more appropriately conducted by an RCP or a representative from the HME provider. An assessment of the home may include any of the following, depending on the type of therapy:

- Accessibility
  in and out of home
  bathroom
  bedroom
  kitchen
  between rooms
  wheelchair mobility (width of doors, flooring, thresholds, stairways)
- Equipment
  required versus available space
  electric power supply (amperage, grounded outlets, and use of a backup generator)
- Environment
  temperature and humidity
  type of heating and ventilation system
  lighting
  living space

Attention should also be given to the presence of any hazardous appliances, storage of flammable or oxidizing agents, and whether individuals smoke in the home (Gilmartin, 1991). Respiratory home care can be administered safely and effectively only when the home meets or exceeds the basic standards for accessibility, equipment, and environment. Any violations, problem areas, or potential safety hazards must be addressed properly and corrected before patient discharge.

The second consideration deals with the family and social climate in which the patient must live. Home-care providers must be sensitive to the existence of a supportive and caring environment and the possibility of physical or emotional abuse. Often family reactions and attitudes toward a patient cannot be completely and correctly ascertained until after patient discharge. Living conditions, patient and family demeanor, and patient status and progress help the health-care provider to assess this aspect of the home environment.

A third and final consideration involves qualifying patients for various types of therapeutic modalities through diagnosis, secondary conditions, specific circumstances, or testing parameters. Qualifying for home oxygen through Medicare is an excellent example of this consideration. To qualify, patients must demonstrate a PaO_2 of 55 torr or less or an oxygen saturation of 88 percent or less. Secondary conditions must exist if the PaO_2 is between 56 and 59 torr or the oxygen saturation is 89 percent. These qualifications are discussed further in Chapter 12. Medicare also specifies conditions for other types of respiratory-care equipment.

The discharge planning process, as outlined in this chapter, is depicted in the following case studies, which illustrate the areas that must be considered for the safe and successful discharge of home-care patients.

CASE STUDY

How to Discharge a Home-Care Patient

M.E. is a 52-year-old black male with a traumatic spinal cord injury. His inability to ventilate adequately has necessitated a tracheotomy and placement on positive pressure mechanical ventilation. M.E. has a spouse, a caring family, and substantial health-care coverage. The decision was made to discharge M.E. to home, where he could be cared for by family members and other caregivers.

The discharge planning team included M.E.'s primary and consulting physicians, his spouse and primary caregiver, the RCP designated as care coordinator, a social-service provider, a physical therapist, an HME provider, and nursing. The plan was to discharge M.E. on a target date with a portable ventilator and any required supportive equipment. Training was initiated with M.E., his family members, and caregivers, and return demonstrations of all major skills and competencies were documented. The home was inspected before M.E.'s discharge by the RCP and the HME provider. A safety check discovered faulty electrical wiring, which an electrician replaced. A patient care plan involving nursing care, physical therapy, and routine follow-up by an RCP through the HME company was developed. After M.E.'s discharge, periodic assessments revealed he was stable with no undesired outcomes.

1. What factors contributed to the success of this case?
2. What specific roles or functions can the RCP fulfill as care coordinator?
3. Identify several unique traits or skills RCPs have that make their role as care coordinators for respiratory patients possible.

CASE STUDY

How Not to Discharge a Home-Care Patient

J.T. is a 76-year-old white female with a long history of COPD and subsequent hospitalizations. Her condition has been deteriorating, with increasing levels of dyspnea and hypoxemia on room air with a PaO_2 of 52 torr and a $PaCO_2$ of 51 torr. J.T.'s primary physician decided to discharge her with an H cylinder for home oxygen therapy at 2 LPM using a nasal cannula and a compressor/nebulizer system for aerosolized bronchodilator treatments Q6H. J.T. has Medicare coverage and lives alone with no immediate family members available.

Social service contacted an HME provider for the home oxygen and aerosol therapy. A driver technician delivered and set up the equipment as prescribed. After 2 weeks, because of increased oxygen use, an oxygen concentrator replaced the H cylinder. However,

J.T. constantly called the HME company complaining that the concentrator was not working properly and that the alarm on the system was being activated. She was also unsure about the proper use of her aerosol treatments. J.T. called her physician and indicated she was experiencing increasing levels of dyspnea and ankle edema. Three weeks after discharge, J.T. was readmitted with congestive heart failure.

1. What glaring omissions in the discharge planning process led to the unsuccessful outcome of this seemingly routine case?
2. What specific roles or functions could an RCP have managed?
3. How could J.T. have been managed and cared for more effectively?

SUMMARY

It has been apparent that stable but chronic respiratory patients can be effectively treated and cared for within the home environment. The types of therapeutic modalities currently available for home use are as varied as the numbers and types of respiratory conditions and range from routine care to high-tech therapy. Safe and effective delivery of patient care requires a carefully designed and implemented discharge plan and a multidisciplinary team. Once the patient is discharged, a comprehensive plan of care can be implemented. Outcomes can be assessed periodically to modify patient care as necessary, correct any problem areas, determine patient progress, and evaluate the success of the care plan.

Review Questions

1. What three conditions or situations qualify an individual as homebound?
2. What three criteria must be satisfied before a patient can be discharged to the home-care environment?
3. Name eight patient conditions appropriate for respiratory home care.
4. Describe the discharge planning process as it pertains to respiratory home care.
5. Identify six members of the discharge planning team who should be involved with the discharge planning process for the homebound respiratory patient.
6. What are five characteristics or attributes which make RCPs ideal care coordinators?
7. What is the difference between a care coordinator and a case manager?

References

American Association for Respiratory Care. (1995a, December). AARC clinical practice guideline: Discharge planning for the respiratory care patient. *Respiratory Care, 40*(12), 1308–1312.
American Association for Respiratory Care. (1995b, December). AARC clinical practice guideline: Long-term invasive mechanical ventilation in the home. *Respiratory Care, 40*(12), 1313–1320.
American Thoracic Society. (1977, Summer). Skills of the health team involved in out-of-hospital care for patients with COPD. Position paper approved by the ATS's Scientific Assembly on Clinical Problems and Its Section on Nursing. *ATS News.*

Anguzza, R. (1991, August). The respiratory care practitioner as case manager. *AARCTimes, 15*(8), 50–51.

Gilmartin, M.E. (1991, March). Long-term mechanical ventilation: Patient selection and discharge planning. *Respiratory Care, 36*(3), 205–213.

Gilmartin, M. (1994, May). Transition from the intensive care unit to home: Patient selection and discharge planning. *Respiratory Care 39*(5), 464.

Giordano, S.P. (1994, April). Current and future role of respiratory care practitioners in home care. *Respiratory Care, 39*(4), 323–324.

Health Care Financing Administration. (1991, June). *Medicare and Medicaid guide.* Part B benefits. Commerce Clearing House, Inc.

Joint Commission on Accreditation of Healthcare Organizations. (1996). *1997–98 Comprehensive accreditation manual for home care.* Oakbrook Terrace, IL: Joint Commission on Accreditation of Healthcare Organizations.

May, D.F. (1991). *Rehabilitation and continuity of care in pulmonary disease.* St. Louis, MO: Mosby-Year Book, Inc.

Saposnick, A. (1995, April). Opportunities abound for RCPs in home care. *AARCTimes, 19*(4), 69.

Sorbello, J., Fluck, R., & Wiezalis, C. (1988, November). Respiratory therapists: Vital members of the home-care team. *AARCTimes, 12*(11), 52–53.

Stewart, K. (1995, December). Striving for quality. *Advance for Managers of Respiratory Care, 4*(10), 43–44.

Tierney, J.R. (1996, Spring). Planning respiratory home care. *Home Care Section Bulletin, (1),* 9. American Association for Respiratory Care.

Suggested Readings

Brown-West, C. (1996, May). Respiratory home-care services are expanding. *AARCTimes, 20*(5), 8, 88.

Bunch, D. (1991, August). Making home care a reality for technology-dependent patients. *AARCTimes, 15*(8), 38–42.

Cartwright, G. (1995, October). Home care RCPs play important role in patient and family education. *AARCTimes, 19*(10), 34–35, 50.

Cherney, A. (1995, March). Tips for working effectively with case managers. *HomeCare, 17*(3), 68.

Engen, C. (1995, March). Assuring quality in case management. *HomeCare, 17*(3), 61–62, 64.

Munderloh, B.J. (1996, June). Managing COPD using respiratory therapists as primary case managers. *AARCTimes, 20*(6), 22–28.

Nesterick, E. (1995, March). Joining the home-care team. *HomeCare, 17*(3), 53–54, 56.

Novoselski, D. (1995, March). Tearing down the myths. *HomeCare, 17*(3), 67–68, 70.

Pertelle, V.R. (1996, June). Managing COPD through case management: An RCP's perspective. *AARCTimes, 20*(6), 27.

Scanlan, C. (Ed.). (1995). *Egan's fundamentals of respiratory care* (6th ed.). St. Louis, MO: Mosby-Year Book, Inc.

Zimbel, V. (1996, Spring). Home care RCPs can win business and improve outcomes with asthma management programs. *Home Care Section Bulletin, (1),* 6–8. American Association for Respiratory Care.

CHAPTER NINE

HOME RESPIRATORY EQUIPMENT AND THERAPEUTICS

David A. Gourley

KEY TERMS

long-term oxygen therapy (LTOT)

negative pressure ventilation

nocturnal oxygen therapy trial (NOTT)

noninvasive positive pressure ventilation (NIPPV)

oxygen conserving device

positive pressure ventilator

transtracheal oxygen therapy (TTOT)

OBJECTIVES

Upon completing this chapter, the reader will be able to:

- Describe the three major oxygen-delivery systems used in the home.
- Identify three oxygen-conserving devices or systems presently available.
- Differentiate between the use of continuous positive airway pressure (CPAP) and bilevel pressure therapy equipment.
- Identify three key factors in the development of home mechanical ventilation.
- Describe patient selection, including major disorders, for home mechanical ventilation.
- Identify five positive pressure ventilators currently used in the home.
- Describe the use of negative pressure ventilation in the home.
- List the advantages and disadvantages of noninvasive positive pressure ventilation (NIPPV).

INTRODUCTION

Home respiratory care has evolved into a subspecialty of respiratory care for several reasons, as discussed previously. Certainly, one of the major driving forces of the development of home respiratory care has been technical advances. Before 1970, most respiratory care equipment was pneumatic, rendering it difficult, if not impossible, for home use (Scanlan, 1995). The equipment was also complex, because it was developed for use by health-care professionals. As home care developed, equipment was simplified to allow patients and caregivers of all ages and educational levels to operate it easily. Advances in the design of portable equipment have caused the availability of home respiratory equipment to grow dramatically.

Another force behind the growth of home respiratory care is the increase in chronic pulmonary disorders as a result of cigarette smoking and environmental factors. This increase has produced a large population of patients needing respiratory care (Burton & Hodgkin, 1984). The "graying" of America, with the baby boom generation reaching retirement age, will produce an increasingly growing population who are living longer with chronic disorders. The combination of technical advances and the increase in respiratory diseases is creating the increased need for home respiratory equipment.

OXYGEN THERAPY

Oxygen therapy equipment is by far the most common modality in home respiratory care. The benefits of **long-term oxygen therapy (LTOT)** were established clearly in 1980 by a **nocturnal oxygen therapy trial (NOTT)** study group that documented the long-term survival of the COPD patient (National Institutes of Health [NIH], 1980). In 1985, the HCFA developed criteria for reimbursing home oxygen equipment in an effort to curtail the indiscriminate use of home oxygen equipment. The HCFA requires that the prescribing physician complete a certificate of medical necessity (CMN) for home oxygen therapy (see Figure 12–3 of Chapter 12). The results from the blood gas analysis (PaO_2) or oximetry (SpO_2) must be within the specified HCFA guidelines for the patient to qualify for home oxygen. These guidelines are discussed in detail in Chapter 12. The physician must also specify the oxygen flow rate or concentration and the frequency of use.

Oxygen therapy is provided in the home by one of three systems:

1. oxygen concentrators;
2. liquid oxygen (LOX); or
3. compressed gas cylinders.

The HME provider may, depending on projected patient needs and use, select the appropriate system for the home-care patient. However, the prescribing physician, if familiar with these units, may also specify the supply and delivery system.

OXYGEN CONCENTRATORS

Oxygen concentrators are the most frequently used home-oxygen system today. The concentrator is an electrically powered device that physically separates the oxygen from the nitrogen in room air. There are two types of concentrators: molecular sieve and membrane oxygenators. The molecular sieves are more common. Membrane oxygenators are also called oxygen enrichers.

The molecular sieve concentrator operates by having an air compressor deliver room air to one of two sieve beds. One sieve bed contains zeolite pellets made of sodium-aluminum silicate. The pellets absorb nitrogen, carbon dioxide, carbon monoxide, and water vapor, while oxygen, and a small amount of argon, flows through them. The sieve beds alternate pressurization to produce oxygen and depressurization to purge waste gases by what is called the pressure swing cycle. The oxygen is stored in an accumulator until delivered to the patient through a flowmeter. A schematic of a typical molecular sieve oxygen concentrator is found in Figure 9–1.

An oxygen concentrator (Figure 9–2) typically produces 95 percent oxygen at 1 to 2 liters per minute (lpm). The oxygen concentration decreases as liter flow increases. The highest liter flow available on a concentrator today is 6 lpm. Concentrators are most appropriate for oxygen delivery by nasal cannula or for titrating oxygen into other systems, like high-humidity tracheostomy collars. Originally concentrators had to be serviced frequently. The oxygen concentration being produced had to be analyzed according to manufacturer's specifications, usually every 30 to 60 days. Today, concentrators have built-in oxygen sensors that sound if the oxygen concentration drops below a specified or predetermined level (usually 90 percent). This eliminates the need for frequent home visits to verify equipment operation (Lucas et al., 1988; Scanlan, 1995).

Membrane oxygenators, or oxygen enrichers, use a plastic membrane approximately 1μ thick. Oxygen and water vapor diffuse easily across the membrane, providing an enriched output of approximately 40 percent oxygen. Flows must be adjusted to a normal

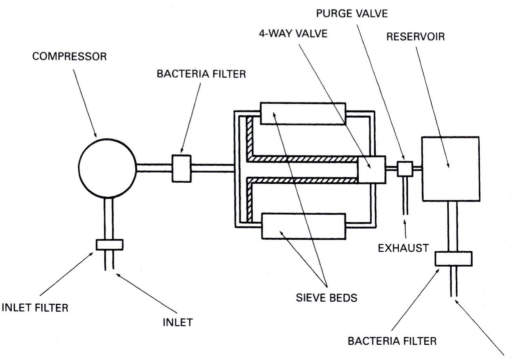

Figure 9–1 *A molecular sieve oxygen concentrator*

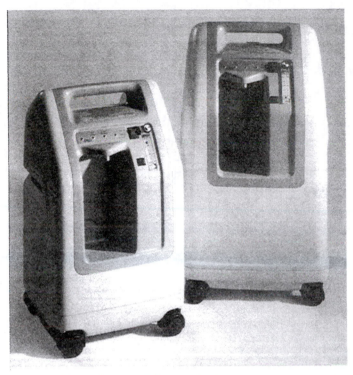

Figure 9–2 *(Left) DeVilbiss SolAiris™ series 3-liter and (right) 5-liter oxygen concentrators. (Courtesy of DeVilbiss Health Care, Inc., Somerset, PA.)*

100 percent oxygen source. Enrichers are available to deliver high humidity. A heated tube allows adjustable levels of absolute humidity up to 38 mg H_2O/liter. These units are used to provide adequate humidity for good tracheobronchial toilet (Scanlan, 1995).

LIQUID OXYGEN

The LOX systems, though not as prevalent as oxygen concentrators, are frequently used in the home and are preferred by many patients and physicians. LOX is ideal for high-flow oxygen users, like patients receiving oxygen via masks and patients requiring porta-bility. The home LOX system, which resembles a thermos (Figure 9–3), is like the hospital bulk oxygen system. The inner container of the thermos, which holds the LOX, is sepa-rated from the outer container by a vacuum to prevent heat transfer and evaporation of the LOX. Oxygen is liquid at or below –297°F (–147°C). Oxygen is a gas above the liquid within the inner container at a pressure of 20 to 25 pounds per square inch (psi). When the flowmeter is opened, oxygen travels through warming coils, vaporizes into gas, and is delivered to the patient. Because gaseous oxygen occupies approximately 860 times the space of liquid oxygen, the duration of liquid systems is much greater than compressed gas cylinders. Due to ambient heat, liquid oxygen slowly vaporizes, even when the unit is not in use. A typical LOX reservoir may require 4 to 6 weeks to empty by evaporation. A

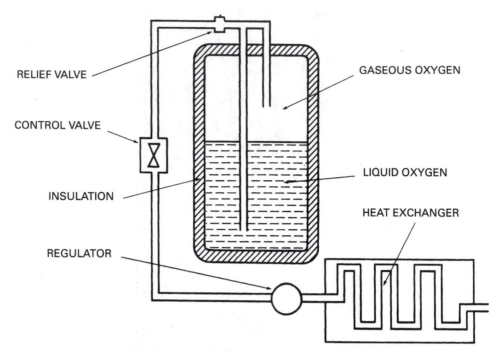

Figure 9–3 *Schematic of a liquid oxygen (LOX) system*

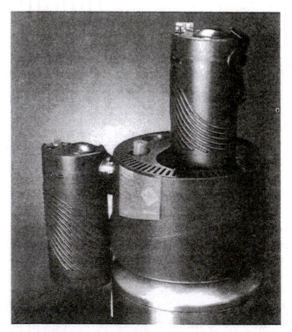

Figure 9–4 *A contemporary liquid oxygen (LOX) system, including reservoir and portable unit*

portable LOX system may empty in approximately 24 hours. This is a disadvantage when compared to other oxygen sources (McPherson, 1988). Figure 9–4 depicts a typical LOX system.

COMPRESSED GAS SYSTEMS

Compressed-gas cylinders of oxygen are the least frequently used system for the home-care patient due to their relatively low volume, weight, bulkiness, and inherent dangers. The intermittent oxygen user can be supplied with an H or T cylinder. These cylinders provide an adequate oxygen supply when required with no loss if not used for prolonged periods. Portability is a major reason for using cylinders at home. Patients who use concentrators for their stationary oxygen systems can be provided with D or E cylinders so they can ambulate and travel. Cylinders are also provided to concentrator patients as a safety measure. In the event of a power failure or a mechanical breakdown, the patient would use the oxygen cylinder until power is restored or the supplier provides a replacement concentrator (Lucas et al., 1988).

Comparing the Three Oxygen Delivery Systems.   There is no perfect home oxygen delivery system. Each has advantages and disadvantages. Table 9–1 takes a closer look at concentrators, LOX, and cylinders in terms of their benefits and liabilities. Ultimately, patient condition, need, physical and mental ability, and caregiver support determine which system is selected and used for home oxygen therapy.

OXYGEN-CONSERVING DEVICES

Several **oxygen conserving devices** are available to reduce the amount of oxygen a patient is using and thereby prolong the duration of the portable system. The two least expensive conserving devices are the reservoir or mustache cannula (Figure 9–5) and the pendant cannula (Figure 9–6). The reservoir cannula functions by storing a small volume of oxygen in the reservoir during exhalation. This oxygen is added to the next inspiration, increasing the volume of oxygen delivered and decreasing the flow of oxygen needed to achieve the desired F_IO_2. The reservoir cannula can be used at about one third to two fifths the flow required for a standard cannula (Scanlan, 1995). The pendant cannula functions like the reservoir cannula, except the reservoir pendant hangs below the neck and can be covered by clothing. This feature makes the pendant cannula more aesthetically pleasing and more accepted by patients, which leads to greater patient compliance.

A more expensive but very successful conserving device is the demand flow or pulsed-dose oxygen system (Figure 9–7). Because most of the effective oxygen delivery occurs during the first half of inspiration, a large portion of the oxygen delivered during late inspiration and expiration is wasted. The demand flow device, which can be used with liquid systems or compressed gas, senses the start of inspiration and immediately delivers a bolus of oxygen. Based on the prescribed liter flow, the bolus volume or the interval for delivery of the bolus changes. In addition to cost savings and prolonged duration of portable systems, patients experience less nasal drying with demand flow systems because the drying effects of oxygen delivery during the expiratory phase are eliminated (White, 1996).

TABLE 9–1 A comparison of the three major home oxygen delivery systems

System	Advantages	Disadvantages	Safety Measures*
Oxygen concentrator	Low pressure system	Requires electric power	Do not place unit on its side
	Does not require deliveries	Requires backup cylinder when power fails	
	Can be moved if on a wheel base	Has limited flowrate capability (maximum 6 lpm)	
	Economical	Concentration decreases at higher flowrates	
Liquid oxygen (LOX)	No need for electric power	Loss of supply if not used routinely	Do not tip reservoir or place portable on its side
	Low pressure system	LOX can cause burns if mishandled	Fill portable unit with care
	Large quantities of gaseous oxygen available in a relatively small container	Requires deliveries	Do not keep portable in car in summer
	Can refill portable unit from reservoir		
Compressed gas	No loss of supply when not in use	Heavy and cumbersome	Secure cylinders with base or cart
	No need for electric power	Requires deliveries	Do not lubricate regulator with oil
		High-pressure unit can be hazardous if cylinder is dropped	Do not keep near sources of heat or cold
			Do not keep in car in summer

*For all systems—Do not smoke or place open flames in area of use, and do not store oxidizing or flammable agents with oxygen. Do not place any system in confined areas such as closets or cabinets.

Transtracheal oxygen therapy (TTOT) is another method for oxygen conservation, but it is not yet used widely. Developed by Dr. Henry Heimlich in 1982, TTOT involves inserting a catheter directly into the trachea between the second and third tracheal rings. Oxygen is then delivered through this catheter from a standard oxygen system, usually a

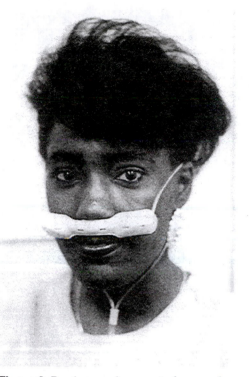

Figure 9–5   *A reservoir or mustache cannula*

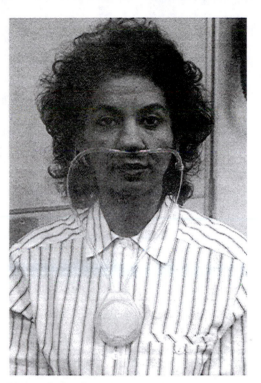

Figure 9–6   *A pendant cannula*

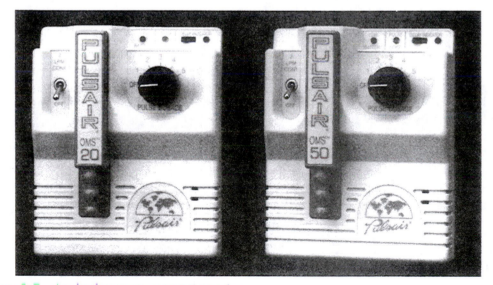

Figure 9–7   *A pulse-dose oxygen-conserving system*

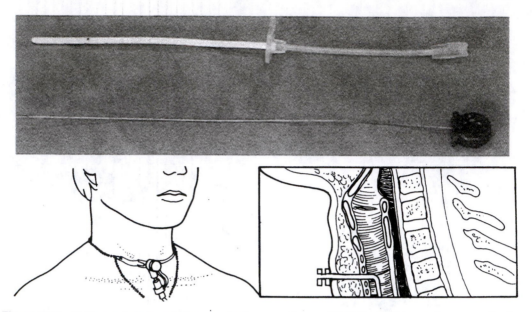

Figure 9–8 *Delivery of oxygen via transtracheal oxygen therapy (TTOT). As illustrated, an example of a transtracheal oxygen catheter, stylet, and correct placement and insertion.*

liquid demand flow. Figure 9–8 illustrates this system. TTOT is not indicated for all patients on long-term oxygen therapy. The most frequent indications for TTOT include:

- inadequate oxygenation with standard methods;
- poor compliance with other devices;
- complications from nasal cannula use;
- cosmetic or aesthetic reasons; and
- need for increased mobility (White, 1996).

Oxygen usage can be reduced by 50 to 75 percent compared to a standard cannula. The major benefits of TTOT include:

- increased mobility;
- avoidance of nasal and ear irritation;
- improved compliance;
- enhanced personal image;
- better sense of taste, smell, and appetite; and
- increased exercise tolerance (Scanlan, 1995)

AEROSOL THERAPY

The increase of incidence of COPD and asthma has increased the demand for equipment used for aerosol delivery in the home. A variety of devices are available to patients, each with specific advantages for its target population.

METERED DOSE INHALER

Metered dose inhalers (MDI) are small canisters of powdered medication and chlorofluo-rocarbon (CFC) or other propellants that are used to deliver bronchodilators, anticholiner-gics, and steroids. To activate the MDI, the patient depresses the canister in the actuator, releasing a specific dose of medication and propellant. Most of the medication is deposited in the upper airway and gastrointestinal tract. The major factor for efficient deposition of medication is patient inhalation technique. Spacers and holding chambers are inhalation accessory devices (IADs) used with the MDI to increase the deposition of medication in the lower airway and eliminate the need for patient coordination in activat-ing the MDI. Upon activation, medication from the MDI is discharged into the spacer or chamber. The spacer or chamber acts as a reservoir until the patient inhales from the device. Larger particles of medication impact the spacer and are removed from suspen-sion, thereby decreasing the amount of medication that would deposit in the upper air-way (White, 1996).

The MDIs are easy to use, compact enough to be carried in a purse or jacket pocket, and about as effective as a handheld nebulizer when used with a spacer. These features have increased frequency of MDIs' home use.

SMALL VOLUME NEBULIZER

Aerosolized medication is frequently administered with a handheld or small volume nebulizer (SVN). The SVNs are usually operated with an electrically powered air com-pressor. Numerous manufacturers produce air compressors. One of the most common is the DeVilbiss Pulmo-aide®. These compressors are easy to operate, extremely dependable, and require little maintenance other than periodic filter changes or cleaning. The hand-held nebulizer should be cleaned according to each manufacturer's specifications and replaced as needed.

There are several battery-operated compressors on the market today. These devices run from a 12-volt automobile battery using a cigarette-lighter attachment. They can be a great advantage to children for use in school and other activities and for the active adult patient. The cost of these units has prevented them from widespread usage and acceptance.

The need for increased portability and use away from the home has sparked the devel-opment of several ultrasonic nebulizers for medication delivery. These devices are also battery operated and have cigarette-lighter attachments. They operate quietly, unlike the air-compressor versions, and are very lightweight. Cost and long-term durability are two concerns with the ultrasonic nebulizers.

CONTINUOUS AEROSOL THERAPY

Delivery of continuous and/or intermittent bland aerosol, most frequently used for patients with tracheostomies, can be achieved with an air compressor. The air compressor for this function is a diaphragm compressor. Air is drawn into a cylinder through an intake valve. A rod moves the diaphragm upward and downward within the cylinder. Air exits the cylinder through an exhaust valve. The compressor must be capable of achieving a maximum pressure of 50 psi. A large volume nebulizer is attached to the compressor for aerosol delivery (McPherson, 1988).

INTERMITTENT POSITIVE PRESSURE BREATHING THERAPY

The IPPB is still used on a limited basis in the home. The electrically powered Bennett AP-5 is the most common device for home IPPB therapy. IPPB is commonly ordered for the dual role of delivering medication and assisting the patient with ventilatory insufficiency. When using IPPB, the clinician must set the inspiratory pressure to ensure an adequate tidal volume is delivered.

SUCTION EQUIPMENT

Good tracheobronchial toilet is essential in the home-care patient. Equipment for suctioning the airway must be available to patients with tracheostomies or those unable to control their airways like patients with CVA or neuromuscular disease. There are two basic types of suction units available for home use. Electrical units, like the one shown in Figure 9–9, operate from any standard home AC outlet. There are also portable units on the market that operate on AC current, on DC current from a cigarette-lighter adapter, or on a

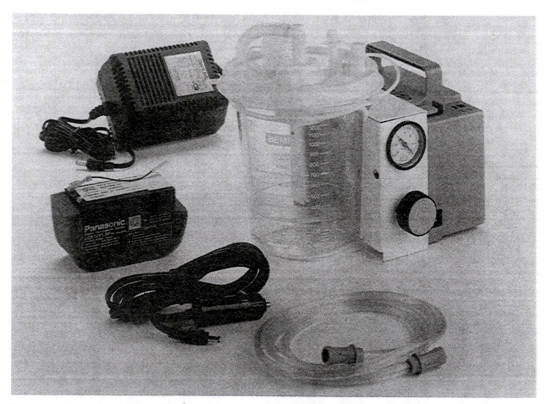

Figure 9–9   *DeVilbiss Vacu-Aide® suction unit. (Courtesy of DeVilbiss Health Care, Inc., Somerset, PA.)*

rechargeable internal battery. The operation of these units is relatively basic and should follow manufacturer's guidelines.

CONTINUOUS POSITIVE AIRWAY PRESSURE AND BILEVEL PRESSURE THERAPY

During the early 1980s, the prevalence of OSA was recognized to be much greater than previously documented. Also at this time, continuous positive airway pressure (CPAP) was recognized as a successful treatment for OSA. This noninvasive technique is less radical than tracheostomy or uvulo-palato-pharyngoplasty (UPPP). The basic home nasal CPAP unit (Figure 9–10) is a flow generator that is set to a prescribed H_2O pressure (usually between 3 and 20 cm). The unit is connected to the patient with smooth, wide bore tubing and a nasal interface, held with Velcro straps. The interface can be a nasal mask, nasal prongs, or a full face mask. A chin strap is used occasionally if air leaks through the mouth excessively. The nasal interface includes or is attached to an adapter with small openings to allow for exhalation and to prevent rebreathing of carbon dioxide. The units usually include a timer or ramp feature that gradually increases pressure to the prescribed level over a preset period. This enhances patient acceptance and tolerance. There are

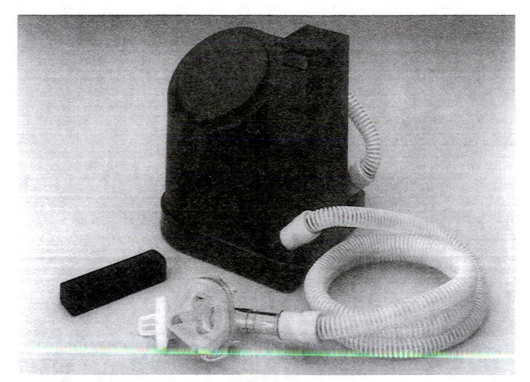

Figure 9–10 *Respironics REMstar® nasal CPAP system*

optional passover humidifiers and heated humidifiers that can be added if nasal drying is a problem. Cleaning and maintaining the unit and accessories, which should follow manufacturer's guidelines, usually include daily cleaning of the nasal interface, periodic cleaning of the other accessories, and periodic cleaning or replacement of the air intake filter (White, 1996).

Bilevel positive airway pressure units were initially developed for use in patients using high levels of CPAP or those patients unable to tolerate CPAP. The bilevel units incorporate an inspiratory positive airway pressure (IPAP) and an expiratory positive airway pressure (EPAP). With the EPAP set lower than the IPAP, the patient can exhale more easily, especially at IPAP pressures greater than 10 cm H_2O. This feature enhances patient tolerance and increases compliance (Scanlan, 1995).

More sophisticated bilevel units, which include a timed backup breath rate, have been developed. These units can function as ventilatory assist devices similar to pressure-limited ventilators but are not approved for life support or for use in patients with tracheostomies. An example of this type of device is displayed in Figure 9–11. Another unit that is currently available is the Quantum PSV (positive support ventilator) by Healthdyne Technologies. Its specific features include a maximum pressure level of 30 cm H_2O, digital displays, special alerts, and a risetime control that adjusts the rate of change from EPAP to IPAP. This control ensures greater patient comfort and compliance with prescribed therapy. Bilevel pressure therapy units have successfully treated both acute and chronic ventilatory insufficiency in patients with a variety of diagnoses, including COPD and neuromuscular disorders. Cleaning and maintaining procedures for the bilevel units are similar to those for standard CPAP units.

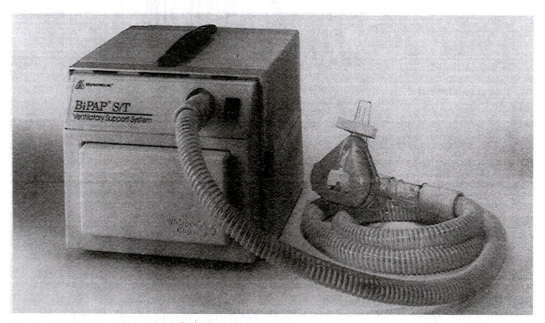

Figure 9–11 *Respironics BiPAP® S/T Ventilator Support System*

HOME MECHANICAL VENTILATION

Though not new, home mechanical ventilation has increased significantly over the past decade. With the polio epidemic of the 1950s, home mechanical ventilation became a necessity. Patients in iron lungs were discharged to homes and long-term facilities due to lack of hospital space and personnel.

Several factors have increased interest in home mechanical ventilation. The development of compact, dependable, portable ventilators and the availability of trained, professional personnel to manage the home ventilator patient occurred almost simultaneously with the development of DRGs and the desire to treat the chronic ventilator patient in a less costly setting.

Patient selection is essential to a successful home ventilator program. The basic criteria for beginning to plan a discharge are:

- patient is clinically stable;
- an adequate number of competent caregivers (family, friends, or professional staff) are available;
- insurance coverage or finances are deemed adequate; and
- home environment is assessed and deemed appropriate and safe.

The patient must be clinically stable, without any acute cardiopulmonary dysfunction, multisystem failure, or acute infections. The following outlines the disorders that are managed most successfully in a home ventilator program:

I. Ventilatory neuromuscular dysfunction
    A. Amyotrophic lateral sclerosis (ALS)
    B. Muscular dystrophy (MD)
    C. Multiple sclerosis (MS)
    D. Poliomyelitis
    E. Diaphragmatic paralysis
    F. Guillain-Barre syndrome
    G. Spinal cord injury
II. Central hypoventilation syndromes
III. Restrictive lung disease
    A. Kyphoscoliosis
    B. Diffuse pulmonary fibrosis
IV. Obstructive lung disease
    A. Chronic obstructive pulmonary disease (COPD)
    B. Bronchopulmonary dysplasia (BPD)

Other diseases and disorders requiring mechanical ventilation can also be managed appropriately in the home environment, but the problems listed here are encountered most frequently and treated effectively (Lucas et al., 1988; O'Ryan, 1987).

POSITIVE PRESSURE VENTILATORS

The most common type of portable mechanical ventilator for home use is the **positive pressure ventilator.** Several manufacturers produce these ventilators, including Lifecare (PLV-100 and PLV-102) (Figure 9–12), Aequitron (LP6, LP6 PLUS, and LP10) (Figures 9–13

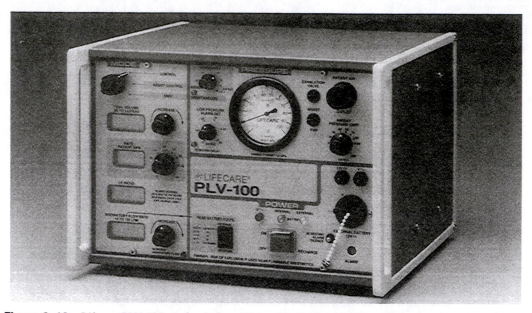

Figure 9–12 *Lifecare PLV-100 mechanical ventilator. (Author's Note: Due to corporate mergers and acquisitions Lifecare is now Respironics.)*

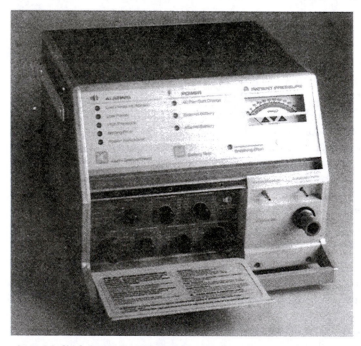

Figure 9–13 *Aequitron Medical, Inc., LP6 PLUS mechanical ventilator. (Author's Note: Due to corporate mergers and acquisitions Aequitron Medical is now part of Nellcor Puritan-Bennett.)*

and 9–14), and BEAR (BEAR 33) (Figure 9–15). Puritan-Bennett once produced the Companion 2800 and 2801 ventilators (Figure 9–16). While they are no longer produced, some Companions are still used in locations across the country.

Mechanical ventilators used in home care have several modes of ventilation, including assist/control, control, and synchronized intermittent mandatory ventilation (SIMV).

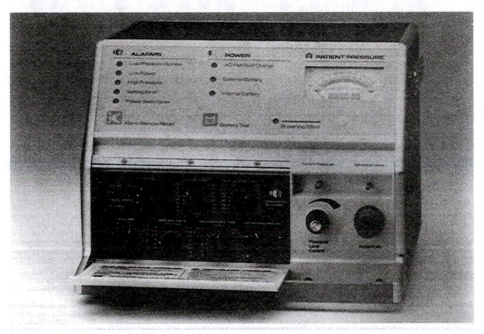

Figure 9–14 *Aequitron Medical, Inc., LP10 mechanical ventilator*

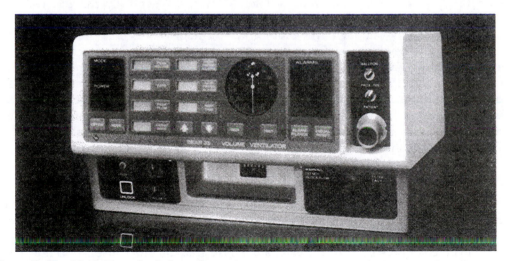

Figure 9–15 *BEAR 33 mechanical ventilator*

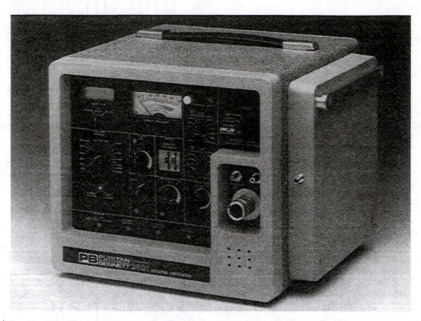

Figure 9–16 *Puritan-Bennett Companion 2801 mechanical ventilator*

They all have adjustable rate settings, tidal volume controls, and inspiratory flow rate or inspiratory time controls. A sigh mechanism is available on the PLV-102 and BEAR 33. The standard alarms that are usually incorporated in these ventilators are high pressure, low pressure, apnea, ventilator malfunction, low power, and power switch over. Oxygen must be bled in from an oxygen source on all units except the PLV-102, which includes a 50 psi oxygen source inlet and allows FIO_2 adjustment between 0.21 and 0.90. The units can operate on AC current, DC current, or internal battery. When fully charged, DC current from an external 12-volt, deep-cycle battery can power the ventilator for up to 24 hours; the internal battery can power the unit for up to 1 hour (Lucas et al., 1988; White, 1996).

The positive pressure ventilator is most commonly used with a tracheostomy. However, a growing number of physicians are implementing **noninvasive positive pressure ventilation (NIPPV)** using a variety of nasal masks and mouthpieces. NIPPV has a promising future in the management of the chronic ventilator patient. Its advantages include reduced risk of infection, improved quality of life, easier phonation, and normal coughing. Disadvantages include difficulty in achieving an airtight seal, skin irritation, and gastric distention (Bach & Alba, 1990).

NEGATIVE PRESSURE VENTILATORS

Negative pressure ventilation (NPV) is another noninvasive technique used in the home. Its operating principle involves generating a negative or subatmospheric pressure outside a patient's chest. This negative pressure is then transmitted through the thorax, causing a drop in alveolar pressure which creates a pressure gradient and causes air to flow into the lung. Time or pressure limits can be set. NPV proved successful during the polio epidemic when iron lungs were used to ventilate hundreds of patients. It has been used successfully

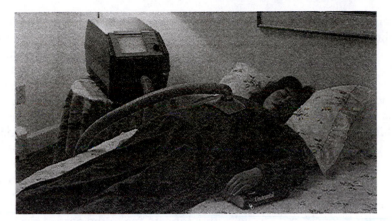

Figure 9–17 *Lifecare NEV-100 negative pressure ventilator used with a pulmosuit. (Courtesy of LIFECARE International, Westminster, CO.)*

since the 1950s on patients with neuromuscular or skeletal disease and central hypoventilation syndromes (Gilmartin & Make, 1980).

NPV includes a ventilator, which can produce negative pressure, and a patient attachment, which encloses the thorax. The iron lung, for example, encased the entire body except the head. In contrast, the cuirass or chest shell fit over the chest or the chest and abdomen. The cuirass is mass produced in various sizes, but customization may be necessary, especially in patients with anatomical deformities like kyphoscoliosis (Fracchia & Ambrosino, 1992; Jackson, 1993).

The pulmowrap is a poncho that covers a shell-like grid which is placed over the patient's chest and abdomen. A back plate may be used for support. Velcro or draw strings fit the poncho snugly on the extremities and around the neck. An elastic belt is used on the hips to provide an airtight seal. The pulmowrap does not have to be customized and is easily applied and removed from the patient. A major problem with the pulmowrap is it leaks substantially around the hips, especially in thin patients. The pneumosuit resembles the pulmowrap but has leggings, which reduces leaks. The pneumosuit is usually custom made and therefore more costly (Gilmartin & Make, 1988).

The negative pressure ventilator is actually a generator with several controls, including peak negative pressure, breath rate, and inspiratory time. While the iron lung is the most familiar negative pressure device, the Lifecare NEV-100 (Figure 9–17) and the Emerson are the most commonly used units today.

ALTERNATIVE DEVICES

The two other alternatives to ventilatory assistance are rarely seen in the hospital but continue to be used in the home. The pneumobelt and the rocking bed are two basic methods of ventilatory assistance that, when used effectively, may eliminate the need for more sophisticated ventilatory support.

The pneumobelt is an inflatable bladder inside a corset which is placed around the patient's abdomen. The bladder is connected to a positive pressure ventilator which inflates the bladder at a preset rate and pressure. The inflation of the bladder compresses the abdomen, raising the diaphragm and causing exhalation. When the bladder deflates, the diaphragm descends and inspiration occurs. The pneumobelt is not effective in the supine position. The patient should be sitting in a 75-degree angle or greater for the pneumobelt to be most effective (Gilmartin & Make, 1980). This device is also used in pulmonary rehabilitation to help patients learn diaphragmatic breathing techniques.

The rocking bed is a platformed mattress over a motor. The motor moves the platform according to a set rate and pitch. The movement of the bed causes abdominal contents to shift and inhalation and exhalation to occur. This motion also seems to mobilize secretions and to reduce the incidence of skin breakdown (Gilmartin & Make, 1988).

VENTILATOR SELECTION

When selecting the appropriate ventilator and ventilatory mode for a patient, a number of factors must be considered. To help practitioners make the correct decision, a ventilator selection decision tree is presented in Figure 9–18. This tree focuses on ventilatory needs, disease progression, lung mechanics, and patient tolerance. Depending on responses dictated by a patient's condition and need, ventilatory support for the homebound patient may be selected and implemented properly.

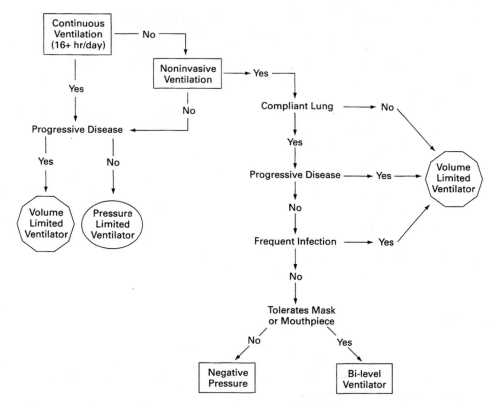

Figure 9–18 *Ventilator selection decision tree. (Courtesy of LIFECARE International, Westminster, CO. Copyright 1994.)*

BASIC NEEDS AND ACCESSORIES

In addition to the ventilator, a wide variety of other equipment and supplies are needed. Table 9–2 reviews the needs and accessories of a typical home ventilator patient. Before a discharge date is set, the patient's home should be inspected by either the HME provider or the RCP involved in the discharge. This helps to ensure the environment is appropriate

TABLE 9–2   Basic needs and accessories for the mechanically ventilated patient in the home environment

Ventilator

Primary ventilator

Secondary ventilator

Ventilator circuit

Ventilator filters

External 12-volt battery

Battery cables

Battery charger

Humidifier or heat moisture exchanger (HME)

Manual resuscitator

Secondary alarm

Tracheostomy Supplies

Spare tracheostomy tubes

One spare tracheostomy tube and another one size smaller

Tracheostomy dressings

Tracheostomy care kits

Disposable inner cannulas

Water-soluble lubricant

Syringe (10 ml)

Tracheostomy ties

Sterile gloves

Speaking valve

Solutions

Sterile water (1,000 ml)

Sodium chloride (1,000 ml)

Unit dose saline

Hydrogen peroxide

Oxygen Source(s)

Concentrator/liquid system

Portable unit

Backup unit

Suction Equipment

Electrically operated unit

Battery-operated unit

Spare suction canisters

Suction connecting tubing

Suction catheters

Gloves

Aerosol Therapy

Compressor/nebulizer

Metered dose inhaler (MDI)

Compressor, 50 psi

Large-volume nebulizer

Tracheostomy masks

Wide-bore tubing

Water traps

Miscellaneous

Hospital bed

Overbed table

Air mattress

Trapeze bar

Bedside commode

Walker

Wheel chair

Pulse oximeter

and safe, which means there should be proper electrical outlets, space for equipment, and overall living comfort. The inspection also allows time for repairs or modifications before discharge.

SUMMARY

This chapter presented and discussed the respiratory-care equipment that is used currently in the home. Knowing this equipment is essential for any clinician providing respiratory home care. Patients and caregivers depend on the equipment provider for education, consultation, and ongoing equipment maintenance. As the next century approaches, home care will continue to embrace more of the respiratory equipment used in the acute-care setting. Pulse oximeters and end-tidal CO_2 monitors are being used on a limited basis. This trend will continue within the parameters of reimbursement. The RCP will continue to play an essential role in managing the respiratory care patient in the home.

Review Questions

1. What three major oxygen delivery systems are used in the home?
2. Name three types of presently available oxygen-conserving devices or systems.
3. What is the difference between CPAP and bilevel pressure therapy equipment?
4. What are three key factors in the development of home mechanical ventilation?
5. How are patients selected for home mechanical ventilation? Name at least eight patient conditions or disorders that are commonly encountered and treated.
6. Name five different positive pressure ventilators currently used in the home.
7. When and how is negative pressure ventilation used in the home?
8. What are the advantages and disadvantages of NIPPV?

References

Bach, J., & Alba, A. (1990, January). Management of chronic alveolar hypoventilation by nasal ventilation. *Chest*, 52–57.

Burton, G., & Hodgkin, J. (1984). *Respiratory care: A guide to clinical practice* (2nd ed.). Philadelphia, PA: J. B. Lippincott.

Fracchia, C., & Ambrosino, N. (1992, August). Spotlighting negative pressure ventilation. *RT International*, 39–42.

Gilmartin, M., & Make, B. (1980). *Problems in respiratory care. Mechanical ventilation in the home: Issues for health care providers.* Philadelphia, PA: J. B. Lippincott. 1988.

Jackson, N. (1993, December/January). Negative pressure ventilation: A review of current use. *RT—The Journal for the Respiratory Care Practitioner*, 95–100.

Lucas, J., Golish, J., Sleeper, G., & O'Ryan, J. (1988). *Home respiratory care.* Norwalk, CT: Appleton and Lange.

McPherson, S. (1988). *Respiratory home care equipment.* Dubuque, Iowa: Kendall Hunt Publishing Company.

National Institutes of Health. U.S. Department of Health and Human Services. (1980, September). Continuous or nocturnal oxygen therapy in hypoxemic chronic obstructive lung disease—A clinical trial. *Annals of Internal Medicine, 93*(3), 391–398.

O'Ryan, J. (1987, March/April). An overview of mechanical ventilation in the home. *Respiratory Management,* 27–35.

Scanlan, C. (1995). *Egan's fundamentals of respiratory care* (6th ed.). St. Louis, MO: Mosby-Year Book, Inc.

White, G. (1996). *Equipment theory for respiratory care* (2nd ed.). Albany, NY: Delmar Publishers.

Suggested Readings

American Association for Respiratory Care. (1991). *A study of chronic ventilator patients in the hospital.* Dallas, TX: American Association for Respiratory Care.

American Society for Testing and Materials. (1993). Standard specification for oxygen concentrators for domiciliary use. *Annual book of ASTM standards.* Philadelphia, PA: American Society for Testing and Materials.

Glenn, K., & Make, B. (1993). *Learning objectives for positive pressure ventilation in the home.* Denver, CO: The National Center for Home Mechanical Ventilation.

Johnson, T. S., & Halberstadt, R. (1995). *Phantom of the night: Overcome sleep apnea syndrome and snoring.* Cambridge, MA: New Technologies Publishers.

Kinnear, W. (1994). *Assisted mechanical ventilation in the home.* Oxford: Oxford University Press.

O'Donohue, W. (1996). *Long-term oxygen therapy: Scientific basis and clinical application.* Marcel Dekker, Inc.: New York, NY.

Petty, T. (1995). *Chronic obstructive pulmonary disease* (2nd ed.). Marcel Dekker, Inc.: New York, NY.

Yuan, L.C., Jun, Z., & Min, L.P. (1995, August). Clinical evaluation of pulse-dose and continuous-flow oxygen delivery. *Respiratory Care, 40*(8), 811–814.

CHAPTER TEN

PROTOCOLS AND PROCEDURES OF CARE DELIVERY

David A. Gourley

David A. Gourley

--- KEY TERMS ---

basic home safety
multidisciplinary team

plan of care
polysomnography

rights and responsibilities

OBJECTIVES

Upon completing this chapter, the reader will be able to:

- Explain the purpose of developing respiratory home-care protocols and procedures.
- List the three components of a protocol or procedure.
- Define *plan of care.*
- Outline the basic procedure for establishing a respiratory home-care modality.
- Identify key variations that may exist between respiratory home-care modalities.
- Identify at least eight respiratory home-care modalities.

INTRODUCTION

Delivering quality respiratory care in the home necessitates specific protocols or procedures to maintain consistency. Consistent, quality care is the basic goal of any respiratory home-care provider. Developing and implementing procedures is labor intensive but necessary if patient care is to be delivered and monitored appropriately. A number of variables affect the composition and complexity of procedures or protocols. This chapter identifies and discusses these variables in an effort to increase both appreciation for and understanding of respiratory care as it is delivered in the home. This chapter also empowers the reader to generate specific home-care policies and procedures following the generic outline provided.

COMPONENTS OF A HOME-CARE PROCEDURE

Procedures should be used when orienting personnel to specific duties and followed when providing care. The procedure should be specific to each task and include brief description of the task, the purpose of the task, and a step-by-step instruction of the setup, operation, patient care, and equipment maintenance. The procedures should be reviewed periodically and updated as needed.

In addition to developing protocols and procedures for all respiratory care modalities, practitioners must develop a **plan of care** for each patient. The purpose of the plan of care is to provide individualized, planned, appropriate care that is directed at care goals and patient needs. The care plan is based on the patient assessment and includes the goals and actions that will resolve the patient's problems or needs. The goals and actions should be implemented and monitored. Patient assessments should be performed periodically and the care plan modified accordingly. This plan of care provides a standardized and efficient format for managing patient information. As such, it serves as a practical communication tool between patient, providers, and prescribing physician. It also serves to minimize the duplication or loss of this information (Joint Commission on Accreditation of Healthcare Organizations [JCAHO], 1995) (Lawlor, 1996).

Procedures or protocols must contain certain details of each modality, and they should follow a basic format. Following is a generic protocol or procedure that can be applied to any respiratory home care modality and related equipment. However, this generic procedure must be tailored to meet the needs of the individual organization or agency providing the care. It must also be targeted to the specifications of the equipment manufacturer.

GENERIC HOME-CARE PROCEDURE

The following outlines the procedure for setting up respiratory home equipment and administering a related modality in a patient's home. Although it is generic, it can be adapted easily to any type of respiratory home care. The three key components of any protocol are description, purpose, and procedure.

DESCRIPTION COMPONENT OF A PROTOCOL

The description of any respiratory home-care procedure or protocol should include:

- a detailed overview or explanation;
- a statement indicating that the delivery of any home-care modality is determined by the referring physician;
- indications for use or delivery (e.g., documented hypoxemia, reversible bronchospasm, or ventilatory support);

- patient diagnosis (e.g., COPD, bronchial asthma, cystic fibrosis, congestive heart failure, sleep apnea syndrome); and
- designation of the appropriate delivery device or method.

In addition, each description should identify any specific requirements or conditions unique to each procedure for:

- Oxygen therapy—appliance, delivered concentration or liter flow, and frequency of use
- Aerosol therapy—appliance, medication and dosage (if applicable), and frequency of use
- Hyperinflation therapy—device, applicable pressure or inspiratory volume, medication and dosage (if applicable), and frequency of use
- Chest physiotherapy—therapeutic mode, delivery site, duration, and frequency
- Airway management—specific type of care and frequency
- CPAP/bilevel therapy—device, pressure(s), and frequency of use
- Ventilatory support—type, mode, volume, respiratory rate, pressure limits, inspiratory flow rate, and/or delivered oxygen concentration

PURPOSE COMPONENT OF A PROTOCOL

The purpose of any therapeutic procedure is to:

- ensure that the patient and/or caregiver understands the safe, correct, and prescribed use of the equipment and accessories;
- ensure that the patient and/or caregiver understands the cleaning and maintenance requirements of the equipment;
- ensure that the patient and/or caregiver understands his or her **rights and responsibilities** in receiving the equipment;
- ensure the patient and/or caregiver can access a health-care professional from the provider at all times; and
- provide the referring physician with ongoing reports of patient assessment, education, goals, and problems.

PROCEDURE COMPONENT OF A PROTOCOL

The procedure component of a protocol includes:

- introduction to patient and/or caregiver;
- perform environmental inspection and assess **basic home safety;**
- set up the prescribed equipment, accessories, and any backup device;
- review indications for prescribed therapy;
- explain the use and operation of the equipment, accessories, and any backup device;
- emphasize the physician's order and the need to follow exact prescription;
- explain safety precautions of prescribed therapy and related equipment;
- explain routine cleaning and maintenance of the equipment and accessories;
- emphasize infection control standards and procedures;

- review troubleshooting of the equipment;
- provide proper telephone contacts of provider;
- perform patient assessment and identify problems and needs;
- provide written instructions to patient and/or caregiver;
- discuss patient's rights and responsibilities;
- complete appropriate documentation; and
- explain schedule for follow-up with patient and/or caregiver.

Key elements of the environmental inspection, including assessment of basic home safety, were covered in Chapter 8. The following protocol for mechanical ventilation is an example of how the generic procedure format may be applied to the development of any home-care protocol.

PROCEDURE FOR HOME MECHANICAL VENTILATION

The procedure for home mechanical ventilation involves setting up a home mechanical ventilator, positive or negative pressure system, to support a ventilator-dependent patient. Preparing for and implementing discharge for a ventilator-dependent patient is a labor-intensive, time-consuming task that is critical to the effectiveness and success of the endeavor. Many health-care providers will be involved in the process, either as members of the discharge team or the home care team. This procedure examines the major areas of concern to the RCP.

DESCRIPTION

The setup and delivery of home ventilation equipment is determined by the referring physician, usually with the input and consultation of a **multidisciplinary team** that includes an RCP, a nurse, a social worker, a discharge planner, a physical therapist, family, other caregivers, and, most importantly, the patient. The indication for a home ventilation setup is primarily the inability to wean a ventilator patient in the acute care setting and the patient's and/or caregivers' desire to discharge to home. Noncontinuous ventilatory support to prevent ventilatory failure is also a common indication for a home ventilation setup.

The more common diagnoses requiring home ventilatory support include ALS, MD, MS, poliomyelitis, diaphragmatic paralysis, Guillain-Barre syndrome, spinal cord injury, central hypoventilation syndromes, kyphoscoliosis, diffuse pulmonary fibrosis, COPD, and BPD.

The multiple types of ventilators and ventilation accessories require that the procedure for each ventilator setup be individualized to the type of ventilation (invasive or noninvasive) and the type of ventilator (positive or negative pressure). The physician's order must include at least the:

- type of ventilator;
- method of ventilation;

- mode of ventilation;
- volume or pressure setting;
- rate setting; and
- F_IO_2

Ideally, planning for the discharge of a home ventilator patient begins at least 2 weeks before the anticipated discharge date. In 1995, the AARC published two CPGs, one dealing with the discharge planning process for the respiratory patient and the other considering long-term invasive mechanical ventilation in the home (American Association for Respiratory Care [AARC], 1995a).

PURPOSE

The purpose of this procedure is to:

- ensure that the patient and/or caregiver understands the safe, correct, and prescribed use of the ventilator and its accessories;
- ensure that the patient and/or caregiver understands the cleaning and maintenance requirements of the equipment;
- ensure that the patient and/or caregiver understands his or her rights and responsibilities in receiving the ventilator and accessories;
- insure the patient and/or caregiver can access a health-care professional from the provider at all times; and
- provide the referring physician with ongoing reports of patient assessment, education, goals, and problems.

PROCEDURE

The procedure component of this program includes:

- introduction to patient and/or caregiver;
- set up ventilator and its accessories in hospital according to the discharging hospital's policy;
- thoroughly inspect the home and completely assess home safety;
- recommend appropriate home repairs and/or modifications;
- review indications for ventilator and accessories and, if applicable, features of the artificial airway;
- explain the use and operation of the ventilator and its accessories;
- demonstrate response to each of the ventilator alarms;
- emphasize the physician's order and the need to follow the exact prescription for care;
- demonstrate proper application of equipment and observe the patient and/or caregiver apply and operate the equipment;
- explain routine cleaning and maintenance of the ventilator and accessories;
- emphasize infection control standards;
- review troubleshooting of ventilator and accessories;

- arrange patient discharge when all team members are satisfied discharge will succeed;
- provide proper telephone contacts of provider;
- perform patient assessment and identify problems and needs;
- provide written instructions to patient and/or caregiver;
- discuss patient's rights and responsibilities;
- complete appropriate documentation;
- as appropriate, continue patient assessment and education in the home;
- explain routine follow-up schedule to patient and/or caregiver; and
- notify appropriate authorities of home ventilation patient (e.g., utilities and emergency medical services [EMS]).

OTHER RESPIRATORY HOME-CARE MODALITIES

In general, a therapeutic modality that can be delivered in the hospital can be modified for home delivery. Following is a general list of respiratory home-care modalities and specific differences or variations.

OXYGEN THERAPY

Home oxygen is available through oxygen concentrators, LOX systems, compressed gas cylinders, or conserving devices. While the major indication for this type of therapy is documented hypoxemia, patient conditions and needs vary. Consequently, these needs must be matched carefully to the appropriate oxygen delivery device. The major difference or variable relates to this delivery device. Concentrators require electrical power and cylinder backup in the event of a power failure. Oxygen delivery to a patient is also limited in terms of the device or appliance that can be used. Portables are usually in cylinder form. LOX requires deliveries but is equipped with a refillable portable system. However, this can be hazardous if a patient does not have manual dexterity or the ability to handle LOX safely. Virtually any patient device or appliance can be used with a liquid system. Oxygen cylinders present delivery, storage, and/or safety problems for high-volume users.

Patients and caregivers must be instructed in the correct and safe use of equipment and oxygen administration. Placing units away from heat sources and high-traffic areas, strictly adhering to no-smoking rules, cleaning and changing patient appliances routinely, caring for equipment properly, and reordering procedures are key items that must be reviewed and reinforced with patients and caregivers alike.

AEROSOL THERAPY

Aerosol therapy may be administered intermittently with a prescribed medication or continuously as a bland aerosol to loosen secretions. The general procedure is similar to that for home oxygen therapy, but the focus is on delivering an aerosol, with or without a prescribed medication. Key concerns involve properly measuring and delivering prescribed aerosolized medications, frequency of use, cleaning and changing contaminated equipment, and promptly identifying and attending to any adverse effects.

HYPERINFLATION THERAPY

While hyperinflation therapy includes incentive spirometry and IPPB treatments, the IPPB form of therapy requires most of the home care provider's attention. While similar in some respects to aerosol therapy, IPPB differs based on the type of equipment and the positive pressure delivered to the patient. Measuring prescribed medication, equipment contamination, proper cleaning routines, and the prompt identification of and attention to any adverse effects are major concerns with this type of therapy.

CHEST PHYSIOTHERAPY

Chest physiotherapy involves postural drainage, chest percussion, vibration, and effective coughing techniques. Postural drainage requires patient positioning using pillows or a hospital bed. Chest percussion and vibration may be performed manually with hands or rubber cups or with a mechanical device. Patients receiving this type of therapy have a problem with chronic secretion production and the expectoration of these secretions. In particular, patients with cystic fibrosis, bronchiectasis, and post-asthma attack are prime candidates for chest physiotherapy.

In addition to RCPs and other trained health-care providers, caregivers can be instructed in the safe and proper administration of chest physiotherapy. Physicians should prescribe the type of therapy, the site of administration, duration, and frequency. An aerosol treatment before chest physiotherapy usually helps to promote expectoration. Oxygen delivery may be required in some patients who desaturate, while orthopnea may be problematic in others.

AIRWAY MANAGEMENT

Airway management procedures routinely include tracheal suctioning, general tracheostomy care, and tracheostomy tube changing. Variations in procedure include indication for therapy, patient type, and underlying diagnosis. Patients requiring airway management have artificial airways, usually tracheostomies. Many are ventilator dependent and suffering from neuromuscular disorders that include ALS, MS, and MD.

Other major concerns regarding airway management focus on safe suction pressures, proper technique involving hyperinflation, and oxygenation before and after suction attempts and after sterilizing technique. This may require intensive training for caregivers. The RCPs changing tracheostomy tubes must be experienced and competent. Equipment maintenance and the availability and use of supplies like suction catheters and tracheostomy tubes are other issues home-care providers must address if this level of patient care is to be performed appropriately.

CPAP AND BILEVEL PRESSURE THERAPY

Specific variations in CPAP and bilevel pressure procedures relate to equipment type and the pressure levels. The referring physician must determine the delivery of any CPAP or bilevel therapy. The indication and diagnosis relate to the presence of OSA as documented by **polysomnography** or sleep study. The physician must specify the CPAP or bilevel pressures (IPAP and EPAP), ramp time, and frequency of use. The RCPs are involved in patient education, equipment setup and use, selection of patient interface, type and size, routine maintenance, patient assessment, and patient compliance monitoring.

DIAGNOSTIC TESTING AND PATIENT EVALUATION

A number of diagnostic procedures used in patient assessment and evaluation are gaining wider acceptance and are being performed more frequently and more accurately. Much of this growth is related to improved technology and equipment portability, coupled with the availability of competent and qualified individuals to perform such testing. In particular, the following procedures can be, and in many instances are, performed routinely within the home:

- spirometry (AARC, 1991b);
- ABG sampling (AARC, 1992);
- capillary blood gas sampling for neonatal and pediatric patients (AARC, 1994);
- pulse oximetry (AARCa, 1991); and
- screening that employs a modified sleep study for OSA determination.

The AARC has developed several CPGs describing the indications, contraindications, hazards, limitations, assessments, resources, monitoring, frequency of use, infection control measures, and settings of these procedures. The home is an accepted setting for the diagnostic and patient evaluation procedures listed. Reimbursement for the performance of these tests may also be available, depending on insurance carrier and coverage type. The RCPs are usually employed to perform these procedures, either by a hospital, a physician's office, or an independent laboratory. However, RCPs connected with an HME provider should not be involved with any assessment of a patient's oxygenation because it is a conflict of interest.

PATIENT REPORTING AND DOCUMENTATION

Several references have been made to the importance of documenting and reporting patient assessments during routine home-care visits. A report form can take many forms as long as it contains certain specific patient data. A general respiratory home-care report should contain patient information (name, address, telephone, age or date of birth, and diagnosis). In addition, the report should identify the attending or referring physician, patient goals and objectives, prescribed therapy, and equipment in use. There should be room for a detailed patient assessment, including response to treatment or therapy. Other comments by the reporting RCP may include appropriate recommendations and the date of the next visit. The form must be signed and dated by the RCP. Forms may also have space for the patient's or caregiver's signature. Figure 10–1 is a basic respiratory home-care visitation form. While this type of report form may suffice for most patient visits, some HME providers prefer to use an additional form for home ventilator patients, one that is more specific to their level of care.

PATIENT HOME VISITATION REPORT

Name _____ DOB _____

Address _____ Telephone _____

Physician _____ Referral _____

Patient diagnosis/history _____

Therapeutic objective(s) _____

Prescribed home care _____

Home care equipment _____

Patient assessment:

Auscultation notes:

Clinical measurements:

	HR	RR	B/P	PEFR	% PRED.
Pre-treatment =	____	____	____	____ LPM	____ %
Post-treatment =	____	____	____	____ LPM	____ %

Pred. pefr = _____ LPM   % improvement = _____ %

Therapeutic plan and related comments:

Next scheduled visit: _____   _____
                              Respiratory Care Practitioner   Date

Figure 10–1 *A standard patient home care report form used to document patient visit, assessment of care, and status of overall condition. (Courtesy of Jarvis & Jarvis Home Health Care, Inc., Hasbrouck Heights, NJ.)*

Essentially, this type of medical record serves as the basis for:

- planning for patient care, including evaluating patient condition and treatment;
- documenting the course of each patient's evaluation, treatment, and key condition changes;
- communicating between providers, other health-care professionals, and any organizations involved in the patient's care; and
- legally protecting the providers of services and care (Lawlor, 1996).

SUMMARY

Written policies, procedures, and protocols have been in use in many arenas for a long time. Home-care providers must use these tools to provide the quality health care that is expected in today's health-care system. Because the home-care provider is an extension of institutional care, the level of care in the home can be no different. All home-care providers must develop policies, procedures, and protocols to meet their particular services and market. All home-care providers must follow the details of these documents to provide consistent, continuous, and complete care. The providers are responsible for ensuring that their policies, procedures, and protocols are realistic and functioning. The procedures in this chapter can serve as a foundation for most home-care providers.

Review Questions

1. What does *plan of care* mean?
2. Why it is important to have respiratory home-care procedures or protocols?
3. What are the essential components of a basic respiratory home-care procedure?
4. Outline the basic procedure for setting up any respiratory home-care modality.
5. Are there any differences or variations in procedure when setting up respiratory care modalities in the home? If so, what are they? To what do they relate?
6. Name at least eight respiratory home-care modalities.

References

American Association for Respiratory Care. (1991a, December). AARC clinical practice guideline: Pulse oximetry. *Respiratory Care, 36*(12), 1406–1409.

American Association for Respiratory Care. (1991b, December). AARC clinical practice guideline: Spirometry. *Respiratory Care, 36*(12), 1414–1417.

American Association for Respiratory Care. (1992, August). AARC clinical practice guideline: Sampling for arterial blood gas analysis. *Respiratory Care, 37*(8), 913–917.

American Association for Respiratory Care. (1994, December). AARC clinical practice guideline: Capillary blood gas sampling for neonatal & pediatric patients. *Respiratory Care, 39*(12), 1180–1183.

American Association for Respiratory Care. (1995a, December). AARC clinical practice guideline: Discharge planning for the respiratory care patient. *Respiratory Care, 40*(12), 1308–1312.

American Association for Respiratory Care. (1995b, December). AARC clinical practice guideline: Long-term invasive mechanical ventilation in the home. *Respiratory Care, 40*(12), 1313–1320.

Joint Commission on Accreditation of Health Care Organizations. (1995). *Accreditation manual for home care*. Oakbrook Terrace, IL: JCAHO.

Lawlor, B. (1996, Fall). The essentials for home care documentation. *Home Care Section Bulletin, (3)*, 7. American Association for Respiratory Care.

Suggested Readings

American Association for Respiratory Care. (1991a, December). AARC clinical practice guideline: Incentive spirometry. *Respiratory Care, 36*(12), 1402–1405.

American Association for Respiratory Care. (1991b, December). AARC clinical practice guideline: Postural drainage therapy. *Respiratory Care, 36*(12), 1418–1426.

American Association for Respiratory Care. (1992a, August). AARC clinical practice guideline: Humidification during mechanical ventilation. *Respiratory Care, 37*(8), 887–890.

American Association for Respiratory Care. (1992b, August). AARC clinical practice guideline: Nasotracheal suctioning. *Respiratory Care, 37*(8), 898–901.

American Association for Respiratory Care. (1992c, August). AARC clinical practice guideline: Oxygen therapy in the home or extended care facility. *Respiratory Care, 37*(8), 918–922.

American Association for Respiratory Care. (1992d, August). AARC clinical practice guideline: Selection of aerosol delivery device. *Respiratory Care, 37*(8), 891–897.

American Association for Respiratory Care. (1993a, May). AARC clinical practice guideline: Directed cough. *Respiratory Care, 38*(5), 495–499.

American Association for Respiratory Care. (1993b, May). AARC clinical practice guideline: Endotracheal suctioning of mechanically ventilated adults and children with artificial airways. *Respiratory Care, 38*(5), 500–504.

American Association for Respiratory Care. (1993c, May). AARC clinical practice guideline: Use of positive airway pressure adjuncts to bronchial hygiene therapy. *Respiratory Care, 38*(5), 516–521.

American Association for Respiratory Care. (1993a, December). AARC clinical practice guideline: Bland aerosol administration. *Respiratory Care, 38*(12), 1196–1200.

American Association for Respiratory Care. (1993b, December). AARC clinical practice guideline: Intermittent positive pressure breathing. *Respiratory Care, 38*(12), 1189–1195.

American Association for Respiratory Care. (1994, August). AARC clinical practice guideline: Delivery of aerosols to the upper airway. *Respiratory Care, 39*(8), 803–807.

American Association for Respiratory Care. (1995, December). AARC clinical practice guideline: Assessing response to bronchodilator therapy at point of care. *Respiratory Care, 40*(12), 1300–1307.

Glenn, K., & Make, B. (1993). *Learning objectives for positive pressure ventilation in the home*. Denver, CO: The National Center for Home Mechanical Ventilation.

Joint Commission on Accreditation of Health Care Organizations. (1993). *Accreditation manual for home care*. Oakbrook Terrace, IL: JCAHO. 1993.

McPherson, S. (1988). *Respiratory home care equipment*. Dubuque, IA: Kendall Hunt Publishing Company.

CHAPTER ELEVEN

HOME CARE ACCREDITATION AND STATE LICENSING REQUIREMENTS

KEY TERMS

accreditation
Accreditation Commission for Home Care (ACHC)
Accreditation Council for Home Medical Services (ACHMS)
Community Health Accreditation Program (CHAP)

Joint Commission on Accreditation of Healthcare Organizations (JCAHO)
legal credentialing
National Committee for Quality Assurance (NCQA)
peer credentialing
scope of practice

OBJECTIVES

Upon completing this chapter, the reader will be able to:

- Define *accreditation* and discuss its importance to home care and HME providers.
- List three organizations that accredit home-care companies.
- Identify one major strength and one major weakness of each accrediting body.
- Identify three of the home-care industry's major concerns with current accreditation programs, and explain how these concerns are being addressed.
- Identify the two levels of accreditation through JCAHO for respiratory home care.
- Describe the JCAHO survey process for respiratory home care.
- Differentiate between peer credentialing and legal credentialing.
- Describe the current and potential impact of legal credentialing or state licensure on the delivery of respiratory home care.

INTRODUCTION

Health-care reform has brought about a greater emphasis on alternate site care, including home care. This emphasis has caused a need for standards and some form of regulation and recognition, particularly for those who deliver and provide various types of home care. A number of organizations are now offering these types of service to the home-care industry in an effort to standardize and legitimize its providers. This chapter looks at these organizations in terms of their focus, standards, and role. This voluntary process of **accreditation** is assuming greater importance in the managed-care environment and provider networks.

Another process that is taking on added significance, especially in home care, is professional recognition. This chapter also considers this issue and its importance to the RCP. Almost every state in the nation has some form of licensure or state credentialing for RCPs. As the focus of patient care shifts from the hospital to the home and other alternate sites, professional recognition of RCPs will play an increasingly important role in ensuring practitioner competency and patient safety. Licensure may be the key to unlocking home-care reimbursement for RCP services.

DEFINITION AND HISTORICAL PERSPECTIVE

Accreditation is the process by which health-care providers, including the HMEs, establish and maintain credibility and acceptance by both the health-care community and the public at large. Accreditation, which is usually voluntary, is the act of determining that an institution, a facility, an agency, or a company has met a certain set of patient care standards. The accreditation concept has been in existence since the early 1900s when Forest Codman, MD, proposed "the end result system of hospital standardization" (Parver & Hildebrandt, 1996). Educational institutions had been involved in a similar system for years. Hospitals were the first to meet a set of standards for professionalism in patient-care delivery and thereby initiated the accreditation process in health care. By the mid-1980s, the focus on patient care began to shift out of the hospital, prompting proposals to include the home-care industry in the accreditation process.

PROFESSIONAL STANDARDS

Although it is not part of the accreditation process, the AARC adopted and published a position statement and set of standards for respiratory home care in 1979 (American Association for Respiratory Care [AARC], 1979). These standards, as discussed in Chapter 7, were the forerunner of respiratory home care accreditation. However, home-care delivery has changed significantly since 1979, especially due to health-care reform and managed care. These home-care standards must be revisited and revised accordingly to reflect the current nature and status of respiratory home care accurately.

JUSTIFICATION FOR ACCREDITATION

Initially, hospitals were the primary target of health-care accreditation, but other facets of the health-care industry expanded. In 1994, close to 7 million patients received services from almost 15,000 home-care providers at a cost of $23 billion (Cathcart, 1995). This produced a growing need to ensure the quality of patient care both in the home and at other alternate care sites.

Following the growth in the patient population, HME providers and home health agencies increased in number. The SMG Marketing Group, a health-care market research firm, reported a 13 percent increase in the number of home health agencies from 1994 to 1995. This growth accounted for long-term care reaching a level of $77 billion (Hamill, 1996). As a result, managed-care organizations began using accreditation as a way to evaluate a health-care provider's performance within their networks while also meeting the requirements of their accreditation through the **National Committee for Quality Assurance (NCQA).** National accreditation is the only performance measure for HME providers recognized by the NCQA, and it is usually obtained through recognized accrediting organizations that set patient-care standards (Hamill, 1996).

ACCREDITING ORGANIZATIONS

The HME providers have criticized accrediting organizations for the time-consuming and rather expensive ordeal that leads to accreditation. However, the present health-care environment makes accreditation a necessity and something HME providers must take seriously. The three organizations accrediting home health agencies and HME providers are the **Joint Commission on Accreditation of Healthcare Organizations (JCAHO),** the **Community Health Accreditation Program (CHAP),** and the **Accreditation Commission for Home Care (ACHC).** Each organization is considered in terms of its focus, format, standards, and importance. Because accreditation fees are usually determined annually and vary based on the organization seeking accreditation, they are not included here. Individuals interested in current fee structures should contact the accrediting body.

JOINT COMMISSION ON ACCREDITATION OF HEALTHCARE ORGANIZATIONS

Because the JCAHO is considered to be the largest and most influential home-care accrediting agency, it is covered in greater detail than the other agencies. Initially, hospitals were accredited by the Joint Commission on Accreditation of Hospitals (JCAH). In 1984, Medicare began using the prospective payment system (PPS), which based length of hospital stay and reimbursement on DRGs. Hospitals were compelled to become more efficient, which led to swifter, and at times hasty, hospital discharges, which in turn increased the need for patient care in the home. Responding to this change in patient care focus from hospital to home, in 1986 the JCAH became the Joint Commission on Accreditation of Healthcare Organizations (JCAHO). Also at this time, the JCAHO initiated a 2-year project to generate a set of comprehensive standards for companies and agencies providing various levels of home care. These standards for home care were published in 1988 but have since undergone a number of significant revisions (Scanlan, 1995).

In 1995, the JCAHO modified the survey process as outlined in its *1995 Accreditation Manual for Home Care (AMHC)—Volumes I and II.* In response to requests from accredited organizations, the JCAHO tried to make its accreditation process more individualized, consistent, and helpful in improving organizational performance. This new process was designed to support patient-centered, performance focused, and functional orientation as instituted in the revised home-care standards. The survey process deviated from the evaluation of specific departments or services and instead focused on assessing the performance of more important patient-focused and organizational functions that support the quality of patient care (Joint Commission on Accreditation of Healthcare Organizations [JCAHO], 1994a).

Consequently, home care accreditation was no longer a "paper-oriented" survey process but instead was one that focused more on outcomes and results. The absence of a policy in a procedure manual was not that significant. Instead, it was more important to determine whether a policy had been implemented, if the staff was aware of such a policy, or if the staff was not following a policy. Complying with standards regularly provided an HME provider with organization and consistency, which resulted in good home care practices becoming the norm (Brinton, 1995).

Problems Associated with the Joint Commission on Accreditation of Healthcare Organizations. Home care accreditation is the JCAHO's fastest growing program, increasing at a rate of 35 percent since 1994 (Cathcart, 1995). In 1995, the JCAHO completed 1,766 home care surveys and planned to complete 2200 in 1996, making home care its largest accreditation segment (Hamill, 1996). Despite this growth, however, the home-care industry continued to view the accreditation standards as unrealistic, unreasonable, and unworkable, mainly because they applied too much to the hospital setting and were irrelevant to home care.

Lack of public disclosure on the quality of a home-care company's services was yet another issue of contention. Some information from the JCAHO is subject to public disclosure upon request or is reportable to responsible government agencies. This information includes accreditation history, accreditation status of an organization, standards under which a survey was conducted, and organizational and operational components in the survey process. The JCAHO treats as confidential any and all information obtained throughout the accreditation process (JCAHO, 1996).

Finally, JCAHO's accreditation fees are considered to be high, even prohibitive for some small organizations. Medicare—Part A may reimburse accreditation fees for some home health agencies (HHAs) but not those for HME providers (Parver & Hildebrandt, 1996). The accreditation fee is based on volume and type of services and the location and length of the survey. The fee is the one that is effective when the survey is conducted. Two payment options are available: (1) pay the full fee when billed or (2) spread payments over 3½ months (JCAHO, 1996).

Current Accreditation Standards. To address the concerns of the home-care industry, the JCAHO again revised its home-care accreditation process and published the changes in 1996 in its *1997–98 Comprehensive Accreditation Manual for Home Care (CAMHC)*. The standards in this manual took effect January 1, 1997. All home-care surveys conducted between this date and December 31, 1998, will be based on this manual (JCAHO, 1996).

The *CAMHC* format includes home-care standards and information on an organization's need for ongoing performance improvement, as well as guidelines for self-assessment and survey preparation. This manual enables organizations to better understand the connection between patient-centered, performance-focused standards and the home-care provider's day-to-day operation. It also enables any organization to better understand the overall accreditation process, facilitate performance self-assessment, and assess its poten-

overall accreditation process, facilitate performance self-assessment, and assess its potential accreditation status before the survey (JCAHO, 1996).

According to the JCAHO, the three key issues any organization striving to achieve excellence must address are:

1. An organization's relationship to the external environment, which in this case is the dynamic health-care environment. To succeed, an organization must anticipate, understand, and proactively respond to its environment's changes.
2. An organization's internal environment, including characteristics and functions relating to excellence in care and services. Specifically, excellence in patient care and services requires factors like professional knowledge; clinical, management governance, and support expertise; and competent technical skills that are effectively integrated and coordinated organization wide to respond to any patient's needs.
3. An organization's method for systematically assessing and improving work functions and outcomes.

Figure 11–1 identifies the major components of the four critical aspects of any health-care organization's internal environment and provides a diagram of the cycle for improving performance (JCAHO, 1996).

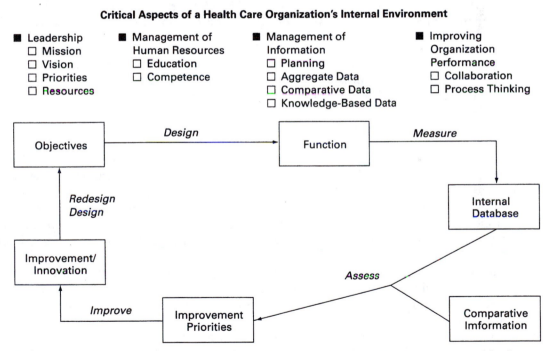

Critical Aspects of a Health Care Organization's Internal Environment

■ Leadership	■ Management of	■ Management of	■ Improving
☐ Mission	Human Resources	Information	Organization
☐ Vision	☐ Education	☐ Planning	Performance
☐ Priorities	☐ Competence	☐ Aggregate Data	☐ Collaboration
☐ Resources		☐ Comparative Data	☐ Process Thinking
		☐ Knowledge-Based Data	

Figure 11–1 *The four critical aspects of any health-care organization's internal environment and a flowchart of the cycle for improving organizational performance. (©1997–98 Comprehensive Accreditation Manual for Home Care. Oakbrook Terrace, IL. Joint Commission on Accreditation of Healthcare Organizations, 1996, page 56. Reprinted with permission.)*

The JCAHO is recognized nationally, enjoys a high profile, and tends to have the greatest status and prestige when it comes to home-care accreditation. Accreditation by the JCAHO is normally valid for 3 years. Accreditation is not automatically renewed, and organizations must apply for and undergo a complete accreditation at the end of each 3-year period. The JCAHO conducts a full accreditation more frequently upon request from an accredited organization (JCAHO, 1996).

Those agencies or organizations eligible for accreditation include:

- home health services on an intermittent or a private-duty basis;
- Medicare-certified home health agencies;
- private duty agencies;
- home infusion therapy services;
- pharmaceutical services;
- equipment management;
- personal care services;
- clinical respiratory services;
- organizations providing rehabilitation technology services; and
- hospice services.

The JCAHO accredits services, not products. Therefore, HME companies applying for accreditation must also provide services in addition to home-care equipment (JCAHO, 1996; Parver & Hildebrandt, 1996).

Respiratory Home Care Standards. To be accredited, respiratory home-care providers must meet standards for home equipment management, clinical respiratory services, or both. The first level of service relates to the use and care of home medical equipment that is sold or rented. This typically involves patients on some form of home oxygen or aerosol therapy. The second level of service relates to clinical respiratory care involving periodic home-care visits with patient assessment. Respiratory providers seeking this type of accreditation are usually involved with home-care that requires routine patient follow-up, like that for ventilator-dependent patients. It appears that patient acuity and company focus are the two factors determing for what level(s) of accreditation a home-care company applies. Home-care companies involved with equipment only pursue the first level of accreditation; those involved only with patient care and assessment seek the second level. Companies providing both levels of service must meet both sets of standards to be accredited.

In 1993, the JCAHO was using a well-defined, separate set of standards to accredit home-care providers. These standards were contained in service-specific chapters of the JCAHO accreditation manual, including two that pertained directly to respiratory home care, "Equipment Management Services" and "Clinical Respiratory Services." However, major revisions in the surveying and accrediting process occurred and became effective on January 1, 1995 (Brinton, 1995), and again on January 1, 1997. Overall, changes in the new *CAMHC* have been minimal and limited to key issues of quality patient care. Accordingly, the number of technical standards was reduced from 505 to 277. These 277 standards, which are basically generic, can be applied at varying levels of intensity to evaluate and accredit all home-care providers. Accreditation standards continue to be grouped into eleven functional chapters that are categorized into two major sections—patient-focused functions and organization-focused functions (Table 11–1) (JCAHO, 1996).

These functions and their respective standards are used to survey and accredit respiratory home care providers. The RCPs involved in accreditation should obtain a copy of the JCAHO's manual and become thoroughly familiar with its format and content. Because it

TABLE 11–1 The functional chapters used by JCAHO in surveying and accrediting home-care providers, including respiratory home care

Patient-Focused Functions

Function	Designation	Goal	Standards
Rights and ethics	RI	To recognize and respect the integral human, civil, constitutional, and statutory rights of each patient during the provision of care to improve patient outcomes	21
Assessment	PE	To determine the services and care to be provided through assessment of each patient's needs	22
Care, treatment, and service	TX	To provide individualized, planned, and appropriate care in settings appropriate to patient-care goals and related patient needs	59
Education	PF	To improve patient health outcomes by appropriately involving patients in their care and care decisions and by promoting recovery, patient comfort, return to function, and healthy behavior through implementation of the patient and family education function	20
Continuum of care and services	CC	To maximize care and services in a continuous, coordinated manner and to use care settings appropriate to the needs of each patient	14
Improving organizational performance	PI	To design processes and systematically measure, assess, and improve performance to improve patient health outcomes	19
Leadership	LD	To provide the framework for planning, directing, coordinating, providing and improving health care and services that respond to the community and patient needs and improve patient health outcomes	32
Environmental safety and equipment management	EC	To promote safe and effective patient care and organization environments, including equipment use, in the delivery of patient care	27

continued

TABLE 11–1   continued

Organization-Focused Functions			
Function	Designation	Goal	Standards
Management of human resources	HR	To identify and provide adequate and competent staff to meet patient needs and fulfill the organization's mission	15
Management of information	IM	To obtain, manage, and use information to improve patient outcomes and individual and organization performance in patient care, governance, management, and support processes	41
Surveillance, prevention, and infection control	IC	To improve patient health outcomes through the identification and reduction of risks for infections in patients and organization staff	7

(Source: Information based on data from the JCAHO's *1997–78 Comprehensive Accreditation Manual for Home Care,* Copyright 1996.)

is beyond the scope of this text to identify each standard, Table 11–2 presents samples of standards that apply to both the equipment management and clinical respiratory services components of respiratory home care accreditation.

The Accreditation Process. The accreditation process can be time consuming, depending on the size and scope of the organization or company and how it has conducted business. Preparing for an initial survey may take 12 to 18 months, but subsequent triennial surveys require less preparation time. The steps toward initial accreditation include:

- The JCAHO application is completed and submitted by the organization. An organization's first full accreditation survey must be scheduled within 1 year of the time the JCAHO receives the application.
- Organization reviews and becomes familiar with the format and content of the current accreditation manual.
- Facility, staff, patients, and work processes are prepared for the survey (all required manuals, forms, and procedures are completed or updated).
- Date of the survey visit is confirmed.
- Following a prearranged agenda, the survey is completed by the assigned surveyor(s).
- A leadership exit conference is conducted and survey findings are sent to JCAHO for analysis and processing.
- The JCAHO provides the organization with an accreditation decision and a request for any required responses or actions in its *Official Accreditation Decision Report.* (JCAHO, 1996)

TABLE 11–2 **Representative standards that apply to the equipment management and clinical respiratory care service components of JCAHO accreditation of respiratory home care providers**

Component	Function	Standard	Definition/Description
Equipment management	Environmental safety and equipment management	EC.7	The delivery processes are appropriate for the equipment provided to meet the patient's needs
		EC.9	The organization provides emergency maintenance, replacement, or backup equipment when appropriate
	Management of human resources	HR.3.1	The numbers, qualifications, and health statuses of staff are appropriate to the scope and services the organization provides
	Surveillance, prevention, and infection control	IC.2	The organization implements and coordinates all components of its infection-control program
Clinical respiratory services	Assessment	PE.2.3	The patient's diagnosis, condition, need, and desire for care or services; response to previous care or services; and the care or service setting determine the scope and intensity of any additional assessments
		PE.3	The organization reassesses each patient periodically during the course of care or services
	Care, treatment, and service	TX.1	The organization uses a care-planning process to ensure care or services are appropriate to each patient's needs
		TX.5	The organization monitors each patient for his or her response to care or services provided

(Information based on data from the JCAHO's *1997–98 Comprehensive Accreditation Manual for Home Care,* copyright 1996.)

To facilitate the survey visit, which may take 1, 2, or more days, the surveyor(s) review all:

- policy and procedure manuals;
- organizational charts;
- educational materials;

- marketing brochures;
- statements of patients' rights and responsibilities;
- employee job descriptions;
- complaint and incident report forms;
- orientation materials;
- emergency preparedness plans;
- on-call logs;
- performance improvement plans;
- copies of written contracts or service agreements; and
- sample patient records.

Also during the survey the surveyor(s):

- tour the facility;
- visit any branch locations;
- interview staff;
- observe equipment deliveries and home visits;
- review equipment and delivery vehicles;
- review home-care records and current patient rental list;
- inspect daily delivery and on-call logs;
- review employee files and any applicable regulatory reports; and
- verify legal permits, licenses, registrations, articles of incorporation, and other related documents.

The best way for an organization to prepare for an accreditation survey is to train its staff to be aware of and in constant compliance with all current home-care standards (Brinton, 1995).

The seven categories of accreditation decisions that can be rendered by the JCAHO are:

1. Accreditation with Commendation—the highest decision possible from the JCAHO, recognizes exemplary performance.
2. Accreditation without Type I Recommendations—organization demonstrates acceptable compliance in all performance areas.
3. Accreditation with Type I Recommendations—organization receives at least one recommendation for addressing an insufficient or an unsatisfactory standards compliance in a specific performance area. Resolution must be completed within a given time through focused survey or written progress report.
4. Provisional Accreditation—organization satisfactorily complies with selected standards as determined during the first of two surveys conducted under the Early Survey Policy. The second or full survey is conducted approximately 6 months after the first to determine the organization's record of performance. Provisional accreditation remains until the second full survey is completed and results in an organization receiving one of the other official accreditation decisions.
5. Conditional Accreditation—organization does not substantially comply with JCAHO standards but is believed able to comply within a given time frame or when the JCAHO finds an accredited organization to have had one or more adverse clinical events for which the organization could reasonably be held responsible. In both instances, corrective action must be demonstrated through a short-term follow-up

survey within 6 months. The organization will be accredited (with or without Type I recommendations) or not accredited.

6. Preliminary Nonaccreditation—organization significantly noncomplies with JCAHO standards or accreditation is withdrawn preliminarily for reasons like falsification of records. This is an appealable decision.
7. Not Accredited—organization is denied accreditation because of significant non-compliance with standards, accreditation is withdrawn for stated reasons, or organization voluntarily withdraws from the accreditation process. This is also an appealable decision. (JCAHO, 1996)

The JCAHO recommendations are of two specific types. A Type I recommendation is a group of recommendations that address insufficient or unsatisfactory compliance with stated standards in a specific area of performance. For an organization to maintain its accreditation, resolution must be completed within a given time frame through focused surveys, written reports, or both. In contrast, a supplemental recommendation does not require formal follow-up but must be dealt with appropriately by the next triennial survey or the accreditation status of an organization may be affected (JCAHO, 1996).

COMMUNITY HEALTH ACCREDITATION PROGRAM

The Community Health Accreditation Program (CHAP) began in 1965 and has focused on community-based health care instead of institutionally based programs. In 1988, CHAP began to develop consumer-oriented outcomes to determine quality in the delivery of patient home care. Through its collection of data from home-care consumers, managers, and staff, CHAP has developed and implemented measurement tools to assess outcomes related to the delivery of home-care services. In 1992, CHAP became the first home-care accrediting body to receive deemed status from Medicare (Parver & Hildebrandt, 1996).

Presently, CHAP accredits the following home-care and community-based organizations, groups, and services:

- voluntary, nonprofit organizations;
- proprietary organizations;
- nursing agencies;
- social-work agencies;
- pharmacies;
- HME providers;
- home infusion therapy;
- homemakers and home-health aides; and
- physical, occupational, and speech therapists.

The two categories of CHAP accreditation are initial accreditation and continued accreditation. Each category is subdivided to include full accreditation, deferred accreditation, continued accreditation, or no accreditation. Home-care organizations seeking accreditation conduct self-assessments and rate themselves based on five "pulse points," namely, financial management, risk management, consumer satisfaction, clinical services, and organizational factors. With this tool, companies and agencies can compare their outcomes with CHAP standards and the Conditions of Participation issued by the HCFA.

Accreditation fees are based on annual case load and respective revenue, including a non-refundable application fee and site-visit fee. CHAP's greatest weakness is lack of recognition. Although it has received deemed status from Medicare, many payors do not know it exists (Parver & Hildebrandt, 1996).

ACCREDITATION COMMISSION FOR HOME CARE

The Accreditation Commission for Home Care (ACHC) is an independent, private, non-profit organization founded in 1986. By 1994, the ACHC had become involved in accrediting home health aides and nursing services, as well as HME providers, home-infusion services, pharmaceutical services, respiratory care, and other allied-health therapy. The ACHC developed and enjoyed growing acceptance when the public grew dissatisfied with other national accreditation programs stemming from the lack of home-care industry's voice, unrealistic standards, and high costs.

The ACHC board of commissioners includes representatives from HME companies, certified home-health agencies, infusion-therapy providers, hospices, private-duty nursing services, county departments of social services, and consumers. As a result, this commission is provider based and ensures a voice for the home-care industry. Standards are similar to those of the JCAHO and consist of thirty-six core standards that are applied to all organizations pursuing accreditation. The four categories of ACHC accreditation are approved, deferred, denied, and nonaccreditation. Positive comments are included in the accreditation summary. An appeals process is also in place. There is a base fee for accreditation, plus a fee for volume and number of home-care services offered. Payment of these fees may be spread over 1 year, which makes ACHC accreditation attractive to smaller companies and organizations (Parver & Hildebrandt, 1996).

ACCREDITATION COUNCIL FOR HOME MEDICAL SERVICES

The **Accreditation Council for Home Medical Services (ACHMS)** was formed in late 1994 by the National Association for Medical Equipment Services (NAMES), the National Alliance for Infusion Therapy, the MED Group, and Van G. Miller & Associates in response to dissatisfaction with JCAHO and CHAP. The ACHMS is exploring alternatives to home-care accreditation and the possibility of establishing another accrediting body. It has concluded that accreditation programs must:

- meet the needs of clients and payors;
- consider limiting the setting in which care and services are rendered;
- foster, motivate, and augment competence within the industry; and
- effectively balance outcomes measures and standards.

The ACHMS is challenging both home-care providers and accrediting bodies to measure and improve their processes based on collected data. A set of reliable performance indicators and organizational goals aimed at meeting or exceeding these indicators must be established. Managed care is making it necessary to standardize quality in the health-care industry as it continues to change and evolve (Hamill, 1996)

The accreditation process is labor intensive, but it benefits an organization in a number of ways. The following case study involving a respiratory home care provider illustrates some of the major issues and concerns that must be addressed in this area.

CASE STUDY

Pursuing Home Care Accreditation

F.G. is an RRT and a state-licensed RCP who is also the president of a small, suburban-based respiratory home-care company with five full-time and two part-time employees, three of whom are RCPs. F.G. has been in business for over 10 years providing basic respiratory home care in the forms of oxygen and aerosol therapy. His attempts at providing a full line of HME services were not profitable. F.G. receives patient referrals from several local hospitals and from a number of dedicated pulmonary physicians who have been extremely satisfied with the service. Although F.G. has considered JCAHO accreditation, he has never submitted an application.

The highly competitive market became more so with the advent of managed care. Several referring physicians became managed-care providers and brought their patients with them. Consequently, F.G.'s company lost several patients when they converted their Medicare coverage to managed-care organizations. It was impossible for F.G. to join a provider network because doing so required some form of accreditation. Hospitals also began asking about F.G.'s accreditation status.

Sensing the urgency of the situation, F.G. decided to pursue JCAHO accreditation for his company. A policy and procedure manual was already used, and the company had updated job descriptions, complete employee files with copies of applicable licenses and credentials, on-call logs, equipment maintenance records, safety inspection reports, and patient files. Because his company provided only respiratory home-care equipment, F.G. decided to apply for accreditation in equipment management. He submitted the application, and a survey visit was scheduled.

1. Why did F.G. finally decide to pursue JCAHO accreditation for his company?
2. How should F.G.'s company prepare for the survey visit? What materials should be collected and prepared for the surveyors' review?
3. What added services or work processes would make this organization eligible for accreditation in clinical respiratory services?

PEER CREDENTIALING

Peer credentialing involves professional recognition of a designated level of competency through documented experience and/or an examination. With regard to respiratory care, the entry level is the certified respiratory therapy technician (CRTT) credential. Advanced practitioner status is designated by the RRT credential. Both examinations and credentials are administered by NBRC in Lenexa, KS.

Before licensure, almost anyone could deliver and administer respiratory home care. However, HME providers sought credentialed RCPs to provide respiratory care in the home as a way of increasing the competency of their service and helping to ensure the delivery of quality care. This also enabled providers to market the value of their organizations to referral sources. The credentialed RCPs legitimized respiratory home care providers and enhanced the safety and quality of the service.

LEGAL CREDENTIALING

Legal credentialing through licensure, state credentialing, or title protection enhances legitimacy because it involves governmental regulation of the respiratory care profession. By mid-1996, only eight states lacked any form of legal credentialing in respiratory care. All states are expected to attain some form of legal credentialing in the next few years (Eicher, 1996a). While peer credentialing is generally voluntary, legal credentialing is mandatory. It allows practitioners to function within a defined **scope of practice,** one that identifies a specific set of procedures that can be performed legally. Care settings and circumstances governing the delivery of care may also be identified. Legal credentialing of RCPs is obtained through the NBRC examination system. Such an arrangement fosters the creation of viable mechanisms for reciprocity between neighboring states, which is advantageous to RCPs who live on or near the borders of two states.

Legal credentialing defines and validates a profession's scope of practice, increases professional recognition, and helps to secure insurance reimbursement. Because insurance carriers recognize and reimburse licensed professionals for home-care services, it became essential for the respiratory-care profession to seek legal credentialing. With it, home-care reimbursement remains possible. Ultimately, state licensing of RCPs should positively affect home-care reimbursement as discussed further in Chapter 12.

Respiratory care licensure appears to be impacting one particular area of home care, namely the role of service or driver technicians who deliver oxygen and other respiratory-care equipment for home use. Two questions have arisen. The first addresses when equipment delivery ends and patient care begins. The second addresses whether these individuals can legally instruct, set up, and administer oxygen or other forms of respiratory care to a patient. Florida and states with similar statutory language have laws that do not prohibit driver technicians from assembling, setting up, testing, and demonstrating oxygen and other forms of prescribed breathing therapy for home use. Most practitioners contend that the responsibilities, as outlined in these exemption clauses, do not constitute a definition of scope of practice. Other state regulations, as in South Dakota's respiratory care licensure law, indicate not only what is not prohibited but also what is prohibited under the law (Eicher, 1995). Still other states, like New Jersey, allow driver technicians to set up and administer home oxygen therapy, but only after they have received documented training in this area and a licensed RCP conducts a follow-up visit within 24 hours (Eicher, 1996b).

The issue remains controversial. Most states agree that driver or service technicians cannot perform patient assessment, provide patient education, or evaluate a patient's response to therapy. Nonetheless, disparity continues over the set up of home oxygen and other therapeutic modalities. Model language may be difficult because of the discrepancy that exists from state to state pertaining to the meaning of terms like *set up, instruction,* and *demonstration.* States debating this issue can refer to the guidelines relating to the delivery and administration of respiratory home care as outlined in the current accreditation manual of the JCAHO. The AARC supports these guidelines and has also been working with NAMES to try to generate a joint policy statement of the role of driver or service technicians in respiratory home care. This input enables states to address this matter effectively (Eicher, 1995c).

In the interim, the Regulatory Committee of NAMES released a position statement entitled, "The Scope of Responsibility of Home Medical Equipment Services Drivers/ Technicians in the Delivery of Oxygen Equipment in the Home Setting." The language is similar to the joint statement considered by the AARC. Essentially, the NAMES statement addresses the state licensure issue and the areas in which driver/technician activities appear to overlap those of the RCPs. NAMES views home oxygen therapy as a modality that is self-administered following the order of a physician or another qualified healthcare practitioner as allowed under state law. It also identifies the specific roles of driver/technicians in the home while asserting that these individuals may not "conduct patient assessments, make clinical recommendations, or otherwise modify or comment on the client's prescribed respiratory care." On a state level, both AARC-chartered affiliates and HME associations should be prepared to work together for a workable resolution to this issue (Eicher, 1996c).

OTHER LEGISLATION IMPACTING RESPIRATORY HOME CARE

On the federal level, in 1995 Senator Orrin Hatch of Utah introduced an extensive nursing home reform bill (S-1177) that would remove the transfer agreement restrictions for respiratory care and allow respiratory care to be a covered nursing-home service. These restrictions are outdated. Their removal would place respiratory care on a level similar to that of physical, occupational, and speech therapy. S-1177 has yet to become law (Eicher, 1995).

Other legislation revolves around state licensing of HME providers in an effort to standardize and validate the home-care industry and protect consumers from possible fraudulent practices. If state agencies are given the power to regulate HME companies, the home-care industry hopes this will increase professionalism, improve its public image, and be instrumental in gaining the respect of both payors and policy makers. Consequently, it is in the best interest of home-care companies to seek accreditation and licensure, if available (Kemper & Sellers, 1996). To assist states in this process, NAMES has drafted a model state licensure bill. It focuses on home-care companies that provide sophisticated medical devices, like oxygen concentrators, mechanical ventilators, respiratory disease management devices, apnea monitors, and infusion-therapy equipment.

According to this model, states will be able to conduct mandatory, ongoing, and random inspections of HME providers to help ensure compliance of all designated rules and regulations. Consumer complaints can also lead to inspections, along with fines or license revocation if noncompliance is determined. An appeal process has also been incorporated as part of the model. States pursuing home-care legislation should advocate a HME advisory council to provide input, data, and education on home medical equipment and assist in the development of related standards (Benner, 1996). All RCPs involved in respiratory home care are encouraged to be vigilant regarding legislation that may affect home care, the practice of respiratory care, and the availability of respiratory home-care services.

--- **SUMMARY** ---

Managed care is significantly impacting the delivery of health care across the nation, including patient home care. Accreditation and legal credentialing are attempts by home-care providers to document organizational effectiveness, validate competency of employees, and ensure quality of care by meeting certain prescribed requirements and standards. Providers of respiratory home care are especially interested and involved because of the professional recognition, acceptance, and insurance reimbursement that are at stake. Although there are three major home care accrediting bodies, each of which has advantages and disadvantages, JCAHO accreditation is the most sought after by respiratory home care providers.

The home-care industry in general has expressed specific concerns of the accreditation process. While problems do exist, most HME providers, including those offering respiratory home care, believe it is in their best interests and those of the industry to obtain some level of accreditation. Legal credentialing of RCPs and HME companies also serve to advance the home-care industry in a managed care environment.

Review Questions

1. What is accreditation, and why is it important to home care and HME providers?
2. Name three organizations that presently accredit home-care companies.
3. What is a major strength and weakness of each accrediting body?
4. What are three major concerns the home-care industry has with the current accreditation programs, and how are these concerns being addressed?
5. What are the two levels of JCAHO accreditation for respiratory home-care services?
6. Describe the major steps in the JCAHO survey process for respiratory home care.
7. What is the difference between peer credentialing and legal credentialing?
8. What impact has legal credentialing or state licensure had on the delivery of respiratory home care?

References

American Association for Respiratory Care. (1979, November). Standards for respiratory therapy home care. An official statement by the AARC. *Respiratory Care, 24*(11), 1080–1082.

Benner, M. (1996, May). The making of a model. *HomeCare, 18*(5), 66, 68.

Brinton, K. (1995, October). The "new" home care accreditation survey. *AARCTimes, 19*(10), 36–38, 41–42.

Cathcart, M. (1995, October). Managed care offers opportunities for home care practitioners. *AARCTimes, 19*(10), 28.

Eicher, J. (1995, October). State regulatory issues in respiratory home care. *AARCTimes, 19*(10), 8, 11.

Eicher, J. (1996a, Spring). New Jersey board rules on HME delivery personnel. *Home Care Section Bulletin, 1,* 6. American Association for Respiratory Care.

Eicher, J. (1996b, June). 1996 state licensure update. *AARCTimes, 20*(6), 10.

Eicher, J. (1996c, Fall). NAMES statement on the role of HME truck driver/technicians. *Home Care Section Bulletin, 3,* 11. American Association for Respiratory Care.

Hamill, T. (1996, May). Council challenges accrediting bodies. *HomeCare, 18*(5), 38, 154.

Joint Commission on Accreditation of Healthcare Organizations. (1994a). *1995 Accreditation manual for home care—Volume I.* Oakbrook Terrace, IL: Joint Commission on Accreditation of Healthcare Organizations.

Joint Commission on Accreditation of Healthcare Organizations. (1994b). *1995 Accreditation manual for home care—Volume II.* Oakbrook Terrace, IL: Joint Commission on Accreditation of Healthcare Organizations.

Joint Commission on Accreditation of Healthcare Organizations. (1996). *1997–98 Comprehensive accreditation manual for home care.* Oakbrook Terrace, IL: Joint Commission on Accreditation of Healthcare Organizations.

Kemper, K., & Sellers, P. (1996, May). Accreditation & licensure: Double standards. *HomeCare, 18*(5), 44, 46.

Parver, C., & Hildebrandt, S. (1996, May). Are three a charm? *HomeCare, 18*(5), 61–62, 64.

Scanlan, C. (Ed.). (1995). *Egan's fundamentals of respiratory care* (6th ed.). St. Louis, MO: Mosby-Year Book, Inc.

Suggested Readings

Cartwright, G. (1995, October). Home care RCPs play important role in patient and family education. *AARCTimes, 19*(10), 34–35, 50.

Eicher, J. (1995, Winter). State regulatory update. *Home Care Section Bulletin, (4),* 5–6. American Association for Respiratory Care.

Lawlor, B. (1996, Spring). The essentials of homecare documentation. *Focus—Journal for Respiratory Care Managers and Educators, 20.*

Stewart, K. (1995, December). Striving for quality. *Advance for Managers of Respiratory Care, 4*(10), 43–44.

CHAPTER TWELVE

REIMBURSEMENT FOR RESPIRATORY HOME CARE

KEY TERMS

capped rental
certificate of medical
necessity (CMN)
durable medical
equipment regional
carrier (DMERC)
home health agency
(HHA)

physician information
sheet (PHYIS)
Six-Point Plan
unique physician
identification number
(UPIN)

written confirmation of a
physician's order (WCPO)
written confirmation of a
verbal order (WCVO)

OBJECTIVES

Upon completing this chapter, the reader will be able to:

- Explain the current mechanism, including coding procedures, for reimbursement of respiratory home-care equipment.
- Present three reasons home-care services rendered by RCPs are not reimbursed by Medicare or other insurances.
- Describe the components of the Six-Point Plan and its impact on home-care equipment reimbursement.
- Define *capped rental* and identify its impact on the home-care industry.
- Define the role of durable medical equipment regional carriers (DMERCs) in the reimbursement of home-care equipment.
- Discuss the importance of the certificate of medical necessity (CMN) with regard to insurance reimbursement.
- Identify the Medicare qualifications for home oxygen therapy.
- Explain managed care's impact on the home-care industry.

INTRODUCTION

As with any organizational function, financial considerations, including a positive cash flow, are essential to continued operation and growth. It is no different with home-care and HME providers. Insurance reimbursement for equipment and services has been and continues to be of major interest and concern to home-care RCPs and those who provide equipment used in the home. Third-party reimbursement for health care has been and continues to be both intricate and controversial, especially in the managed-care environment the health-care industry is presently facing. Annually, billions of dollars continue to be paid by private, state, or federal insurance programs to providers delivering a myriad of medical and health-care services and benefits, including home-care equipment to patients (May, 1991). While Medicare and other insurance carriers recognize and reimburse companies for the rental or purchase of this equipment, they generally do not reimburse RCPs for the home-care services they render. The respiratory care profession has been trying to resolve this issue through the efforts of the AARC in Washington, DC, and on the state level.

Reimbursement for respiratory equipment in the home continues to be the target of increased scrutiny by both Congress and the insurance industry. Changes in reimbursement patterns and rates are occurring and will continue to do so in the foreseeable future. All this is influenced by a number of variables. This chapter explores a number of these reimbursement concerns, namely covered versus noncovered items and services, the cost-effectiveness of respiratory home care, equipment categories, the issue of **capped rental** for home-care equipment, qualifications for reimbursement, Medicare and Medicaid payments, reimbursement by private insurance companies, and the impact of managed care on the home-care industry and respiratory home care in particular.

COVERED HOME-CARE SERVICES

Health insurance carriers, including Medicare and Medicaid, recognize and reimburse providers for the rental or purchase of most home-care equipment and related supplies. This equipment is grouped as:

- durable medical equipment, prosthetics, orthotics, and supplies (DMEPOS), including frequently and substantially serviced items;
- items with capped rentals;
- home oxygen equipment;
- transcutaneous electrical nerve stimulation (TENS) units, glucose monitors, IV pumps, and related supplies;
- parenteral and enteral nutrition (PEN); and
- immunosuppressive drugs.

In terms of provider services, insurance carriers recognize and reimburse nursing, physical therapy, occupational therapy, and speech therapy for home-care visits and services rendered within the home.

REQUIREMENTS FOR COVERAGE

Reimbursement for any item of home-care equipment or service requires a physician's prescription, a qualifying diagnosis and, in certain cases, a **certificate of medical necessity (CMN)** that contains essential patient information and specifies certain qualifying conditions. The CMN and its importance to reimbursement is discussed later in this chapter. The prescription for home-care equipment serves as a CMN provided it contains all necessary information. However, these requirements vary from carrier to carrier, including Medicare. Any errors or omissions when processing an insurance claim can delay processing or result in denial of payment for equipment and supplies used by a home-care patient. The HME providers must be thoroughly familiar with all current procedures and standards for filing insurance claims, including appropriate coding for billed items or services, and should file in a timely fashion.

CODING PROCEDURES

As with diagnostic, therapeutic, and rehabilitative services, billing for any home medical device or appliance must include a correctly coded patient diagnosis in accordance with the fourth edition of the *International Classification of Diseases, 9th Revision, Clinical Modification* or *ICD-9-CM*. As discussed in Chapter 6, this classification system is recommended for use in all clinical settings, including the home. It is required for reporting diseases and diagnoses to the federal government, in particular the U.S. Public Health Service and HCFA.

Currently, patient billing revolves around two systems of approved procedural coding from the AMA and HCFA. In 1992, HCFA proposed a plan to promote cross-coding between the AMA's CPT and the HCPCS. However, there appears to be little need for cross-coding between these two systems. The CPT coding focuses on procedures and services, while HCPCS focuses mostly on equipment and supplies. One area of the CPT coding system that may have a pivotal impact on RCPs' ability to bill for and receive reimbursement for respiratory home care involves the use of the "evaluation and management services" code 99351 for home services—established patient (home visit). A modifier to this code has been suggested to indicate that the services were rendered by an RCP (Molle, 1993a). No action has yet been taken on this recommendation, and equipment continues to be the only reimbursable component involving respiratory care. To receive payment for home-care equipment, only diagnostic coding using the *ICD-9-CM* and equipment coding using the HCPCS system are required by Medicare and other insurance carriers.

Because HCPCS coding, as briefly discussed in Chapter 6, had only minor application to pulmonary-rehabilitation reimbursement, it is more appropriate to elaborate on it here. The HCPCS is a collection of codes representing the procedures, supplies, products, and services provided to Medicare beneficiaries and to individuals enrolled in private health insurance with the purpose of promoting uniform reporting and statistical data collection. Published annually, the *HCFA Common Procedure Coding System* manual outlines these reimbursable services, including patient transportation, DME, oxygen, and related respiratory equipment and supplies. Codes contained in this manual are grouped into three different levels:

Level I   Codes found in the *Physicians' Current Procedural Terminology* manual are copyrighted by the AMA and consist of five position numeric codes describing physician and non-physician services.

Level II   Codes approved and maintained by the Alpha-Numeric Editorial Panel (HCFA, the Health Insurance Association of America, and the Blue Cross and Blue Shield Association). These are five position alpha-numeric codes describing primary items and nonphysician services not covered in Level I. For example, the HCPCS Level II alpha-numeric code for a percussor (electric or pneumatic home model) is E0480. Special administrative coverage instructions usually apply to most respiratory home-care equipment.

Level III Codes developed by Medicare carriers for use at the local level. These are five position alpha-numeric codes in the W, X, Y, or Z series depicting physician and nonphysician services not covered in Level I or Level II.

Other examples of HCPCS Level II codes for respiratory-care equipment include:

A4618   breathing circuits

A4620   variable concentration mask

E0424   stationary compressed gaseous oxygen system, rental; includes contents (per unit), regulator, flowmeter, humidifier, nebulizer, cannula or mask, and tubing (1 unit = 50 cubic feet)

E0450   volume ventilator, stationary or portable

E0460   negative pressure ventilator, portable or stationary

E0500   IPPB machine, all types, with built-in nebulization; manual or automatic valves; internal or external power source

E0575   nebulizer, ultrasonic (Health Care Financing Administration [HCFA], 1995)

The HCPCS coding is used most frequently by hospitals, physician offices, and home-care companies supplying DME, oxygen, and other forms of respiratory-care equipment. Primary coding revisions or updates are published annually in each year's manual, but newsletters may be required to inform providers of any major changes that occur during the course of any given year. Because these codes are subject to change, it is important for practitioners involved in this process to keep current with any revisions, modifications, or deletions by referring to updates or newsletters that publicize proposed or enacted coding changes (Molle, 1993b).

The AARC's ad hoc Committee on Procedural Coding has been working with HCFA regarding proposed coding revisions, especially in the sections of the HCPCS coding system pertaining to Supplies for Oxygen and Related Respiratory Equipment and Durable Medical Equipment (Molle, 1994). Since 1993, this ad hoc committee has also been responding to concerns about cross-coding. It has been reviewing and studying the coding systems in an effort to make recommendations pertaining to:

- codes that require clarification and/or redefinition;
- respiratory-care services, equipment, and supplies needing codes; and

- methods that could be used in revising these systems to accurately reflect patient care services being provided by RCPs.

The AARC remains actively involved with both the AMA and HCFA regarding any proposed changes in procedure coding in an effort to obtain recognition of RCPs and the health-care services they provide (Molle, 1993b).

NONCOVERED HOME CARE SERVICES

While home medical equipment is covered by medical insurance plans, respiratory care is not covered as a specific home health benefit. Of course, respiratory care services are reimbursed fully in the hospital. There is also reimbursement for respiratory care in an SNF and through a **home health agency (HHA),** which is a public agency or private organization engaged primarily in providing skilled nursing care and other therapeutic services, including respiratory care. Examples of HHAs include visiting nurse associations (VNAs), official health agencies, and hospital-based home-care programs. These agencies must be licensed by state regulatory boards and certified under the Medicare Conditions of Participation if Medicare reimbursement is sought for homebound beneficiaries (Dunne, 1994).

Finally, to a very limited degree, there is also reimbursement for respiratory care in the home, but not to the degree that services are covered in the hospital or other facilities. One question that continues to be asked is, "Why aren't respiratory-care services reimbursed in the same manner in all sites like other forms of therapy and nursing care?" The answer to this question involves timing, the evolution of other health-care professions, and the political and clinical environments in which respiratory care has existed. The reasons respiratory home-care services were not recognized or covered by Medicare and other health care-insurers may be summed as:

1. Respiratory care was in its infancy and not well-established in the early 1960s when the Conditions of Participation governing Medicare and Medicaid were drafted. At that time, there were fewer than 5,000 RCPs, fewer than 1,000 respiratory-care departments, and fewer than 20 respiratory-care programs nationwide.
2. In the 1960s, respiratory physiology and pathology were not fully understood nor appreciated. In addition, there was little physician involvement in this area.
3. Legislators were unaware of the potential value of respiratory care.
4. Other health-care professions began to emerge and compete for available health-care dollars. Well-established professions, like nursing and physical therapy, were recognized for the types and levels of care they provided and continued to receive reimbursement for the patient services they rendered.
5. Reimbursement has become a highly charged political issue, demanding a strong presence both in Washington, DC, and on the state level (AARC, 1989). Political attention requires leadership, direction, and money. The respiratory-care profession, through the AARC, its state and federal directors, and its political action committee (AARCPAC), has been striving for recognition, acceptance, and reimbursement. The profession must continue to be "politically savvy" (Giordano, 1987).

HCFA has underscored two major points the federal government will continue to use to keep RCPs from receiving any home-care reimbursement: (1) the estimated cost of expanding Medicare coverage and (2) reliance on nonrespiratory care personnel to provide respiratory home care (Cotton, 1987). These points have continued to cause problems for RCPs receiving reimbursement for home care or pulmonary rehabilitation. While to many health-care providers it appears logical and cost-effective to recognize and cover RCPs for these services, respiratory care is simply not mentioned in the Medicare legislation. Congress would have to pass amendments to change any reimbursement mechanism. For this to occur, Congress would have to be convinced of the cost-effectiveness of respiratory care provided at alternate sites, including the home.

COST-EFFECTIVENESS OF RESPIRATORY HOME CARE

With health-care costs continuing to rise and placing the nation's health-care system in a financial crisis, home care is one of the bright spots. It remains to be seen what long-term impact health-care reform and managed care will have on health-care delivery and health-care costs in general. In the meantime, home health care continues to show only modest increases in annual expenditures. Of the total $850 billion spent for all health-care services in 1991, home care represented only 2.5 percent ($11.1 billion) (Cerne, 1993). The U.S. Department of Commerce identified home health care as the fastest growing segment of the health-care industry, with a market reaching $20 billion by 1996 (Dunne, 1994). Of particular interest is the role respiratory home care is playing in this growth and cost-effective outcome.

A number of studies have been conducted to help demonstrate the role and the cost-effectiveness of respiratory home care. These studies have demonstrated unequivocally that respiratory home care improves patient care and reduces health-care costs. For example, in 1994 Aetna Insurance Company reported a cost-per-month savings from home care compared to traditional hospital care. In particular, there was a $6,589 monthly savings for a ventilator-dependent child (monthly hospital care at $15,742 versus $9,153 for home care), a $15,448 savings for a patient requiring respiratory support (monthly hospital care at $24,715 versus $9,267 for home care), and a savings of $24,500 for care of respiratory distress with oxygen dependency (monthly hospital care at $36,000 versus $11,500 for home care). Other findings show that ventilator-dependent individuals can be cared for at home effectively at a savings of more than $150,000 per patient (Saposnick, 1995).

APCO Associates, working on behalf of the Home Care Coalition, has been involved in research to inventory data on the cost-effectiveness of home care. Specific findings from this research include:

- A 1994 Government Accounting Office (GAO) study entitled, "Medicaid Long-Term Care, Successful State Efforts to Expand Home Services While Limiting Costs," found that Oregon, Washington, and Wisconsin were able to provide more services to more people with the same dollars by shifting patient care to the home.
- Of the caregivers to the elderly 49 percent were elderly (over 65). Reimbursement

from the federal government must take a lead in the use of trained and cost-effective home-care service providers to ease the burden on elderly populations.

- Significant savings continue to be realized with increased home care for low birth-weight infants. (APCO Associates, 1995).

A 1991 report entitled, "Economic Analysis of Home Medical Equipment Services," which was prepared for the home-care industry, evaluated the cost-effectiveness of home care for three patient populations: patients with hip fractures, patients with ALS, and patients with COPD. In particular, this report cited that COPD patients who increasingly relied on home care enjoyed an annual savings of $520. Based on the current prevalence of COPD, these savings total nearly $48.5 million per year (APCO Associates, 1995).

The National Association for Home Care's "Basic Statistics About Home Care, 1994" reported that ventilator-dependent adults cared for at home enjoyed a $14,520 per month savings ($21,570 per month hospital costs versus $7,050 per month home-care costs). The same report stated that oxygen-dependent children cared for at home netted an average $6,810 savings per month ($12,090 per month per patient hospital costs versus only $5,250 per month home-care costs). A study reported in *Chest* in 1991 found that COPD patients cared for at home experienced a $328 per month savings based on costs for hospitalizations, emergency-room visits, and home care. Also in 1991, the *American Journal of Diseases of Children* reported that potential savings for all fifty technology-dependent children in the program (those on oxygen or ventilatory support) could approximate $4 million per year (AARC, 1996a; APCO Associates, 1995).

Other studies continue to demonstrate the cost-effectiveness of respiratory home care. A 1990 Gallup survey found that over 11,500 ventilator-dependent patients were being cared for in U.S. hospitals at a cost of over $9 million per day. The survey also reported that it took an average 35 days to place a ventilator-dependent patient in an alternate care site like the home or an SNF. This delay results in over $27,000 in unnecessary hospital costs per patient. It may be concluded that outdated reimbursement policies that limit a patient's access to respiratory services at alternate sites, including the home, contribute to these discharge delays and resulting excess costs (Dunne, 1994). It is hoped that both HCFA and Congress will realize that savings and effective patient care will result from recognizing and reimbursing RCPs who provide home-care services.

EQUIPMENT RENTAL AND PURCHASE

Home-care equipment rental has been criticized greatly simply based on economics. For example, a simple commode or quad cane can be purchased for under $100, but HME providers were renting these items at a higher cost. Similarly, Medicare was paying monthly rental fees on these items for years for many patients. Something had to be done to reduce this waste.

This "something" was the Six-Point Plan that was part of the Omnibus Budget Reconciliatory Act of 1987 and was signed into law by President Ronald Reagan on December 22, 1987. The measure, which took effect on January 1, 1989, solved some of the Medicare reimbursement problems that had been plaguing the home-care industry (Novoselski, 1989). The Six-Point Plan sought to simplify and improve reimbursement for home-care equipment and devices covered under Medicare—Part B; establish a stable reimbursement environment so the industry could focus on quality, affordable patient care; and devise a method for calculating reimbursement fee schedules (Segedy, 1989). The Six-Point Plan specifically addressed a number of home-care equipment items that were grouped into the following six classes:

1. Inexpensive or other routinely purchased DME. The plan would pay for rentals or lump-sum purchases. However, the total payment amount could not exceed the actual charge or the fee for purchase as computed by the published instructions.
2. Items requiring frequent and substantial servicing. This type of equipment was paid for on a monthly rental basis until medical necessity ended.
3. Certain customized items. Because of the unique nature of these items, they cannot be grouped for profiling purposes. Payment is made on a lump-sum purchase basis.
4. Other prosthetic and orthotic devices. Prosthetic and orthotic devices, other than noted exceptions, are paid for on a lump-sum purchase basis.
5. Capped rental items. Payment for these items is made on a rental or purchase basis. For rental items, payment is made on a monthly rental basis not to exceed a 15-month period of continuous use. This point would eventually impact monthly rentals of compressor/nebulizer devices.
6. Oxygen and oxygen equipment. Monthly payments are made to each beneficiary receiving home oxygen. However, when a beneficiary has purchased an item of oxygen equipment, monthly installments are paid equivalent to the fee schedule amounts or until the medical necessity ends or the fee schedule amount for purchase of the equipment has been reached. (HCFA, 1989).

These six points immediately impacted the reimbursement for oxygen and other types of respiratory home-care equipment.

Most home-care equipment continues to be rented monthly. However, in an effort to reduce health-care costs, there is a growing trend among insurance carriers to purchase home-care equipment for patients who plan to use it indefinitely. This is the policy of many private insurers who have elected to reimburse patients for outright purchases of equipment, including compressor/nebulizers, CPAP units, and blood glucose monitors. As mentioned previously, HCFA, through its Six-Point Plan, authorized Medicare carriers to implement a capped rental basis on certain types of home-care equipment (Thomas-Payne, 1994a). The following case study illustrates the capped rental process.

CASE STUDY

Capped Rental on Home-Care Equipment

J.S. is a Medicare beneficiary with chronic bronchial asthma. Because of her inability to use an MDI properly, her physician prescribed a nebulizer with compressor for home use. A local home-care company delivered the equipment and instructed J.S. on its proper use and maintenance. This company billed the regional Medicare carrier for this equipment rental.

For the first 3 months of rental, the company received 100 percent of an established rental fee at the customary 80 percent reimbursement. J.S. was responsible for the 20 percent copayment. After 3 months, because of a built-in payment reduction of 25 percent, the supplier received 75 percent of this established fee reimbursed at the 80 percent rate. After 10 months of continuous use and rental, the company gave J.S. a purchase option and notified the Medicare carrier of its offer. J.S. decided to continue renting the compressor until the 15-month cap was reached. As with other capped rentals, the home-care company will be able to bill Medicare for a maintenance and service fee on this compressor every 6 months.

1. What is the major purpose of capped rental equipment?
2. Does the patient receive any benefit from having equipment on a capped-rental basis?
3. What impact, if any, does capped rental have on home-care equipment suppliers?

Legislation that took effect on January 1, 1994, moved several home-care equipment items from the "frequent and substantially serviced" category to the "capped rental" category. With regard to respiratory home-care equipment, Medicare classified the following items with (HCPCS codes) under the capped-rental category:

E0670	Nebulizer with compressor
E0585	Nebulizer with compressor and heater
E0452	Intermittent assist device (bilevel system)
E0601	CPAP device
K0193	CPAP device with humidifier
K0194	Intermittent assist device with CPAP with humidifier
E1375	Nebulizer, portable (classified as a routinely purchased item)

Capped rental was also retroactive, which meant that any rental payment made before the implementation date of January 1, 1994, counted toward the payment cap if the item was moved into an equipment category having one (Thomas-Payne, 1994a).

MEDICARE REIMBURSEMENT

The Six-Point Plan and the capped rental policy are some of the recent changes in the way Medicare reimburses providers for home-care equipment. However, the creation of Medicare itself was one of the most significant changes affecting health-care coverage in the United States. Federal legislation was written and introduced in 1965 to create the Medicare and Medicaid programs under the Social Security Act. Medicare was to operate on the federal level, while Medicaid was designed to function statewide with federal assistance. This federal legislation also created HCFA under the auspices of the U.S. Department of Health and Human Services (then, the Department of Health, Education and Welfare) to administer the Medicare and Medicaid programs and other federal insurance programs.

Medicare is the federal insurance program for the elderly and the disabled. Coverage consists of Part A and Part B. Part A provides reimbursement for care in hospitals and

SNFs, while Part B provides health-care services through home-care agencies and HME providers. These services include home-care equipment and supplies, nursing care, and physical, occupational, and speech therapy. Because respiratory care is not mentioned in the Social Security Act, there is no provision for coverage of respiratory care services under Medicare. Respiratory-care equipment, included as part of the DME category, is covered. Payment to RCPs for any services provided is made routinely by the home-care companies from the equipment rental fees these HME providers receive from Medicare and other insurance carriers. Naturally, any reductions in reimbursement for home-care equipment will adversely affect a home-care company's ability to employ RCPs.

In addition to DME rentals, eligible patients may also qualify for home health benefits under Medicare. These benefits must be obtained through a home health agency or others through an arrangement with an HHA, and the beneficiary must also:

- be confined to home; or
- be under the care of a physician; or
- need intermittent skilled nursing services; or
- need physical, occupational, or speech therapy.

In addition, a plan of care must be established by a physician and reviewed periodically by that physician (HCFA, 1990a).

DURABLE MEDICAL EQUIPMENT REGIONAL CARRIERS

Handling medical and health-care claims for approximately 39 million beneficiaries and reimbursing providers for home-care equipment and services has been a difficult and complicated process for Medicare. Medicare had been using a system of thirty-four designated local carriers throughout the United States to manage the growing number of claims it was receiving. To streamline the large number of local carriers, HCFA proposed in 1991 to establish a system of four **durable medical equipment regional carriers (DMERCs)** to handle claims for medical care, health-care services, and home-care equipment. The four carriers would pay claims based on a beneficiary's residence instead of the point of sale. The proposal also required a new provider number application for home-care businesses (Oakland, 1991). In 1992, HCFA released its transition plan for consolidating to four regional carriers (Oakland, 1992). These four DMERCs have been designated A, B, C, and D and represent four regions or areas within the United States. Figure 12–1 and Table 12–1 identify the states, commonwealths, and U.S. possessions that comprise the four regions (Oakland, 1993).

Official DMERC transition began on October 1, 1993, with early boarders in any of the four regions. This was followed in November 1993 by states in which a DMERC was based. State-by-state transfer began on December 1, 1993 (Oakland, 1993). Contained in the new DMERC medical policies were descriptions of the conditions for Medicare coverage, new billing codes, revised product descriptions, new forms, bundling edits, and utilization guidelines. Grandfathering was also a part of this DMERC transition. Grandfathering was simply a process to extend coverage to any patient who was covered by a

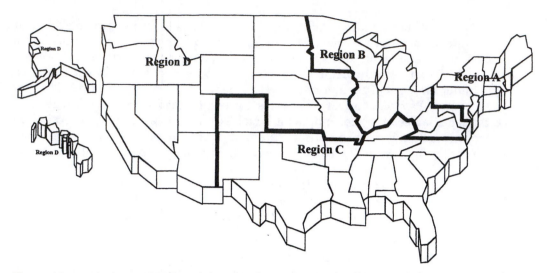

Figure 12–1 *The four DMERCs and the states they cover. The District of Columbia is in Region B, while Puerto Rico and the U.S. Virgin Islands are in Region C. American Samoa, Guam, and the Marianna Islands are in Region D. (Based on data from HomeCare News, HomeCare, November 1993.)*

local carrier before the changeover to DMERCs. Its purpose was to protect both supplier and beneficiary when the DMERC's coverage criteria were more restrictive than the previous carrier's rules. Eligibility for grandfathering required a CMN to have been filed with the previous local carrier for that item of coverage.

However, rules differed according to the item supplied. Specifically, only the following items were grandfathered:

- Capped rental items—until the patient no longer needed the item or the patient's needs changed or a different item was prescribed. Providers were required to bill these items under the code the previous carrier used.
- Frequently and substantially serviced items—until the patient no longer needed the equipment or changed equipment. Coverage included related supplies or medications.
- Oxygen—until the existing CMN expired, at which time the patient had to be recertified under the new DMERC policies.
- Supplies for TENS units, glucose monitors, and IV pumps—only as long as the equipment with which the supplies were used was covered by a previous local carrier. Some equipment, like IV pumps, were capped rental items and subjected to related policies. Other equipment was rented or purchased.
- Parenteral and enteral nutrition—services were covered until the existing CMN expired or May 1, 1994, whichever came first.
- Immunosuppressive drugs—coverage continued until the benefit period, 1 year from the date of discharge following a transplant was exhausted.

TABLE 12–1 The four DMERCs and their corresponding states, commonwealths, and possessions

DMERC	States, Commonwealths, and U.S. Possessions
Region A	Connecticut, Rhode Island, Maine, New Hampshire, Vermont, Delaware, New Jersey, Pennsylvania, Massachusetts, and New York
Region B	Maryland, District of Columbia, Virginia, West Virginia, Indiana, Ohio, Illinois, Michigan, Wisconsin, and Minnesota
Region C	North Carolina, South Carolina, Georgia, Florida, Kentucky, Tennessee, Alabama, Mississippi, Louisiana, Arkansas, Texas, Oklahoma, Colorado, New Mexico, the U.S. Virgin Islands, and Puerto Rico
Region D	Kansas, Missouri, Iowa, North Dakota, South Dakota, Nebraska, Utah, Idaho, Montana, Wyoming, Washington, Oregon, California, Nevada, Arizona, Alaska, Hawaii, American Samoa, Guam, and the Marianna Islands

(Based on data from HomeCare News, *HomeCare*, November 1993.)

This grandfathering applied only to the basic coverage of an item. It was important to HME providers who were concerned about maintaining a positive cash flow during the DMERC transition process and to patients who were concerned about their home care and related coverage (Thomas-Payne, 1993).

CERTIFICATE OF MEDICAL NECESSITY

The role of the CMN in home-care equipment reimbursement has been discussed. In general, CMNs contain information about the patient, the prescribing physician, and the description of service. They existed long before the conversion to DMERCs, but this conversion has presented HME providers with new challenges in medical documentation. Because the content of CMNs appears to change constantly, it has been difficult in some cases to develop written versions. However, several DMERC CMNs are currently used. They cover equipment like:

- hospital beds;
- alternating pressure pads and air-fluidized beds;
- wheelchairs;
- CPAP systems;
- suction units;
- prosthetics, orthotics, and lymphedema pumps;
- surgical dressings and urological supplies;
- TENS units;
- seat-lift mechanisms;
- motorized scooters;
- immunosuppressive drugs;

- infusion pumps and glucose monitors; and
- PEN and home oxygen systems.

Home oxygen requires the new DMERC 484.2 form, which must be completed by the prescribing physician or the physician staff member (Thomas-Payne, 1994b). Home-care suppliers who complete restricted CMNs risk civil penalties of $1,000 for each violation. This includes anyone who has a financial arrangement with a home-care provider (Thomas-Payne, 1994c).

Although CMNs vary, they require the following basic information:

- type and date of certification (initial, revised, or recertified);
- patient information (name, address, telephone number, and health insurance claim number [HICN]);
- supplier information (name of company, address, telephone number and Medicare supplier number provided by the National Supplier Clearinghouse [NSC]);
- place of service and, if applicable, facility name and address;
- all applicable HCPCS codes;
- physician name, address, telephone number, and **unique physician identification number (UPIN)**;
- diagnosis codes according to the *ICD-9-CM*;
- estimated length of service;
- any clinical information to determine medical necessity;
- narrative description of equipment and cost; and
- physician attestation, signature, and date (signature and date stamps are not acceptable).

Figure 12–2 is the new CMN for home oxygen therapy and Figure 12-3 provides instructions for completing this CMN.

Because only physicians and physician office staff are legally permitted to complete CMNs for home oxygen, HME providers usually send CMNs to physicians accompanied by informational cover letters. These cover letters attempt to explain how a CMN should be completed and signed. Now that DMERCs are specifying which items require a CMN and which CMNs must be completed by the physician or physician staff, care must be taken when drafting a cover letter. A supplier's cover letter can include the physician's verbal order, a description of the patient's need, a complete description of the equipment ordered, and the charge submitted for any prescribed item. More important, the following restrictions apply to supplier-generated cover letters:

- the format cannot look like a DMERC CMN;
- the substance of the physician's order cannot be changed;
- templates and sample forms cannot be used, and physicians cannot be counseled regarding completing the form or the verbiage to use to achieve coverage; and
- instructions cannot indicate by box number exactly what answer or information should be put on the CMN (Thomas-Payne, 1994c).

To eliminate the need for, or at least supplement, these supplier-generated cover letters, HME providers have devised a type of form known as a **written confirmation of a verbal order (WCVO).** In 1995, DMERCs released drafts of a **written confirmation of a**

U.S. DEPARTMENT OF HEALTH & HUMAN SERVICES
HEALTH CARE FINANCING ADMINISTRATION

FORM APPROVED
OMB NO. 0938-0534

CERTIFICATE OF MEDICAL NECESSITY

DMERC 484.2

OXYGEN

SECTION A   Certification Type/Date: INITIAL ___/___/___   REVISED ___/___/___   RECERTIFICATION ___/___/___

PATIENT NAME, ADDRESS, TELEPHONE and HIC NUMBER	SUPPLIER NAME, ADDRESS, TELEPHONE and NSC NUMBER
(___)___-____ HICN _____	(___)___-____ NSC # _____

PLACE OF SERVICE _____	HCPCS CODE	PT DOB ___/___/___ ; Sex ___ (M/F) ; HT.____(in.) ; WT.____(lbs.)
NAME and ADDRESS of FACILITY if applicable (See Reverse)	———— ———— ———— ————	PHYSICIAN NAME, ADDRESS, TELEPHONE and UPIN NUMBER (___)___-____ UPIN # _____

SECTION B   Information In This Section May Not Be Completed by the Supplier of the Items/Supplies.

EST. LENGTH OF NEED (# OF MONTHS): _____ 1-99 (99=LIFETIME) | DIAGNOSIS CODES (ICD-9): _____ _____ _____ _____

ANSWERS	ANSWER QUESTIONS 1-10. (Circle **Y** for Yes, **N** for No, or **D** for Does Not Apply, unless otherwise noted.)
a) _____ mm Hg b) _____ % c) ___/___/___	1. Enter the result of most recent test taken <u>on or before</u> the certification date listed in Section A. Enter (a) arterial blood gas PO$_2$ and/or (b) oxygen saturation test. Enter date of test (c).
Y N	2. Was the test in Question 1 performed EITHER with the patient in a chronic stable state as an outpatient OR within <u>two</u> days prior to discharge from an inpatient facility to home?
1 2 3	3. Circle the one number for the condition of the test in Question 1: (1) At Rest; (2) During Exercise; (3) During Sleep
XXXXXXXXXXXXXXX XXXXXXXXXXXXXXX XXXXXXXXXXXXXXX	4. Physician/provider performing test in Question 1 (and, if applicable, Question 7). Print/type name and address below: NAME: ADDRESS:
Y N D	5. If you are ordering portable oxygen, is the patient mobile within the home? If you are <u>not</u> ordering portable oxygen, circle D.
_____ LPM	6. Enter the highest oxygen flow rate ordered for this patient in liters per minute. If less than 1 LPM, enter a "X".
a) _____ mm Hg b) _____ % c) ___/___/___	7. If greater than 4 LPM is prescribed, enter results of most recent test <u>taken on 4 LPM</u>. This may be an (a) arterial blood gas PO$_2$ and/or (b) oxygen saturation test with patient in a chronic stable state. Enter date of test (c).
	IF PO$_2$ = 56–59 OR OXYGEN SATURATION = 89%, AT LEAST ONE OF THE FOLLOWING CRITERIA MUST BE MET.
Y N D	8. Does the patient have dependent edema due to congestive heart failure?
Y N D	9. Does the patient have cor pulmonale or pulmonary hypertension documented by P pulmonale on an EKG or by an echocardiogram, gated blood pool scan or direct pulmonary artery pressure measurement?
Y N D	10. Does the patient have a hematocrit greater than 56%?

NAME OF PERSON ANSWERING SECTION B QUESTIONS, IF OTHER THAN PHYSICIAN (Please Print):
NAME: _____   TITLE: _____   EMPLOYER: _____

SECTION C   Narrative Description of Equipment and Cost

(1) <u>Narrative</u> description of all items, accessories and options ordered; (2) Supplier's charge and (3) Medicare Fee Schedule Allowance for <u>each</u> item, accessory and option. *(See instructions on back.)*

SECTION D   Physician Attestation and Signature/Date

I certify that I am the treating physician identified in Section A of this form. I have received Sections A, B and C of the Certificate of Medical Necessity (including charges for items ordered). Any statement on my letterhead attached hereto, has been reviewed and signed by me. I certify that the medical necessity information in Section B is true, accurate and complete, to the best of my knowledge, and I understand that any falsification, omission, or concealment of material fact in that section may subject me to civil or criminal liability.

PHYSICIAN'S SIGNATURE _____   DATE ___/___/___   (SIGNATURE AND DATE STAMPS ARE NOT ACCEPTABLE)

FORM HCFA 484 (5/97)

Figure 12–2   *The new oxygen certificate of medical necessity (CMN). U.S. Department of Health and Human Services, Health Care Financing Administration, May 1997.*

SECTION A:	**(May be completed by the supplier)**
CERTIFICATION TYPE/DATE:	If this is an initial certification for this patient, indicate this by placing date (MM/DD/YY) needed initially in the space marked "INITIAL." If this is a revised certification (to be completed when the physician changes the order, based on the patient's changing clinical needs), indicate the initial date needed in the space marked "INITIAL," and also indicate the recertification date in the space marked "REVISED." If this is a recertification, indicate the initial date needed in the space marked "INITIAL," and also indicate the recertification date in the space marked "RECERTIFICATION." Whether submitting a REVISED or a RECERTIFIED CMN, be sure to always furnish the INITIAL date as well as the REVISED or RECERTIFICATION date.
PATIENT INFORMATION:	Indicate the patient's name, permanent legal address, telephone number and his/her health insurance claim number (HICN) as it appears on his/her Medicare card and on the claim form.
SUPPLIER INFORMATION:	Indicate the name of your company (supplier name), address and telephone number along with the Medicare Supplier Number assigned to you by the National Supplier Clearinghouse (NSC).
PLACE OF SERVICE:	Indicate the place in which the item is being used, i.e., patient's home is 12, skilled nursing facility (SNF) is 31, End Stage Renal Disease (ESRD) facility is 65, etc. Refer to the DMERC supplier manual for a complete list.
FACILITY NAME:	If the place of service is a facility, indicate the name and complete address of the facility.
HCPCS CODES:	List all HCPCS procedure codes for items ordered that require a CMN. Procedure codes that do not require certification should not be listed on the CMN.
PATIENT DOB, HEIGHT, WEIGHT AND SEX:	Indicate patient's date of birth (MM/DD/YY) and sex (male or female); height in inches and weight in pounds, if requested.
PHYSICIAN NAME, ADDRESS:	Indicate the physician's name and complete mailing address.
UPIN:	Accurately indicate the ordering physician's Unique Physician Identification Number (UPIN).
PHYSICIAN'S TELEPHONE NO:	Indicate the telephone number where the physician can be contacted (preferably where records would be accessible pertaining to this patient) if more information is needed.
SECTION B:	**(May not be completed by the supplier. While this section may be completed by a non-physician clinician, or a physician employee, it must be reviewed, and the CMN signed (in Section D) by the ordering physician.)**
EST. LENGTH OF NEED:	Indicate the estimated length of need (the length of time the physician expects the patient to require use of the ordered item) by filling in the appropriate number of months. If the physician expects that the patient will require the item for the duration of his/her life, then enter 99.
DIAGNOSIS CODES:	In the first space, list the ICD9 code that represents the primary reason for ordering this item. List any additional ICD9 codes that would further describe the medical need for the item (up to 3 codes).
QUESTION SECTION:	This section is used to gather clinical information to determine medical necessity. Answer each question which applies to the items ordered, circling "Y" for yes, "N" for no, "D" for does not apply, a number if this is offered as an answer option, or fill in the blank if other information is requested.
NAME OF PERSON ANSWERING SECTION B QUESTIONS:	If a clinical professional other than the ordering physician (e.g., home health nurse, physical therapist, dietician) or a physician employee answers the questions of Section B, he/she must print his/her name, give his/her professional title and the name of his/her employer where indicated. If the physician is answering the questions, this space may be left blank.
SECTION C:	**(To be completed by the supplier)**
NARRATIVE DESCRIPTION OF EQUIPMENT & COST:	Supplier gives (1) a narrative description of the item(s) ordered, as well as all options, accessories, supplies and drugs; (2) the supplier's charge for each item, option, accessory, supply and drug; and (3) the Medicare fee schedule allowance for each item/option/accessory/supply/drug, if applicable.
SECTION D:	**(To be completed by the physician)**
PHYSICIAN ATTESTATION:	The physician's signature certifies (1) the CMN which he/she is reviewing includes Sections A, B, C and D; (2) the answers in Section B are correct; and (3) the self-identifying information in Section A is correct.
PHYSICIAN SIGNATURE AND DATE:	After completion and/or review by the physician of Sections A, B and C, the physician must sign and date the CMN in Section D, verifying the Attestation appearing in this Section. The physician's signature also certifies the items ordered are medically necessary for this patient. Signature and date stamps are not acceptable.

According to the Paperwork Reduction Act of 1995, no persons are required to respond to a collection of information unless it displays a valid OMB control number. The valid OMB control number for this information collection is 0938-0534. The time required to complete this information collection is estimated to average 15 minutes per response, including the time to review instructions, search existing resources, gather the data needed, and complete and review the information collection. If you have any comments concerning the accuracy of the time estimate or suggestions for improving this form, please write to: HCFA, P.O. Box 26684, Baltimore, Maryland 21207 and to the Office of Information and Regulatory Affairs, Office of Management and Budget, Washington, D.C. 20503.

Figure 12–3 *Instructions for completing the new oxygen certificate of medical necessity (CMN). U.S. Department of Health and Human Services, Health Care Financing Administration, May 1997.*

physician's order (WCPO) form and a **physician information sheet (PHYIS)** form to be used by suppliers in lieu of a cover letter. These documents are acceptable provided they contain all relevant information and avoid the problems associated with cover letters. Presently, either cover letter, WCVO, or WCPO may be used when submitting a CMN for physician completion (Thomas-Payne, 1995). While most CMNs are mailed directly to the physician, some suppliers prefer to hand carry their forms to the physician's office so that if any problems or questions arise, they can be addressed immediately. Any physician-office staff person is permitted to complete a CMN for a physician's review and signature, which helps to make the process less cumbersome and time consuming (Morselander & Thomas-Payne, 1992).

REIMBURSEMENT FOR HOME OXYGEN THERAPY

While a variety of respiratory-care equipment is eligible for reimbursement by Medicare and other health-care insurance, oxygen is the most widely used and the one subject to most scrutiny. From 1985 to 1994, Congress or HCFA have reduced payments for home oxygen therapy thirteen times, including freezes in the consumer price index (CPI). In addition, the HCFA has made five other program changes that reduced payment (AARC, 1996c). A number of proposals to cut oxygen reimbursement loom on the horizon (Kim, 1996; Pitts, 1996a). However, the Home Oxygen Services Coalition (HOSC) has been working closely with Congress to limit pending cuts in the Medicare home oxygen benefit to 10 percent, and combine it with a 7-year freeze in the CPI. Some members of Congress appear to agree, but additional Congressional support is needed (Clark, 1996). Until some type of action is taken, with the present financial status of the Medicare program some reduction in the reimbursement for home oxygen was inevitable. On January 1, 1998, a 25% cut in the home oxygen reimbursement rate was implemented along with a 5-year freeze in the CPI. Another 5% cut in the oxygen reimbursement rate took effect on January 1, 1999.

On another front, to ensure that any pending cuts in HME reimbursement are appropriate, HCFA proposed a competitive bidding project that would involve bidding on five product categories, including home oxygen systems. Region C DMERC was selected as the site for this project. Product and service standards were recommended by the National Technical Expert Panel (NTEP) with the suggestion that any oxygen bidders have a strong RCP presence or access to an RCP. While accepting most of the product and service standards for home oxygen, the Region C DMERC carrier did not accept the NTEP recommendation that oxygen providers employ or have access to a licensed RCP. In 1996, the HCFA decided to put the entire competitive bidding project on hold until 1997 (Saposnick, 1996).

Any drastic cuts in the home oxygen benefit will have a devastating impact on HME suppliers and respiratory home care. Measures to maintain supplier profitability, in the event of reimbursement cuts, include reducing operating overhead, diminishing roles for RCPs, reducing preventive maintenance, changing delivery schedules, lessening patient interaction, changing equipment-purchase patterns, and using oxygen transfilling systems (Pitts, 1996b). Transfilling oxygen cylinders is one cost-saving method providers are pursuing in the face of potential reductions in the Medicare home oxygen benefit and the lower payments offered by MCOs. Transfilling equipment can be expensive and requires compliance with local building and fire codes and the repackaging codes of the Food and Drug Administration (FDA). However, any decision to use transfilling systems should be based on safety and business concerns and not simply possible reimbursement cuts (Pitts, 1996c).

Currently, Medicare and other health-care insurers recognize home oxygen in the forms of compressed gas cylinders (stationary and portable), LOX systems, and oxygen concentrators. In 1989, under the OBRA 1987 legislation, all charges for home oxygen therapy were "bundled," reduced by 5 percent, and then divided by the number of beneficiaries in an effort to determine an average monthly payment for all oxygen modalities. Under this legislation, reimbursement was adjusted for those patients receiving liter flows greater than 4 lpm and reducing reimbursement by 50 percent for patients using home oxygen at flowrates less than 1 lpm.

Also in 1989, HCFA eliminated the "prn" provision for home oxygen and tightened its coverage criteria for oxygen by requiring testing for all Medicare oxygen beneficiaries. This was followed with the implementation of Form HCFA-484 in 1990, the Attending Physician's Certificate of Medical Necessity for Home Oxygen Therapy.

To qualify for the home oxygen benefit under Medicare, patients must satisfy one of the following diagnosis requirements:

- severe primary lung disease, including COPD, cystic fibrosis, bronchiectasis, diffuse interstitial lung disease, or pulmonary neoplasm (primary or metastatic);
- hypoxia-related conditions or symptoms that may improve with oxygen therapy, including recurring congestive heart failure (CHF), pulmonary hypertension, or erythrocythemia (hematocrit is 57 percent or higher); or
- conditions subject to medical review but are not always covered, including orthopnea, severe arrythmia, morning headache, cardiomyopathy, impaired cognitive process, or nocturnal restlessness.

Patient conditions that are not covered include shortness of breath without hypoxia, angina pectoris without hypoxia, severe peripheral vascular disease resulting in oxygen desaturation in one or more extremities, and terminal disease that does not affect the lungs. Specific patient testing involves ABG analysis or measurement of oxygen saturation (SpO_2) via pulse oximetry no more than 30 days before oxygen therapy is initiated (Pennsylvania Blue Shield, 1992). Current qualifications for home oxygen therapy are summarized in Figure 12–4.

Portable or ambulatory oxygen is also a reimbursable item provided the physician specifies on the CMN the type of activity or exercise to be performed and the amount and frequency of ambulation or exercise. The patient must regularly pursue the activity in the home, and the activity cannot be met by a stationary system. An example of an exercise prescription for portable oxygen follows.

Patient to ambulate with oxygen at 2 lpm for 15 minutes, three times a day. Patients who qualify are eligible to receive portable oxygen cylinders. Medicare will reimburse home-care providers monthly for this portable oxygen based on a set monthly fee (HCFA, 1990b).

HOW DO PATIENTS QUALIFY FOR HOME OXYGEN UNDER MEDICARE?

PATIENTS MUST HAVE AN ACCEPTABLE DIAGNOSIS:

Severe lung disease, including chronic obstructive pulmonary disease, diffuse interstitial lung disease, cystic fibrosis, bronchiectasis and widespread pulmonary neoplasm

OR

Hypoxia-related symptoms or findings that have an expected improvement with oxygen therapy, including pulmonary hypertension, recurring congestive heart failure, chronic cor pulmonale, erythrocytosis, impairment of the cognitive process, nocturnal restlessness and morning headaches

PATIENTS DO NOT QUALIFY WITH ANY OF THE FOLLOWING:

Angina pectoris in the absence of hypoxemia, severe peripheral vascular disease or terminal illnesses without lung involvement

ACCEPTABLE BLOOD GAS OR OXYGEN SATURATION VALUES INCLUDE:

Arterial PO_2 at or below 55 mmHg or an oxygen saturation at or below 88%

PROVISIONAL COVERAGE IS OFFERED IF TEST RESULTS DEMONSTRATE:

Arterial PO_2 between 56 mmHg and 59 mmHg or an oxygen saturation at 89% with a secondary diagnosis including any of the following conditions:

- dependent edema, suggesting congestive heart failure (CHF)
- cor pulmonale or
- erythrocythemia with a hematocrit 57% or higher

However, another blood gas analysis or oxygen saturation must be performed between 60 and 90 days after the initiation of oxygen therapy

PATIENTS DO NOT QUALIFY WITH THE FOLLOWING TEST RESULTS:

Arterial PO_2 60 mmHg or higher or an oxygen saturation 90% or higher

Figure 12–4 *Medicare guidelines for home oxygen therapy. (Based on data from the U.S. Department of Health and Human Services, Health Care Financing Administration, May 1990.)*

REIMBURSEMENT FOR OTHER RESPIRATORY HOME-CARE EQUIPMENT

Medicare requirements for other forms of respiratory home-care equipment are less strict. While Medicare reimburses providers for most forms of respiratory equipment, some items are now covered by capped rental. Other health-insurance carriers also rent home-care equipment on a monthly basis and purchase the equipment if extended use is anticipated. Items covered under the Medicare capped rental policy include nebulizers with compressors, suction units, nasal CPAP devices, and bilevel pressure systems. Portable nebulizers are categorized as a routinely purchased item. Chest percussors, IPPB devices, and mechanical ventilators, on the other hand, are classified as items that require frequent and substantial servicing and are therefore rented indefinitely. Home mechanical ventilation (invasive and noninvasive) is a critical area of involvement for RCPs. The role of an RCP with ventilator-dependent patients at home is not only cost-effective, but it greatly enhances the quality and level of patient care (Briskorn, 1994). Most RCPs are reimbursed for these home-care services by the HME supplier through equipment rentals.

Of particular interest are nebulizers with compressors. Commonly referred to as compressor/nebulizers or pump/nebulizers, these devices have recently experienced substantial changes in reimbursement. Growing pressure to control health-care costs, new technology, and improved service in alternate care sites has led many health-care industry analysts to depict the $1.9 billion respiratory home-care market as very promising. Despite trends indicating a 6 to 12 percent increase in the demand for respiratory products resulting from an increased elderly population, the $115 million compressor/nebulizer market in the United States appears to be in transition.

Spearheading this transition was the move of compressor-driven nebulizers from the frequently and substantially serviced category to one that includes capped rental items. This has resulted in a significant drop in the reimbursement paid to HME providers (Gruenwedel, 1996). In addition, the DMERCs originally proposed MDIs over compressor/nebulizers and required all patients to go through a trial period with an MDI before considering the possibility of a nebulizer with compressor. However, comments from the AARC, physicians, and equipment manufacturers led to new language. The revised policy in draft form states that nebulizers with compressors may be used instead of MDIs in the following cases:

1. A pulmonologist has advised the use of a nebulizer with compressor to avoid hospitalization; or
2. A treating physician has decided (based on pulmonary function testing and a patient's condition) that it is medically imperative to forego an MDI trial and immediately resort to a compressor/nebulizer (AARC, 1995).

Because of the reimbursement cuts and price restructuring, the value of nebulizers with compressors has changed drastically. As a result, fewer HME providers are supplying this type of equipment to Medicare patients. Some are referring patients to local pharmacies that provide compressor/nebulizers on a rental or purchase basis. Other suppliers are still providing this item hoping that increased rental volume will help to offset reductions in payment. Manufacturers of compressor-driven nebulizers, on the other hand, are either exiting the market or striving to reduce their costs in an effort to compete. The result is a growing number of patients who are no longer being instructed in the proper use and maintenance of this equipment. Consequently, the quality of service and patient care in this area are being affected (Gruenwedel, 1996).

MEDICAID REIMBURSEMENT

Medicaid was part of the 1965 legislation that also established the Medicare program as part of the Social Security Act. Medicaid, with federal assistance, is administered on the state level to provide medical and health-care services and benefits to the economically disadvantaged. Depending on the extent to which a state covers hospital stays, respiratory-care services are covered. However, coverage for respiratory care provided outside the hospital is a different issue.

There are considerable differences in how state Medicaid programs recognize and cover respiratory-care services. Medicaid in some states provides a limited benefit for RCP services, while other Medicaid programs consider it a part of HME or a nursing-home benefit. In the mid-1980s, Congress passed legislation permitting state Medicaid programs to exercise the option of covering respiratory-care services for chronic ventilator patients at home. Currently, fourteen states have exercised this option to provide this level of coverage. Texas, in particular, has formally amended its Medicaid law and incorporated respiratory care into state statute. California has also amended its Medicaid program (MediCal) to extend coverage for respiratory-care services to all qualified Medicaid recipients, not just those who are ventilator dependent. Nationwide, under Medicaid's early and periodic screening, diagnostic and treatment benefit (EPSDT), individuals under 21, may be eligible to receive respiratory-care services covered by the "other necessary health care" provision (AARC, 1996b).

PRIVATE INSURANCE CARRIERS

Private insurers tend to follow Medicare's lead by not recognizing respiratory care as a covered benefit. However, private carriers reimburse providers for respiratory-care equipment that is rented or purchased. The tendency is not to rent equipment indefinitely, as has been the practice, but to purchase items for patients who will be using equipment for extended periods. Both compressor/nebulizer units and nasal CPAP systems fall into this rental to purchase or direct purchase category. Depending on policy and coverage, after payment of an annual deductible, private insurers cover 75 to 80 percent of an eligible item. The balance or copayment is the patient's responsibility and may be satisfied if another policy is in effect.

IMPACT OF MANAGED CARE

As discussed in Chapter 1, managed care is significantly impacting the delivery and reimbursement of medical and health-care services. In particular, both Medicare and state Medicaid programs have seen increasing numbers of individuals being enrolled as beneficiaries in managed-care programs. Many HME providers are scrambling to become involved in or recognized members of managed-care provider networks, while others have opted to "ride the storm" and see what the future brings. Usually, HMOs and other managed-care plans have instituted fee schedules for home-care equipment rental and purchase, which providers agree to accept.

In many cases, these fees are lower than prevailing fees charged by Medicare and traditional insurance carriers. Network providers in managed-care plans rely on patient volume to help offset the lower fees. However, some industry observers are concerned that HME providers will also try to cut operating costs if managed-care provider fees are too low. This may influence some home-care companies to offer older, less expensive equipment; dispense fewer supplies; provide less frequent equipment maintenance; use unlicensed or untrained personnel; and reduce the overall level of patient services.

Until reimbursement for home-care services is secured, RCP employment in home care will be linked directly to equipment reimbursement. Any substantial reductions in reimbursement, including any by Medicare, would significantly impact this employment. Both the federal government and the home-care industry must be able to monitor and respond appropriately to any negative impact all this might have on patient care. Nevertheless, it remains safe to say that health-care reform and its offshoot, managed care, have and will continue to have a significant influence on health-care delivery and particularly, home health care in the years to come.

SUMMARY

Reimbursement for home-care equipment and services continues to be a controversial and closely monitored issue, not only by the respiratory-care profession but by the entire home-care industry. With increased emphasis on home care, significant attention is being paid to what can be done in the home, by whom, and at what cost. Reimbursement remains a highly charged and politically involved economic concern. Ever since the 1960s, with the introduction of Medicare and Medicaid, respiratory care has sought recognition and reimbursement. While oxygen and other respiratory home-care equipment are covered items, respiratory home-care services are not. However, changes that may bring about a different, more positive reimbursement picture for RCPs are on the horizon. Demonstration projects, realization of the cost-effectiveness of respiratory home care, the impact of managed care, and Congressional action may all result in the eventual recognition of and coverage for respiratory home care.

Review Questions

1. What mechanisms, including coding procedures, are currently in place for the reimbursement of respiratory home-care equipment?
2. Why are home-care services rendered by RCPs not reimbursed by Medicare or other insurances?
3. What is the Six-Point Plan, and what impact has it had on home-care equipment reimbursement?
4. What does *capped rental* mean, and what impact has it had on respiratory home care?
5. What are DMERCs, and what is their function in the reimbursement of home-care equipment?
6. What is a CMN, and why is it essential to insurance reimbursement?
7. What are the qualifications, according the Medicare, for home oxygen therapy?
8. What impact is managed care having on the home-care industry?

References

American Association for Respiratory Care. (1989). *Final report of the consensus meeting on home respiratory care equipment*. Dallas, TX. AARC.

American Association for Respiratory Care. (1995, February). DMERCs listen to concerns of their communities of interest. *AARCTimes, 19*(2), 39.

American Association for Respiratory Care. (1996a, March). Cost-effectiveness of respiratory care. *Home Care* (a compilation of articles and statements prepared by the AARC). Dallas, TX. AARC.

American Association for Respiratory Care. (1996b, March 25). Medicaid coverage for respiratory care. *Home Care* (a compilation of articles and statements prepared by the AARC). Dallas, TX. AARC.

American Association for Respiratory Care. (1996c, Summer). Summary of oxygen cuts/freezes from 1985 to 1994. *Home Care Section Bulletin,* (2), 7–8. American Association for Respiratory Care.

APCO Associates. (1995, May). *A data and literature survey on the cost-effectiveness of home care* (conducted for the Home Care Coalition). APCO Associates, Inc.

Briskorn, C.N. (1994, April). Ventilator variables. *HomeCare, 16*(4), 89–90.

Cerne, F. (1993). Homeward bound: Hospitals see solid future for home health care. *Hospitals, 67,* 52–54.

Clark, L.J. (1996, Summer). Challenges of the Home Oxygen Services Coalition in 1996. *Home Care Section Bulletin,* (2), 7. American Association for Respiratory Care.

Cotton, R.D. (1987, March). Will respiratory care professionals ever be reimbursed? *AARCTimes, 11*(3), 51.

Dunne, P. (1994, April). Demographics and financial impact of home respiratory care. *Respiratory Care, 39*(4), 311, 314.

Giordano, S. (1987, March). Why aren't the respiratory care professional's services reimbursed? *AARCTimes, 11*(3), 53–54.

Gruenwedel, E. (1996, April). Nebulizers impacted by policy changes. *HomeCare, 18*(4), 90–91.

Health Care Financing Administration. (1989, January). Six-point plan: The final document. *HomeCare, 11*(1), 62–70.

Health Care Financing Administration. (1990b, October). Home health services. *Medicare and Medicaid guide.* U.S. Department of Health and Human Services.

Health Care Financing Administration. (1990a, May). *Form HCFA-484.* U.S. Department of Health and Human Services.

Health Care Financing Administration. (1995, January). *HCFA Common Procedure Coding System (HCPCS 1995).* U.S. Department of Health and Human Services.

Kim, H. (1996, January). Respiratory distress. *HomeCare, 18*(1), 73–74, 76, 120.

May, D.F. (1991). *Rehabilitation and continuity of care in pulmonary disease.* St. Louis, MO: Mosby-Year Book.

Molle, C.J. (1993a, October). More than Morse . . . Procedure coding for the respiratory cryptographer—Part I: CPT coding. *AARCTimes, 17*(9), 74.

Molle, C.J. (1993b, October). More than Morse . . . Procedure coding for the respiratory cryptographer—Part II: HCPCS coding. *AARCTimes, 17*(10), 52–54.

Molle, C.J. (1994, October). More than Morse . . . Procedure coding for the respiratory cryptographer—Part II: Update on HCPCS coding recommendations. *AARCTimes, 18*(10), 18–21, 23–26.

Morselander, K., & Thomas-Payne, L. (1992, September). Reimbursement literacy. *HomeCare, 14*(9), 61–62.

Novoselski, D. (1989, January). Viewpoint. *HomeCare, 11*(1), 13.

Oakland, K. (1991, December). HCFA proposes four carriers, provider number restrictions. *HomeCare, 13*(12), 27.

Oakland, K. (1992, April). HCFA releases transition plan for regional carrier consolidation. *HomeCare, 14*(4), 30, 34.

Oakland, K. (1993, November). HomeCare News. DMERC transition delayed again. *HomeCare, 15*(11), 20, 22.

Pennsylvania Blue Shield. (1992, September 30). Home oxygen therapy certification and recertifica-
tions. *Medicare Special Bulletin, 3,* 7–9. Camp Hill, PA: Pennsylvania Blue Shield.

Pitts, M: (1996a, May). A breath ahead. *HomeCare, 18*(5), 95–96, 98.

Pitts, M. (1996b, August). Oxygen transfilling issues explained. *HomeCare, 18*(8), 56.

Pitts, M. (1996c, August). Rising to the occasion. *HomeCare, 18*(8), 52, 54, 56.

Saposnick, A. (1995, April). Opportunities abound for RCPs in home care. *AARCTimes, 19*(4), 68.

Saposnick, A. (1996, Summer). Notes from the chair. *Home Care Section Bulletin,* (2), 1–2. American
Association for Respiratory Care.

Segedy, A. (1989, January). Six-point plan: Carriers, dealers say new HME rates too low. *HomeCare,
11*(1), 59–62.

Thomas-Payne, L. (1993, November). Grandfather clause. *HomeCare, 15*(11), 133–134.

Thomas-Payne, L. (1994a, January). A recipe for confusion. *HomeCare, 16*(1), 81–82.

Thomas-Payne, L. (1994b, February). Breathing easier. *HomeCare, 16*(2), 77–78.

Thomas-Payne, L. (1994c, March). Dealing with documentation. *HomeCare, 16*(3), 109–110.

Thomas-Payne, L. (1995, November). They're baaackk! *HomeCare, 17*(11), 162.

Suggested Readings

American Association for Respiratory Care. (1993, November). Home care reimbursement guidelines change under DMERCs. *AARCTimes, 17*(11), 46–47, 49.

American Association for Respiratory Care. (1996, May). AARC makes unprecedented commitment
to documenting the RCP's impact on patient care. *AARCTimes, 20*(5), 16–17.

Gruenwedel, E. (1996, Feburary). Why liquid O_2 is worth its costs. *HomeCare, 18*(2), 70–71.

Public Health Service. (1991, October). *International classification of diseases, 9th revision, clinical modification,* U.S. Department of Health and Human Services Publication No. (PHS) 91–1260, V(1), iii,
xiii-xvi, xxiii, 419–420.

Rowell, J.C. (1996). *Understanding medical insurance—A step-by-step guide* (3rd ed.). Albany, NY: Delmar Publishers.

CHAPTER THIRTEEN

SUBACUTE CARE AT SKILLED NURSING AND LONG-TERM CARE FACILITIES

William F. Clark

KEY TERMS

carve-out
homogenous patient characteristics

medical subacute
outcome oriented
postacute care

prospective payment system (PPS)
rehabilitation subacute

OBJECTIVES

Upon completing this chapter, the reader will be able to:

- Define *subacute* or *postacute care.*
- Describe how managed care and capitated care are influencing subacute care.
- List and describe the core elements of an ideal subacute-care program.
- Describe how subacute care can have positive patient outcomes and lower health-care costs.
- Describe how RCPs will integrate into the subacute-care market.

INTRODUCTION

In the past there was a clear boundary between acute care and long-term or home care. Hospitals were paid for the number of procedures. The more complex the procedure, the higher the reimbursement. Hospitals invested heavily in high technology because the cost could be shifted to the consumer. Patients remained in the hospital until they were able to walk out or the hospital needed the bed for a more acutely ill patient. Long-term care and home care were simple adjuncts to acute care with very little technical or complicated patient care. The national debate on health care changed the health-care environment because the cost of health care was increasing at an alarming rate. To try to decrease the cost of health care, DRGs were introduced. Instead of being paid by the procedure, which seemed to encourage hospitals to keep patients as long as possible, the institution is paid a flat rate depending on the discharge diagnoses. If the institution can treat and discharge the patient before the cost of treatment exceeds the amount received for the diagnoses, the institution would make money. The DRGs encouraged hospitals to discharge patients sooner and to discharge patients with more acute-care needs than in the past. These acute care needs could not be met by existing long-term and home-care programs. Therefore, a new category of care arose, subacute care.

WHAT IS SUBACUTE CARE, AND HOW CAN RESPIRATORY CARE FIT IN?

In the rapidly evolving field of subacute care, no strict definition is possible. The *PDR Medical Dictionary* defines *subacute* as "between acute and chronic; denoting the course of a disease of moderate duration or severity." Many look at subacute care or **postacute care** as something repackaged for the consumer. In her article, "What's New in Subacute Care?," Kelly Shriver (1996) states that subacute care "has come to be used to refer to a level of care—skilled care for patients with complex needs—that some nursing facilities, home-care providers, and others have been providing for years under a variety of different names. . . ." Subacute care can be classified as the traditional high-end, skilled nursing care that was delivered in the hospital and is now delivered in an alternative site or as serving patients who require less intensive care than the traditional acute care but more attention than traditional nursing-home care.

In their report to the federal government entitled *Subacute Care: Policy Synthesis and Market Area Analysis, Lewin-VHI* offers a picture of the subacute-care industry. The report shows that subacute care has encompassed all the traditional postacute-care services. However, Barbara Manard (1995), principal author, also points out that the term *subacute care* promises more. "The term 'subacute care' was in the past used to describe hospitalized patients who failed to meet established criteria for a medically necessary acute stay, but is now used almost exclusively to refer to patients treated in settings other than acute-care beds" (ES-1). The report also indicates that providers are not using time trying to define *subacute*, they are pushing ahead and experimenting with ideas to see what is successful in their market.

The JCAHO has established accreditation criteria and standards for this evolving field. The American Health Care Association in Washington, DC, and the JCAHO in Oakbrook Terrace, Illinois, have jointly approved the following definition of subacute care:

> Subacute care is comprehensive inpatient care designed for someone who has an acute illness, injury, or exacerbation of a disease process. It is goal-oriented treatment rendered immediately after, or instead of, acute hospitalization to treat one or more specific, active, complex medical conditions or to administer one or more technically complex treatments, in the context of a person's underlying long-term conditions and overall situation.
>
> Generally, the individual's condition is such that the care does not depend heavily on high-technology monitoring or complex diagnostic procedures. Subacute care requires the coordinated services of an interdisciplinary team including physicians, nurses, and other relevant professional disciplines who are trained and knowledgeable to assess and manage these specific conditions and perform the necessary procedures. Subacute care is given as part of a specifically defined program, regardless of the site. (Medicare and Medicaid Guide. 820:9/22/94, #42,645)

This definition, instead of limiting subacute care to the traditional elderly patient population, allows for a wide range of patients including almost all age brackets and many traditional acute-care procedures. In her article, "Riding the Express," Cathy Tokarski (1995) states that the "range of services considered subacute can include infusion therapy; respiratory care; cardiac services; wound care; rehabilitation services; postoperative recovery programs for knee and hip replacements; and cancer, stroke, and AIDS care" (p. 22).

CORE ELEMENTS OF AN IDEAL SUBACUTE-CARE PROGRAM

The Lewin-VHI report lists the core elements of an ideal subacute-care program. The first ideal core element is:

> First, ideal subacute care is an organized program. It is more than "any type of care provided to high-end Medicare patients." Some programs are organized around specific disease categories (e.g., stroke or cancer), others are organized around specific interventions (e.g., pain management or wound care), and some are organized around other more or less **homogenous patient characteristics** (e.g., pediatrics or "medically complex"). In general, providers tend to distinguish between **"rehabilitation subacute"** patients, which include conditions such as hip replacement, spinal cord injuries, and brain injuries. These patients tend to require more rehabilitation services, such as physical, occupational, and speech therapies. Conversely, **"medical subacute"** patients tend to have conditions that require intensive medical and nursing care, but fewer other therapies. These groups of patients include those with cardiovascular diagnoses, cancer, ventilator care, wounds, and IV therapy (ES-2). (Manard, 1995)

A recent survey done by the Moore Group confirms this split in subacute care. The Moore survey also shows that long-term care facilities most often provide rehabilitation subacute care and that hospitals and freestanding nursing homes have both claimed the medical subacute-care area. Respiratory care has definitely found a **carve-out** in medical subacute care. Its ability to assess and treat complex cardiopulmonary problems and its knowledge of cardiopulmonary physiology makes it the logical choice when the patient has intensive medical care involving the respiratory system. However, respiratory care must find a place in the **rehabilitative subacute-care** area. This area involves patient and family education, patient retraining, and pulmonary rehabilitation.

The Lewin-VHI report lists the second core element as:

> In the ideal, a subacute-care program is intensely focused on achieving specified, measurable outcomes. The outcomes or goals may (some say must) vary for each patient (e.g., healing a wound or resorting the patient to a particular level of functioning). Some argue that **outcome-oriented** programs are nothing new; that, in fact, part of the definition of any medical and nursing care includes preserving and/or restoring some aspect of physical functioning. While true, subacute programs in the ideal stress an intensity of focus on outcomes, as well as achieving outcomes in a particularly efficient and lower cost manner. For example, the American Health Care Association includes "efficient and effective utilization of health-care resources" in its short definition of subacute care (ES-2). (Manard, 1995)

Respiratory care must rise to this challenge. Too many practitioners still "count procedures" instead of measuring outcomes. Measuring patient outcomes and understanding outcome-oriented programs enable respiratory care to help subacute-care facilities maintain "efficient and effective utilization of health care resources." Table 13–1 shows how outcomes measurement will affect subacute care.

The third core element listed in the Lewin-VHI report is:

> Special resources are also included in the ideal. These generally include physical plant features such as a distinct unit (highly recommended by the National Subacute Care Association [NSCA]), and more and better trained staff (than a "traditional" NF), especially physicians and nurses. The exact degree of physician and licensed nurse involvement required is a matter of some debate, particularly since increasing involvement of highly trained staff increases costs (ES-3). (Manard, 1995)

With the integrated health networks discussed later in this chapter, respiratory-care practitioners can find a definite place in this ideal subacute unit. The AARC research initiative has demonstrated that respiratory-care practitioners are "better trained" in cardiopulmonary patient assessment and treatment and can provide quality care with positive outcomes at a lower cost.

The fourth and final core element in the Lewin-VHI report is:

> Finally, ideal subacute care encompasses a set of techniques thought essential to achieving stated goals. These techniques include the use of interdisciplinary teams to plan and provide patient care and case managers, whose jobs involve both resource use monitoring and more traditional care-coordination activities. Care techniques in the ideal also include the use of "care maps" and/or critical pathway protocols, program evaluation based on measured outcomes, and an emphasis on continuous quality improvement (ES-3). (Manard, 1995)

TABLE 13–1   The effects of outcomes measurement on subacute-care services

Outcomes Measurement Components for Subacute Services	
Outcomes are one aspect of quality	Measured outcomes are favored while process measures are less a measure of health-care quality.
Increased interest in patient outcomes in all health-care modalities	Increased interest in the ability to compare outcomes within similar types of patients, as well as across different types of settings.
Outcome measures specific to subacute care are being developed	Functional Independence Measure (FIM) best known measure for rehabilitation patients are being used. Other outcome measures must be developed.
Outcome measures will play an important but as yet undetermined role	Monitoring quality is costly. Current emphasis on outcomes measurement might provide strong and effective incentives for CQI.

(Adapted from Manard, B. et al., *Subacute Care: Policy Synthesis and Market Area Analysis,* Lewin-VHI, 1995.)

In SNFs, on-site case managers who are highly trained, skilled clinical professionals are vital when communicating with physicians, clinical team members, patients, and family. Respiratory-care practitioners would be logical case managers for a subacute care unit that is organized around intervention dealing with cardiopulmonary disease or a unit that is devoted to ventilator care. Managed-care organizations are pressing for critical pathways as timed sequencing of interventions in the care plan of the patient to achieve positive outcomes. Respiratory care, again with the leadership of the AARC, has provided the most thorough listing of clinical practice guidelines to date. These guidelines are the cornerstone of clinical/critical pathways and protocols.

WHAT IS FUELING THE GROWTH OF THE SUBACUTE-CARE INDUSTRY?

Subacute-care providers are being helped by several trends in the health-care market. These trends include managed-care organizations, whose growth is being facilitated by the federal government asking hospitals and physicians to reduce costs, and the caps being placed on reimbursement for services in the acute-care setting. Long-term care and SNFs have benefited initially by gearing up for the more complex medical care and switching their signs from long-term to subacute care. Hospital executives are beginning to realize that converting acute-care units to subacute care units may help to control costs by providing care in a less expensive setting.

Managed-care organizations, private insurance companies, and even the federal government are continuously seeking alternate sites for health care. The alternate sites must exhibit both cost savings and quality. As the population of America continues to age, acute-care facilities will experience a gap in care. The elderly patient's acute illness may resolve, but the patient may be too weak to be discharged home, even with visiting nurses and home care. This transitional gap is perfect for subacute care to provide a continuum of care.

The postacute-care arena has grown rapidly since the mid-1980s. This growth seems to be fueled by several factors. The primary factors fueling this growth are managed care and Medicare's **prospective payment system (PPS)** for inpatient hospitals. These factors are followed closely by the development of integrated health networks. Finally, the lack of regulations on post acute or subacute care has helped to expand the market.

Many claim that managed care has been the most important driving force behind alternative site care like subacute care. The introduction of capitated care payments to institutions and physicians has generated the aggressive search for less expensive health care. The financial pressures of capitated care, which limits the amount of health-care dollars paid over the patient's life, has fueled the two aspects of subacute care: lower cost and higher quality. Capitation is moving rapidly into the Medicaid market. Managed-care organizations understand that money can be made if the patient is kept out of the acute-care hospital. Discharging a patient to a subacute-care facility instead of home can help to prevent costly readmissions if the subacute-care institutions provide quality care.

In her article, "Is subacute care worth your money?," Lisa Maher (1995) states, "Patients often get transferred from acute to subacute care by case managers who work for the insurers" (p. 19). Maher points out the financial advantages that occur when alternate site of care is used. Table 13–2 shows that these savings also occur if a patient can be transferred to a subacute-care setting instead of remaining in an acute-care facility or even in a long-term or rehabilitation hospital setting. This table also shows that an SNF receiving $95 to $150 per day for a bed can charge between $175 to $800 per day for the same bed in a subacute-care facility.

While managed care may be thought to be the most aggressive driving force behind the expansion of subacute care, many feel that it has not reached the mainstream of health care. However, subacute-care expansion has dominated all market areas. To explain this, many feel that one must look to Medicare and the advent of prospective payment. Medicare is still the dominant payor across all aspects of health care. With the advent of prospective payment, Medicare has forced acute-care institutions to discharge patients as soon as possible. This is especially challenging when hospitals are treating an increasing number of elderly patients who are stable and do not require acute care but cannot be placed in extended-care facilities due to the level of care needed or a lack of space. While

TABLE 13–2 Postacute care—where subacute care fits in

	Postacute Care				
	Long-Term Hospital	Rehabilitation Hospital or Unit	Subacute Care	Nursing Home (Skilled Nursing Facility)	Outpatient Rehabilitation
Typical patient	Medically unstable	Medically fragile with severe functional limitations	Sick or injured; stable	Medically stable	Stable
Nursing/ therapy (hours per day)	8 to 9 nursing/ 3 to 4 therapy	More than 5.5 nursing/ more than 3 therapy	3 to 8 nursing/ 1 to 5 therapy	1 to 5 nursing/ therapy 3 to 5 times a week	1 to 5 nursing/ therapy 2 to 3 times a week
LOS (days)	60 to 300 (average 90)	10 to 40	20 to 90	More than 180	N/A
Physician involvement	Contact several times a day; on site	Contact daily; two or more specialists involved	On call; at least once a week	On call	Periodic
Cost (per day)	$650 to 1,200	$400 to 1,000	$175 to 800	$95 to 150	$50 to 100

(Source: Maher, L., "Is Subacute Care Worth Your Money?" *Business and Health*, Vol. 13, Issue 7, July 1995, p. 24.)

Medicare is limiting the reimbursement of acute-care facilities, it has provided a 3-year exemption to subacute-care providers from the cost limits used to determine reimbursement levels. These two forces are making acute-care institutions either contract with subacute-care facilities to form an integrated heath-care network or, if the census is consistently down, convert some of the acute-care beds to subacute-care beds. Tokarski (1995) states, "There may be a very strong incentive for new providers . . . to develop subacute-care programs with Medicare patients and build up their costs as high as they can so they reap inflated reimbursement levels once the 3-year exemption ends" (p. 22). Shriver (1996) also points out that, "By forming DRG-exempt skilled-nursing units, hospitals in some cases are legally billing Medicare twice for the same service: once through the DRG for the acute care service and once for post-acute services" (p. 36).

The health-care industry seems to be moving to integrated health networks. A 1994 survey showed that 71 percent of hospitals and SNFs either had initiated or were investigating the initiation of integrated health networks. The market forces detailed previously show the financial advantages of this move. If acute-care facilities cannot convert beds to subacute care, many companies are eager to help them form alliances with SNFs with subacute-care beds to provide a continuum of care. Because hospitals have a much higher cost base due to the needs of acute-care patients, the ability to move stable patients out of the costly environments can help hospitals save money.

In his article, "License to Steal," Joseph Epstein (1995) states "Health-care industry experts are predicting that managed-care companies, with 40 to 45 percent of their costs stuck in in-patient hospital care, will drive increasing numbers of hospital patients into the subacute-care beds in nursing homes" (p. 34). Table 13–3 demonstrates the savings of using subacute care for twelve common DRG procedures. This table shows considerable savings using subacute care, but it does not show the increase revenue that can be generated by charging for the subacute care as well. Management companies have started to contract with hospitals and SNFs to help upgrade the skilled nursing beds to subacute-care level. The management company provides the expertise on subacute-care reimbursement and regulations that may be lacking in the partner institutions.

The lack of regulatory barriers seems to be the final driving force behind the expansion of subacute care. Many states do not require a certificate of need (CON), which has encouraged the proliferation of subacute-care facilities. A bill was introduced in New Jersey in 1995 to exempt hospitals from securing a CON to convert acute-care beds to subacute-care ones. The rationale is that the institution is not adding beds, only converting existing ones to a lower level of acuity. In addition, the industry is largely unlicensed and unregulated, which allows for liberal interpretation of subacute care's potential. Although there seems to be a lack of regulations, managed-care companies find the need to place patients in acute-care institutions unreasonable. Tokarski (1995) says, "One incentive that nursing-home providers of subacute services want to dump is the requirement that subacute-care patients undergo a 3-day hospital stay prior to their transfer to a subacute facility" (p. 23). This requirement comes from the Social Security Act under post-hospital extended-care services, which states:

> The term "post-hospital extended care services" means extended care services furnished an individual after transfer from a hospital in which he [she] was an inpatient

TABLE 13–3   Subacute saves the day—and the dollars

DRG Procedure	Current Hospital Days	DRG Payment	Required Hospital Days	Potential Subacute Days	Savings per Procedure
Respiratory infection and inflammation	12 to 13	$12,125	4	8 to 9	$3,922
Simple pneumonia and lung inflammation	9	$7,747	4	5	$1,933
Cardiac valve procedure with pump	22 to 23	$63,505	14	8 to 9	$4,345
Coronary bypass	16	$40,092	7	9	$5,334
Heart failure and shock	8	$4,054	3	5	$1,494
Major joint and limb reattachment procedures of lower extremity	11 to 12	$16,199	3	8 to 9	$4,943
Hip and femur procedure	10 to11	$9,418	3	7 to 8	$4,268
Fracture of femur	14 to 15	$9,021	4	10 to 11	$3,183
Fracture of hip and pelvis	12	$7,744	3	9	$3,063
Skin graft for skin cancer or cellulitis with complications	22 to 23	$19,547	7	15 to 16	$6,948
Kidney and urinary tract infection with complications	9	$7,061	3	6	$2,725
Rehabilitation	21 to 22	$15,630	3	18 to 19	$6,552

(Source: Epstein, J., "License to Steal." Reprinted from *Financial World*. Copyrighted 1996. All rights reserved.)

for not less than 3 consecutive days before his [her] discharge from the hospital in connection with such transfer. For purposes of the preceding sentence, items and services shall be deemed to have been furnished to an individual after transfer from a hospital, and he [she] shall be deemed to have been an inpatient in the hospital immediately before transfer therefrom, if he [she] is admitted to the skilled nursing facility (A) within 30 days after discharge from such hospital, or (B) within such time as it would be medically appropriate to begin an active course of treatment, in the case of an individual whose condition is such that skilled nursing facility care would not be medically appropriate within 30 days after discharge from a hospital; and an individual shall be deemed not to have been discharged from a skilled nursing facility if, within 30 days after discharge therefrom, he [she] is admitted to such facility or any other skilled nursing facility. (Social Security Act paragraph 16,961, section 1861)

Managed-care companies also wish to eliminate this requirement. Maher (1995) states, ". . . some large, fully capitated medical groups that contract to staff hospital emergency rooms have directives to transfer any patient who doesn't require acute-care services—invasive procedures or complex diagnostics, for example—directly from the ER to a subacute unit" (p. 19).

WHAT WILL RESPIRATORY CARE'S INVOLVEMENT BE IN SUBACUTE CARE?

As respiratory-care practitioners provide more evidence that they can provide high-quality care with positive patient outcomes at a lower cost than other health-care providers, they will become an integral part of subacute care. In his 1996 article, "Subacute

TABLE 13–4   Various levels of care included in subacute care

Levels of Subacute Care and Respiratory-Care Involvement

	Traditional	General	Chronic	Long-Term Transitional
Location	Within hospital or freestanding	Nursing home	Chronic-care facility	Long-term care hospital
Length of stay	15 to 20 days	20 to 30 days	60 to 90 days	40 to 80 days
Percentage of patients returning home	80 to 90 percent	60 to 80 percent	Very few	60 percent
Where patient is transferred if not transferred home	N/A	Chronic subacute-care facility, most home patients require home care	Long-term facility or stay until hospice/death	Another subacute-care setting, long-term care or hospice/death
Daily nursing	5.5 to 6.5 hours	3.5 to 5 hours	3.5 to 5 hours	N/A
Respiratory-care practitioner utilization	High—provides same level as acute care with interdisciplinary team work and patient education	Teaching and training functions —can be extended to long-term or home with patient leaves	Consultant role to nurses due to reimbursement limits	More intensive than acute care —most patients have some type of respiratory problem

(Source: Bunch, D., "Phenomenal Growth of Subacute Care Offers New Opportunites for RCPs," *AARCTimes,* Vol. 20, No. 3, March 1996, p. 48.)

Respiratory Care," Robert Taraszewski explains that presently, "Programs in subacute respiratory care generally follow three basic acuity levels, each with its own appropriate level of RCP and equipment commitments" (p. 33). These three levels are ventilator-dependent patients, which is the highest acuity level; airway-management patients; and complex ventilator patients. All these patients require frequent respiratory assessment to ascertain the need for respiratory procedures like suctioning, bronchodilator therapy, oxygen therapy, pulmonary toilet, and airway management. This involvement was further outlined by Kathleen Griffin in the 1996 article, "Phenomenal Growth of Subacute Care Offers New Opportunities for RCPs," by Debbie Bunch. Griffin describes four levels of subacute care and the implications they have for respiratory care. Table 13–4 shows these four levels and breakdowns of the type of care and respiratory involvement.

WHERE IS THE SUBACUTE-CARE INDUSTRY GOING?

Until there are scientific studies to show that subacute care saves money by shifting patients from the acute-care setting and studies on quality in subacute-care facilities to show positive patient outcomes, the industry will be hard-pressed to justify the tremendous growth. The Lewin-VHI report indicates that while many regional or local studies with anecdotal evidence are available, "a national study of the potential savings to Medicare of subacute care is based on several questionable and critical assumptions. Unless these assumptions proved true, simply moving patients to SNFs could be more costly to Medicare than the current situation" (ES-10) (Manard, 1995). In their article entitled "Long-Term Care," Robert Kane and Rosalie Kane (1995) expand on this situation by stating, "Because Medicare pays hospitals a fixed fee per admission, the hospital, not Medicare, enjoys the financial benefit of more aggressive postacute care. Thus, Medicare is more likely to consider some form of bundled payment, which combines coverage for hospital and posthospital care, rather than a special rate for subacute care" (p. 1690). If this prediction should occur, the growth of subacute care would rapidly end. However, if the industry can show that there are cost savings and positive patient outcomes from subacute care, the value of subacute care would be proven and the industry would continue to expand. Money and quality are the driving forces that can assure subacute care's position in health care.

SUMMARY

Because subacute or postacute care is such a new field, it is impossible to define. In this infancy of its existence, the subacute field is trying to find its niche in the health-care arena. It would be difficult to predict how the field will evolve or what role respiratory-care practitioners will play. Subacute care is simply trying to adapt to the changing health-care environment.

Review Questions

1. What is *subacute* or *postacute care?* Is there any difference between the two?
2. How are managed care and capitated care influencing subacute care?

3. What are the core elements of an ideal subacute-care program?
4. How can subacute care have positive patient outcomes and lower health-care costs?
5. How will RCPs integrate into the subacute-care market?

References

Bunch, D. (1996, March). Phenomenal growth of subacute care offers new opportunities for RCPs. *AARCTimes, 20*(3), 46–49.

Epstein, J. (1995, September 26). License to steal. *Financial World, 164*(20), 34–35.

Fogel, L., & Grossman-Klim, K. (1995, October). Getting started with subacute care. *Healthcare Financial Management, 49*(10), 64–74.

Kane, R., & Kane, R. (1995, June 7). Long-term care. *Journal of the American Medical Association, 273,* 1690–1691.

Lenckus, D. (1995, February 20). Subacute care market offers alternative to hospital care. *Business Insurance, 29, 3,* 6+.

Maher, L. (1995, July). Is subacute care worth your money? *Business and Health, 13*(7), 18–24.

Manard, B. et al. (1995). *Subacute care: Policy synthesis and market area analysis.* Lewin-VHI.

Medicare and Medicaid Guide. (1994). Washington, DC: Commerce Clearing House.

PDR Medical Dictionary (1st ed.). (1995). Montvale, NJ: Medical Economics.

Shriver, K. (1995, January 22). What's new in subacute care? *Modern Healthcare, 26,* 1996, 34–38.

Social Security Act. (1991). Post-hospital extended care services. 42 U.S.C. 1395x(I) 16,961:1861. Washington, DC: Commerce Clearing House.

Taraszewski, R. (1996, March). Subacute respiratory care. *Advance for Managers of Respiratory Care, 5*(3), 30–33.

Tokarski, C. (1995, July 5). Riding the express. *Hospitals and Health Networks, 69,* 20–23.

Suggested Reading

Subacute care. (1996). Dallas, TX: American Association for Respiratory Care.

CHAPTER FOURTEEN

CLINICAL AND REGULATORY ASPECTS OF SUBACUTE CARE

KEY TERMS

arranged-for services
extended-care services

incident to physician
services

length of stay (LOS)
transfer agreement

OBJECTIVES

Upon completing this chapter, the reader will be able to:

- Describe the discharge planning process involving the placement of patients in subacute-care beds.
- Identify four patient-related criteria for placing a patient in a subacute-care facility.
- Identify eight diagnostic categories that can be managed effectively at the subacute-care level.
- Identify eight respiratory care modalities or procedures administered at subacute-care facilities.
- Describe the accreditation mechanism for and government regulation of subacute-care facilities.
- Define the phrase *incident to physician services.*
- Describe how respiratory care and RCPs are recognized and reimbursed for involvement at the subacute-care level.

INTRODUCTION

Efforts to reduce rising health-care costs through the PPS and managed care have pressured, and continue to pressure, hospitals to discharge patients to their homes or, if appropriate, to alternate sites of care. Subacute care at alternate sites like SNFs and extended-care facilities has helped to curtail these increasing health-care costs while providing patients with quality medical care. As a result, long-term and subacute care have grown rapidly. This growth has been advantageous for many RCPs who have been reengineered or downsized out of employment at acute-care hospitals throughout the United States (Daus, 1995). This chapter looks at the type and level of care provided at subacute-care sites, as well as accreditation of these sites, other regulatory issues, and reimbursement for services provided, particularly those provided by RCPs.

PATIENT SELECTION AND DISCHARGE PLANNING

Patients requiring subacute care have a broad spectrum of medically complex problems, many of which involve respiratory-related complications. Placing a patient in a hospital subacute-care unit, an SNF, a comprehensive rehabilitation hospital, or another type of preferred nonacute care facility is based on clinical considerations and the preference of the patient, family, or both. The discharge planning team should be multidisciplinary and involve RCPs, especially when considering the placement of a ventilator-dependent individual. Other members of the multidisciplinary discharge team may include a physician, a nurse, a case manager, a physical therapist, other health-care providers, and family. The discharge plan should include the following elements:

- evaluation of the patient for the appropriateness of the discharge;
- determination of the optimal site of care;
- determination of the optimal resources for patient care; and
- determination that financial resources are adequate.

The selected alternate-care site may provide a higher or lesser level of care depending on the patient's overall condition. The discharge plan should always be developed and implemented as early as possible before patient transfer (AARC, 1995e).

Common subacute-care referrals from hospitals include needs for physical, occupational, and speech therapy and rehabilitation; IV therapy; ventilator and pulmonary rehabilitation; cardiac rehabilitation; wound care; pain management; dialysis; and chemotherapy (Walton & Heidegger, 1993). Consequently, most patients discharged to subacute-care facilities fall into one of the following diagnostic categories:

- strokes or cerebrovascular accidents (CVAs);
- congenital anomalies;
- major multiple trauma;
- polyarthritis, including rheumatoid arthritis;
- neurological disorders, including MS, motor neuron disease, polyneuropathy, MD, and Parkinson disease;
- brain injuries (traumatic and nontraumatic);
- spinal cord injuries;
- amputations;
- joint placements;
- fracture of the femur, including hip fractures; and
- burns.

Other than the specific need for and focus on rehabilitation, the criteria for inpatient placement to a subacute-care facility reflect those for placement into a rehabilitation hos-

Other than the specific need for and focus on rehabilitation, the criteria for inpatient placement to a subacute-care facility reflect those for placement into a rehabilitation hospital and include:

- medical supervision;
- 24-hour nursing;
- relatively intense level of support services;
- a multidisciplinary approach to the delivery of patient care;
- significant improvement in a given period; and
- realistic goals of self-care or independence in ADL.

Patients placed in subacute-care facilities receive, based on their conditions and needs, a spectrum of **extended-care services.** These services include care, aid, and assistance that inpatients at subacute-care facilities, like SNFs, require. Specifically, the items and services furnished by SNFs include:

- nursing care under the supervision of a professional RN;
- bed and board;
- physical, occupational, and speech therapy furnished at the facility or by others through contractual arrangements;
- medical social services;
- drugs, biologicals, supplies, appliances, and equipment for use in the care and treatment of inpatients;
- medical services provided by interns or residents-in-training of a hospital with which the SNF has a **transfer agreement;** and
- other services necessary to the health of patients, including respiratory care.

RESPIRATORY CARE MODALITIES

Respiratory care provided at the subacute-care level involves routine bedside care, support of the ventilator-dependent patient, emergency measures, and patient monitoring and assessment. The RCPs play an important role in overall patient care, and their involvement in subacute care has been integral to its rapid growth and acceptance. To help promote the cost-effective delivery of an optimal level of respiratory care in SNFs, the AARC and AHCA issued a joint statement entitled, "Guidelines for Respiratory Care Services in Skilled Nursing Facilities," in 1985. This document defined the scope and requirements for respiratory-care delivery at subacute-care sites and looked specifically at staffing, quality assurance, infection control, physical facilities and equipment, medical gas systems, and record keeping (AARC/AHCA, 1985).

BEDSIDE RESPIRATORY CARE

Specific routine therapy administered to patients at the bedside include:

- oxygen therapy (AARC, 1992c);
- selection of an appropriate aerosol delivery device (AARC, 1992e);
- bland aerosol administration (AARC, 1993d);
- delivery of aerosols to the upper airway (AARC, 1994a);

- assessing the response to bronchodilator therapy (AARC, 1995c);
- incentive spirometry (AARC, 1991a);
- IPPB (AARC, 1993e);
- postural drainage therapy (AARC, 1991b);
- use of positive airway pressure adjuncts to bronchial hygiene therapy (AARC, 1993c);
- directed cough (AARC, 1993a); and
- nasotracheal suctioning (AARC, 1992b).

The AARC has developed specific CPGs for each of these procedures. For each, SNFs and extended-care facilities have been identified as settings in which these procedures may be performed and modalities administered.

VENTILATORY SUPPORT

Caring for the ventilator-dependent patient is one of the most important and demanding patient-care modalities rendered at the subacute-care level. The role and responsibility of the RCP are essential to effective and safe patient care. With technology and teamwork, RCPs are improving outcomes for ventilator-dependent patients in subacute-care units and at subacute-care facilities. Acute-care facilities manage patients during acute episodes with an average **length of stay (LOS)** of 4 to 7 days. Subacute facilities focus on long-term outcomes with an average LOS of 60 to 90 days. Besides routine ventilatory care, nutrition, and psychosocial issues, weaning, swallowing, and ambulation are also emphasized. To provide adequate ventilatory support, a subacute-care facility should be equipped with piped-in oxygen, air, vacuum, and ventilators and appropriate patient monitors (Thompson, 1995).

Specific procedures related to ventilatory support that may be performed at SNFs and extended-care facilities according to the AARC's CPGs include:

- humidification during mechanical ventilation (AARC, 1992a);
- endotracheal suctioning of mechanically ventilated patients (AARC, 1993b);
- ventilator circuit changes (AARC, 1994b); and
- transport of the mechanically ventilated patient (AARC, 1993f).

While ventilators used at subacute-care sites may not be as complex as the units used in acute-care units (e.g., ICUs and CCUs), they can still provide adequate ventilatory support using CMV, SIMV, and/or PSV modes. Weaning should also be attempted if indicated by patient condition and ability.

Some of the specific advantages of subacute ventilator management include reduced health-care costs, similar care and outcomes to acute-care units and facilities, subacute environment is more favorable to patient care, and psychosocial activities are normalized (Thompson, 1995).

EMERGENCY MEASURES

Subacute care may involve a number of patient-related emergencies. The two most common are:

- management of airway emergencies (AARC, 1995b); and
- defibrillation during resuscitation (AARC, 1995a)

The AARC has developed CPGs for these procedures, including procedures for application at subacute-care sites.

PATIENT MONITORING, EVALUATION, AND ASSESSMENT

While not as intensive or extensive as that performed at acute-care settings, patient monitoring, evaluation, and assessment are routinely performed by RCPs to determine patient status and progress. According to the AARC's CPGs, three common methods of patient monitoring and assessment performed at SNFs and extended-care facilities are:

- pulse oximetry (AARC, 1991c);
- sampling for arterial blood gas analysis (AARC, 1992d); and
- capnography/capnometry during mechanical ventilation (AARC, 1995d).

These methods are in addition to any routine physical examination and spirometry that might also be done at subacute-care sites.

STAFFING

Staffing at a subacute-care facility to provide various levels of patient care varies according to the type of facility and the type of patients. Because, by definition, subacute patients are more medically stable, physician interaction or intervention daily is rarely required. Most subacute facilities have a higher ratio of RNs and LPNs to certified nurse assistants than a nursing home. In addition, many of these nurses have acute-care or rehabilitation backgrounds. The availability of physical, occupational, and speech therapy; dietitians; and social service personnel depends on the diagnoses accepted at the facility and the facility's scope and focus. The RCPs will be required at extended-care facilities that manage large numbers of ventilator-dependent cases involving weaning and rehabilitation. Staffing of RCPs depends on the number of respiratory and ventilator patients per day (Walton & Heidegger, 1993).

The SNFs and other subacute-care facilities that provide respiratory-care services outside the hospital are just as responsible for providing quality care as hospital-based respiratory-care departments. To help ensure the quality of care, the services of an active medical director should be obtained. This individual:

- provides the medical perspective of good practices in respiratory care;
- assists with the initiation of any new practices;
- assists with the development of policy/procedure manuals and treatment protocols;
- ensures that individuals providing respiratory care are qualified;
- serves as an educational resource;
- consults with other prescribing physicians when problems occur;
- monitors methods of patient assessment;
- assists with equipment selection;
- ensures compliance with state and federal regulations; and
- is accessible to the staff for direction (AARC, 1990).

INFECTION CONTROL

Implementation of effective infection-control measures remains an important part of patient care at the subacute level. While most of the studies regarding infection control have been aimed at hospital care, no definitive studies of long-term care facilities have been conducted (AARC, 1992c). Infection control depends on patient need, presence and degree of any underlying conditions, and facility policies and procedures. Recommended infection-control measures in subacute care are:

- frequent handwashing on the part of the health-care practitioner;
- implementation of standard precautions (formerly universal precautions), including the use of gloves, protective eyewear, and liquid-barrier gowns;
- observation of all infection-control guidelines for a patient;
- observation of the recommendations from the CDC for the control of exposure to tuberculosis;
- use of sterile solutions in breathing circuits;
- utilization of single-patient-use items;
- routine changing of disposable patient appliances or interfaces, tubing, and circuits, although exact frequency has yet to be determined;
- disinfection or sterilization of equipment between patient use; and
- proper handling and disposal of all contaminated equipment and disposable supplies.

The technique for disinfection or sterilization depends on the method(s) available at the facility. Common methods are steam autoclaving, ethylene oxide gas sterilization, cold or chemical sterilization, and pasteurization. Use of disposables versus reusables is an economic consideration that varies from facility to facility.

ACCREDITATION AND REGULATION OF SUBACUTE CARE

Subacute-care facilities may be accredited by the JCAHO or the Commission on Accreditation for Rehabilitation Facilities.

JOINT COMMISSION ON ACCREDITATION OF HEALTHCARE ORGANIZATIONS

The JCAHO is a private, nonprofit organization that evaluates and accredits more than 5,300 hospitals and more than 3,000 other health-care organizations and institutions, including home-care providers and subacute-care facilities. According to the JCAHO, subacute care is comprehensive inpatient care designed for patients with acute illnesses, injuries, or exacerbations of a disease process. Based on an individual's condition, patient care does not depend heavily on high-technology monitoring or complex diagnostic procedures. Therapy and treatment are goal oriented and administered immediately after, or instead of, acute hospitalization. One or more specific, active, and complex medical condition may be treated in the context of a patient's underlying long-term condition or overall situation (Medicare and Medicaid Guide, 1994).

This serves as the basis for JCAHO standards for subacute-care facilities and institutional accreditation. Complying with all related standards results in a 3-year accreditation. Facilities not in full compliance are awarded conditional accreditation (deficiencies require remediation or corrective action) or no accreditation. As with hospital care, Medicare reimbursement for inpatient care at subacute-care facilities depends on JCAHO accreditation.

COMMISSION ON ACCREDITATION FOR REHABILITATION FACILITIES

Though not as broad as the JCAHO, this agency provides an alternative to JCAHO accreditation with a more specific and extensive focus on the organization and the operation of rehabilitative hospitals and related institutions. Rehabilitative facilities are evaluated based on established criteria and standards. Complying with these standards results in institutional accreditation.

FEDERAL AND STATE REGULATIONS

Federal and state governments have regulated subacute-care facilities and continue to do so as subacute care grows and expands. For example, New Jersey enacted legislation in 1996 limiting the number of subacute-care beds in an institution. This law reduced the number of beds an institution could designate as subacute to 7 percent of the total medical/surgical beds or 12 beds, whichever is greater (New Jersey Senate Bill No. 368, 1996).

It is in the public's interest for states to help develop an effective and efficient spectrum of quality health-care services. To this end, hospitals are converting to less intensive and more appropriate levels of care for postacute patients and creating subacute-care units that ensure optimal quality care, promote the continuity of care, and avoid duplicating health-care facility bed capacity. Consequently, state departments of health have assumed an increasingly active role in this area of health-care growth and expansion. Many believe state regulation will help to control any growth surges and thereby prevent excessive numbers of subacute-care beds.

On the federal level, Medicare intermediaries are beginning to investigate respiratory-care arrangements at the subacute-care level. The basic question revolves around the methods by which respiratory-care services are delivered at SNFs and covered by Medicare. According to the *Health Care Financing Administration (HCFA) SNF Manual*, (HIM12, 1995) for Medicare to reimburse respiratory care to an SNF as an ancillary service, an employee of a transfer hospital with which the SNF has a transfer agreement must provide the service in the SNF. An SNF may not bill separately for respiratory-care services. Some facilities and respiratory practitioners have been looking into possible loopholes in the law covering payment arrangements through Medicare. Any violation of this law is deemed fraudulent and appears to be the cause for concern on the part of the HCFA regional offices and Medicare (Bianculli, 1996).

REIMBURSEMENT FOR SUBACUTE CARE

Health-care insurers, including Medicare and Medicaid, recognize and reimburse the subacute level of care. The HMOs and other managed-care organizations have been moving patients to subacute-care facilities like SNFs because nursing care at the subacute-care level is 40 to 60 percent less than hospital-related, acute-care costs. Institutions, particularly nursing homes, are realizing financial incentives by designating some of their beds as subacute care. Insurance reimbursement for a typical nursing-home bed may range from $95 to $150 per day, while reimbursement for the same bed designated as subacute care can range from $175 to $800 per day (Maher, 1995). Nursing care, physical therapy, occupational therapy, and speech therapy are typically reimbursed at SNFs, extended-care facilities, and other subacute-care sites.

REIMBURSEMENT FOR RESPIRATORY-CARE SERVICES

The RCPs, however, are only reimbursed for their services if the subacute-care facility has a transfer agreement with the hospital. The RCPs must be employees of the transfer hospital. A transfer agreement is a formal arrangement between a hospital and a subacute-care facility to augment the continuity of patient care. A model transfer agreement has been developed to assist interested institutions in this area. In addition to identifying the date of contract between the two institutions, the model also identifies that the subacute facility, to facilitate continuity of care and the timely transfer of patients and records between the hospital and the facility, initiated the arrangement.

One question that has been raised concerns how close the two institutions should be to each other. According to federal requirements, there is no specific distance requirement. However, the Social Security Act envisioned that facilities and transfer agreement hospitals should be close enough to make the transfer of patients feasible. In addition, patients should not be expected to be transferred great distances to enter a subacute-care facility (Ault, 1994).

In the absence of a transfer agreement, respiratory-care services are not reimbursable. The AARC is working with the federal government to have this restriction removed or modified. The Department of HHS appears to favor eliminating the general SNF coverage restrictions on **arranged-for services** to create a consolidated billing requirement for SNFs. The HHS has also developed a more limited legislative proposal that would amend the law to specifically permit SNF coverage of respiratory-care when furnished under arrangements with the SNF by an outside source other than the SNF's transfer-agreement hospital (Hoyer, 1995). While no formal action has been taken on these proposals, studies continue to demonstrate the potential savings for Medicare patients who receive respiratory care in subacute-care facilities (Lewis, 1996).

Reimbursement for care provided by RCPs may also hinge on the fact that the care is **incident to physician services.** This pertains to services or supplies furnished as integral, although incidental, parts of physicians' personal professional services in the course of diagnosing or treating injuries or illnesses. In addition, these services must be rendered by employees of the physician under a physician's direct supervision. In most cases, patient care that is "incident to" services is reimbursable.

OUTLOOK FOR THE RESPIRATORY-CARE PROFESSION

The outlook for respiratory care at the subacute-care level is bright. As subacute care continues to expand, additional roles and responsibilities for RCPs will emerge. While healthcare reform and hospital restructuring may have reduced employment opportunities at acute-care facilities, they have increased jobs at SNFs, extended-care facilities, and other alternate-care sites. The RCPs must strive to become cross-trained and multiskilled and to take a proactive approach to the current career possibilities in subacute care.

SUMMARY

Whether at an SNF, an extended-care facility, a rehabilitation hospital, or another subacute-care site, RCPs are involved actively in providing a wide spectrum of respiratory-care services. In particular, this care involves routine bedside therapy like oxygen and aerosol delivery, hyperinflation and chest physiotherapy, and airway management. Ventilatory support is an essential aspect of respiratory care at subacute facilities and requires RCPs to be active. Emergency procedures tend to involve airway emergencies, but they may also entail CPR in certain cases. While patient monitoring and evaluation are also carried out at the subacute-care level, they vary depending on the type of equipment and personnel at the site. Monitoring may not be as intensive as that performed at acute-care sites, but it still adequately assesses and evaluates patient condition, status, and progress. Ventilator-dependent patients in particular require monitoring that may include pulse oximetry, capnography, blood gas analysis, and cardiovascular testing.

As in other aspects of health-care delivery, there is accreditation, government regulation, and a reimbursement mechanism for subacute care. Because this level of care is growing rapidly, certain changes in regulation and reimbursement have taken place and will continue to do so as subacute care assumes a definitive identity. With this rapid development, employment opportunities for health-care practitioners, including RCPs, have increased significantly. Involvement at this level requires experience, cross-training, and multicompetency. The RCPs with a variety of skills are more likely to take advantage of the opportunities and challenges subacute care is offering.

Review Questions

1. What role does the discharge planning process play in placing a patient in a subacute-care bed?
2. What are four patient-related criteria for placing a patient in a subacute-care facility?
3. Name eight diagnostic categories that can be managed effectively at the subacute-care level.
4. Name eight respiratory care modalities or procedures that can be administered at subacute-care facilities.

5. Are subacute-care facilities subject to accreditation and government regulation? If so, by whom and how?
6. What does *incident to physician services* mean?
7. How are respiratory-care professionals and RCPs recognized and reimbursed for their involvement at the subacute-care level?

References

American Association for Respiratory Care. (1990, February). Medical direction for respiratory-care services provided outside of the hospital. *AARCTimes, 14*(2), 20.

American Association for Respiratory Care. (1991a, December). AARC clinical practice guideline: Incentive spirometry. *Respiratory Care, 36*(12), 1402–1405.

American Association for Respiratory Care. (1991b, December). AARC clinical practice guideline: Postural drainage therapy. *Respiratory Care, 36*(12), 1418–1426.

American Association for Respiratory Care. (1991c, December). AARC clinical practice guideline: Pulse oximetry. *Respiratory Care, 36*(12), 1406–1409.

American Association for Respiratory Care. (1992a, August). AARC clinical practice guideline: Humidification during mechanical ventilation. *Respiratory Care, 37*(8), 887–890.

American Association for Respiratory Care. (1992b, August). AARC clinical practice guideline: Nasotracheal suctioning. *Respiratory Care, 37*(8), 898–901.

American Association for Respiratory Care. (1992c, August). AARC clinical practice guideline: Oxygen therapy in the home or extended-care facility. *Respiratory Care, 37*(8), 918–922.

American Association for Respiratory Care. (1992d, August). AARC clinical practice guideline: Sampling for arterial blood gas analysis. *Respiratory Care, 37*(8), 913–917.

American Association for Respiratory Care. (1992e, August). AARC clinical practice guideline: Selection of aerosol delivery device. *Respiratory Care, 37*(8), 891–897.

American Association for Respiratory Care. (1993a, May). AARC clinical practice guideline: Directed cough. *Respiratory Care, 38*(5), 495–499.

American Association for Respiratory Care. (1993b, May). AARC clinical practice guideline: Endotracheal suctioning of mechanically ventilated adults and children with artificial airways. *Respiratory Care, 38*(5), 500–504.

American Association for Respiratory Care. (1993c, May). AARC clinical practice guideline: Use of positive airway pressure adjuncts to bronchial hygiene therapy. *Respiratory Care, 38*(5), 516–521.

American Association for Respiratory Care. (1993d, December). AARC clinical practice guideline: Bland aerosol administration. *Respiratory Care, 38*(12), 1196–1200.

American Association for Respiratory Care. (1993e, December). AARC clinical practice guideline: Intermittent positive pressure breathing. *Respiratory Care, 38*(12), 1189–1195.

American Association for Respiratory Care. (1993f, December). AARC clinical practice guideline: Transport of the mechanically ventilated patient. *Respiratory Care, 38*(12), 1169–1172.

American Association for Respiratory Care. (1994a, August). AARC clinical practice guideline: Delivery of aerosols to the upper airway. *Respiratory Care, 39*(8), 803–807.

American Association for Respiratory Care. (1994b, August). AARC clinical practice guideline: Ventilator circuit changes. *Respiratory Care, 39*(8), 797–802.

American Association for Respiratory Care. (1995a, July). AARC clinical practice guideline: Defibrillation during resuscitation. *Respiratory Care, 40*(7), 744–748.

American Association for Respiratory Care. (1995b, July). AARC clinical practice guideline: Management of airway emergencies. *Respiratory Care, 40*(7), 749–760.

American Association for Respiratory Care. (1995c, December). AARC clinical practice guideline: Assessing response to bronchodilator therapy at point of care. *Respiratory Care, 40*(12), 1300–1307.

American Association for Respiratory Care. (1995d, December). AARC clinical practice guideline: Capnography/capnometry during mechanical ventilation. *Respiratory Care, 40*(12), 1321–1324.

American Association for Respiratory Care. (1995e, December). AARC clinical practice guideline: Discharge planning for the respiratory care patient. *Respiratory Care, 40*(12), 1308–1312.

American Association for Respiratory Care and American Health Care Association. (1985, November). *Guidelines for respiratory care services in skilled nursing facilities.* Dallas, TX, and Washington, DC.

Ault, T.A. (1994, July 14). (Director, Bureau of Policy Development—HHS). Letter to Kevin R. Barry of Reed, Smith, Shaw, and McClay, Washington, DC.

Bianculli, J.L. (1996, April). Medicare intermediaries crack down on respiratory therapy arrangements in SNFs. *AARCTimes, 20*(4), 68–71.

Daus, C. (1995, April/May). RCPs forge new ground in subacute care. *RT—The Journal for Respiratory Care Practitioners, 8*(3), 87–88.

Health Care Financing Administration. (1995). *Health Care Financing Administration (HCFA) SNF Manual.* HIM 12.

Hoyer, T.E. (1995, August 3). (Director, Office of Chronic Care and Insurance Policy, Bureau of Policy Development—HHS). Letter to Trudy Watson, President AARC.

Lewis, D. (1996, March). Study targets potential savings for Medicare patients receiving respiratory care in SNFs. *AARCTimes, 20*(3), 52.

Maher, L. (1995, July). Is subacute care worth your money? *Business and Health 13*(7), 24.

Medicare and Medicaid Guide. (1994, September 22). Definition of subacute care in skilled nursing facilities. *Medicare and Medicaid Guide, 41.731–41.732.* Commerce Clearing House, Inc.

New Jersey Senate Bill No. 368. (1996, August 19). An Act to Regulate Subacute Care Beds in the State of New Jersey. NJ Public Law 1996, Chapter 102.

Thompson, R.E. (1995, January/February). Ventilator management in subacute care. *Advance for Managers of Respiratory Care 4*(1), 20, 22.

Walton, J., & Heidegger, R. (1993, May). Subacute care: A new opportunity for RCPs. *AARCTimes, 17*(5), 49–50.

Suggested Readings

Brown, C. (1995, September). Seeking Medicare coverage for RCPs in alternate sites. *AARCTimes, 19*(9), 8.

Cornish, K. (1996, March). Integrating subacute services. *Advance for Managers of Respiratory Care, 5*(3), 35–36, 51.

Graham, R. (1996, March). Steps to developing policy and procedure in the subacute setting. *Advance for Managers of Respiratory Care, 5*(3), 23–25.

Guion, L. (1996, March). Expanding our RC department's services to include subacute care. *AARCTimes, 20*(3), 54–56.

Taraszewski, R. (1996, March). Subacute respiratory care. *Advance for Managers of Respiratory Care, 5*(3), 30–33.

Weis, J.M. (1996, March). Developing post-acute service contracts. *Advance for Managers of Respiratory Care, 5*(3), 37–38.

CHAPTER FIFTEEN

ASPECTS OF PATIENT AND FAMILY EDUCATION

William F. Clark

KEY TERMS

affective domain
cognitive domain
diagnostic evaluation

formative evaluation
kinesics
paralinguistics

proxemics
psychomotor domain
summative evaluation

OBJECTIVES

Upon completing this chapter, the reader will be able to:

- Describe why the practitioner must be ready to educate the patient and family and how it is achieved.
- List reasons a patient or a family are not ready to learn, and explain how to remove these barriers.
- Define the evaluation process and explain how it should be used in teaching.
- Describe how the aspects of teaching are exemplified in the National Asthma Education Program.
- Outline the steps of the training process according to the AARC's CPG on providing patient and caregiver training.
- Identify five ways in which RCPs can function as patient educators.

INTRODUCTION

This chapter is divided into two parts. The first describes the patient and the family-educational process. In her book, *Patient and Family Education*, Marcia Hanak (1986) outlined recommendations for patient education. Using those recommendations, this first section is divided into five subsections, which are:

1. Ensure that the practitioner is ready to educate the patient and family.
2. Assess whether the patient and family are ready to learn.

3. When the patient and family are ready to learn, determine what kind of learning activities will be employed.
4. Use as many teaching methodologies as possible.
5. Assess the success of the process with proper evaluation tools.

In demonstration of a nationally known educational process that incorporates these processes, the second section details the National Asthma Education Program instituted by the National Heart, Lung, and Blood Institute of the National Institutes of Health, which is part of the U.S. Department of HHS.

THE EDUCATIONAL PROCESS

Every health-care provider who contacts patients directly provides some patient education. Even the simple task of providing basic therapy requires that patients understand what is expected of them. Most of the time the patient is indirectly responsible for his or her therapy. If the patient does not follow directions or does not understand what the health-care provider wants, the care will be less than effective. If the practitioner does not communicate effectively, for instance, in the use of a nebulizer or an MDI, the patient will not use the therapy effectively. Therefore, everyone who comes into contact with the patient should have a basic understanding of patient education.

Unfortunately, few allied-health programs provide graduates the skills they need to understand the needs and motivations of the patients and caregivers they must educate. Health-care providers know the information and can apply it effectively to any patient situation. However, few practitioners can communicate that same competency to a person with no medical background. Patient education is the most important aspect to helping the patient live a long and productive life. It is time for all health-care providers to learn to teach.

THE PRACTITIONER AND THE PATIENT

Webster defines *teaching* as, "the action of a person who teaches; profession of a teacher; something taught: precept, doctrine or instruction." Vital to this definition is the ability and expertise of the teacher. To be an effective teacher, the practitioner should apply the following principles of education:

1. Know the information and material. Be comfortable with it.
2. Ascertain when the patient and family are ready to learn.
3. Perform a learning-needs assessment.
4. Identify patient objectives and outcomes.
5. Use varied teaching methodologies.
6. Evaluate the process and extent of learning.
7. Revise and refine as necessary.

All this can be integrated into one model. June Dyche (1988), in her book *Educational Program Development for Employees in Health Care Agencies*, diagrams the teaching/learning process effectively (Figure 15–1). The process circles and, if necessary, starts again. The

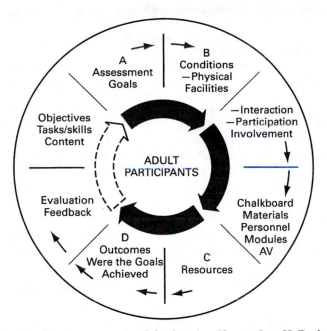

Figure 15–1 *The teaching/learning process in adult education. (Source: June H. Dyche,* Educational Program Development for Employees in Health Care Agencies, *Tri-Oak Educational Division, 1988, p. 33.)*

assessment goals are based on the skills and tasks the patient and family need. These goals and objectives lead to the type of environment that would be optimal for teaching. The environment and the involvement needed for the teaching process dictate the type of materials and the resources needed to complete the learning process. When completed, outcomes must be assessed and evaluation feedback used to ensure the goals and objectives were met. If the feedback indicates the goal and objectives were not met, then the objectives must be altered and the process reinitiated.

Because the patient and the family cannot have a live-in practitioner, the educational process is vital to the patient's continued well-being and ability to live a full life even with a long-term illness. David Rice's (1995) chapter, "Patient, Community, and Staff Education," in Dantzker's *Comprehensive Respiratory Care* states, "Learning is most universally defined as a change in behavior." Practitioners must understand that they must change the behavior of the patient and the family. This behavioral change must be understood by the patient and supported by the family or the learned behavior will not survive. The ultimate goal of this educational process is to provide the patient the tools to live the best life possible and the family the tools to support the patient in the best way possible.

PRACTITIONER READINESS TO TEACH

The first maxim of teaching is, "Know the information." Therefore, a practitioner who wants to enter family and patient education should first read extensively about the area in which he or she wants to teach. Thoroughly understanding the subject allows the practitioner to

---

TABLE 15–1 Comparing helping as a social relationship and helping as a therapeutic relationship

---

Helping as a Social Relationship	Helping as a Therapeutic Relationship
May be an intimate or a personal act. Helper uses a wide variety of resources.	Is a personal but not an intimate act. Helper primarily uses well-defined, specialized professional skills.
Relationship does not necessarily allow participants to realize personal goals. (Can foster constructive or destructive dependence.)	Relationship should always allow participants to realize personal goals. (Should foster constructive dependence.)
Can result in continued interdependence or self-dependence.	Should result in self-dependence; dignity is maintained through professional closeness.

(Purtilo, R., and Haddad, A., *Health Professional and Patient Interaction*, W. B. Saunders Company, 1996. Reprinted with permission.)

---

modify the information to meet the various needs and demands of the patient and family. This point cannot be over emphasized. Many practitioners think they know the material until they are confronted by inquisitive patients and family members.

Practitioners must also understand the attitudes they convey to the patients. Even if the health-care provider is technically competent, the patient may need more than a therapeutic relationship. In their 1996 book, *Health Professional/Patient Interaction*, Ruth Purtilo and Amy Haddad describe the difference between social relationships with patients and therapeutic relationships. Table 15–1 depicts helping as both a social and a therapeutic relationship. The patient may or may not accept the help generated by social relationships. Because social relationships are not specific in content, the patient may look upon the help they generate as an invasion of their privacy. Most practitioners are more familiar with the therapeutic relationship. It is not surprising that most practitioners rely heavily on therapeutic skills and take a clinical attitude when treating patients. Unfortunately, the patient can perceive this as cold and impersonal. The effective teacher finds a way of presenting clinical information in a personal way to keep patients involved in their education (Purtilo & Haddad, 1996).

PATIENT AND FAMILY READINESS TO LEARN

When assessing the patient and family's readiness to begin the learning process, the practitioner must understand that certain barriers to learning must be eliminated or at least minimized. The practitioner must assess the impact of the illness on the lifestyle of the patient and the family and the patient's and family's willingness to change. Life may never return to "normal," so the patient and family must understand the need for change, and they must want to change. The practitioner must also assess what the patient and family know already and ascertain any previous negative experiences, misconceptions, or misinformation that may hinder the learning process. Finally, the practitioner must realistically assess what the patient and family need to know and develop the teaching plan to meet the self-management skills that will provide the best chances for success.

Because most patient education is directed toward a long-term illness or injury, the practitioner will have to address the problems associated with a chronic illness and determine whether the patient and family can benefit from an educational program. An acute illness is easier to address because it usually has a finite length of disability. Chronic illness differs in that the patient usually does not return completely to a healthy condition.

This cycle of physical deconditioning and helplessness was described by Kate Lorig et al. in *Living a Healthy Life with Chronic Conditions* (1994). "Unlike acute illness, chronic illnesses have multiple causes varying over time, and include heredity, lifestyle factors (smoking, lack of exercise, poor diet, stress, etc.), exposure to environmental factors, and physiological factors." The patient and the family develop a sense of helplessness that is reinforced by the physical deconditioning that can occur (Figure 15–2). "Believing nothing can be done is a guarantee that nothing will be done, reinforcing helplessness and perpetuating this vicious cycle" (Lorig et al., 1994). It is important for a practitioner to understand the differences between acute and chronic diseases (Table 15–2) and to provide an environment that will help the patient and family cope with these problems. Practitioners must show their patients and family members that they can live with chronic illness by mastering the physical and psychological problems and achieving the best physical and emotional aspects of life.

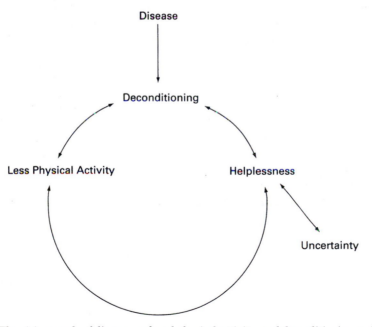

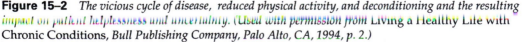

Figure 15–2 *The vicious cycle of disease, reduced physical activity, and deconditioning and the resulting impact on patient helplessness and uncertainty. (Used with permission from* Living a Healthy Life with Chronic Conditions, *Bull Publishing Company, Palo Alto, CA, 1994, p. 2.)*

TABLE 15–2 The differences between acute and chronic disease

	Acute Disease	Chronic Disease
Beginning	Rapid	Gradual
Cause	Usually one	Many
Duration	Short	Indefinite
Diagnosis	Commonly accurate	Often uncertain, especially early
Diagnostic tests	Often decisive	Often of limited value
Treatment	Cure common	Cure rare
Role of professional	Select and conduct partners of therapy	Teacher and patient
Role of patient	Follow orders	Partner of health professionals, responsible for daily management

(Source: Lorig, K. et al., *Living a Healthy Life with Chronic Conditions,* Bull Publishing Company, 1994, p. 3. Used with permission.)

Other emotions patients feel include the loss of self-image, privacy, and independence. If patients have long-term illnesses or injuries when they leave the hospital, these losses may follow them home. Practitioners must try to help patients cope with their feelings and how they see themselves. Most patients must contend with the feeling that they depend on something outside their control, whether it be their conditions, medications, or prognoses. In the hospital, the loss of self-image and privacy can affect how patients react to their situations. Once out of the hospital, the pressures of life also affect the patient. Financial and personal problems that were forgotten in the hospital may now be foremost on the patients' minds. A good practitioner knows when to allow the patient to talk and listens to what the patient has to say. It might be as simple as understanding the patients' needs, confirming the patient is getting better, and convincing the patient that using the skills the practitioner teaches will help the patient to lead a more productive life.

The practitioner must understand that some patients do not want to get well nor acknowledge the progress toward recovery. Some patients like the attention they get when they are sick. Some prefer to escape "real life" to orderly hospital life. The escape from real life sometimes makes it impossible for the health-care provider to educate the patient. The patient will understand, but he or she has decided not to get well (Purtilo & Haddad, 1996).

The practitioner must be careful about patient dependence. There are three types of dependence: detrimental over dependence, constructive dependence, and self-dependence. The practitioner should be particularly watchful for over dependence. Over dependence occurs when the patient depends too much on the practitioner and seems to cling to the practitioner. "When a patient or health professional is seeking more dependence than what is constructive, that person may have a neurotic need to clutch the security he or she believes lies in the relationship. A health professional may desperately need to be liked either to prove his or her competence or to control another person" (Purtilo & Haddad,

1996). The relationship that should be forged between the practitioner and the patient is constructive dependence based on mutual need and respect. The patient must maintain his or her identity while acknowledging the need for the practitioner's skills and knowledge. The patient needs the skills and services of the practitioner, and the practitioner provides them professionally. "If the clinician encourages and facilitates learning by the patient and the patient responds by participating in decisions, a partnership is born. To be most effective, self-management of chronic illness requires such a partnership" (Lorig et al., 1994).

When the patient has obtained enough knowledge and skills to be confident in his or her ability to control the situation, constructive dependence leads to self-dependence. While the practitioner can now be a constant source of encouragement and guidance, the patient has been empowered by the educational process (Purtilo & Haddad, 1996). When patients are empowered to self-manage illnesses, they have the skills to address their illnesses, carry out normal activities, and handle emotional changes (Lorig et al., 1994).

The relationship between patients and their families is also very important for the practitioner to understand. The interaction between patient and family can help or hinder the educational process. When handling a chronic illness, a patient requires changes in the normal family environment. Some family members can adapt to the changes. Some may not and may find the new environment difficult and disruptive. In their 1992 book, *Health Communications: Strategies for Health Professionals*, Peter and Laurel Northouse describe the interaction that occurs between the patient and family members. The authors explain that the health-care professional who is going to try to educate the patient and family must understand the dynamics of the changes in the family roles. Each member of the family has a role that has developed over time. When a chronic illness disrupts the family environment, the practitioner must assess the changes in the roles and how the family is coping with the changes. If the dominate family member is incapacitated suddenly, the practitioner must understand the change. The practitioner must also understand how the changes in the environment may cause some members of the family to become rigid in their roles. "The other role pattern that can be disruptive to families is role rigidity, which occurs when individuals are inflexible or unable to change their roles to meet the demands of a new situation. Role rigidity can limit a family's adaptive potential" (Northouse & Northouse, 1992).

Finally, there should be an assessment and balance of what the patient and family know and what they need to know. Practitioners must help the patient and family assimilate essential knowledge to self-manage the illness. Many practitioners over educate patients and families with many facts that only confuse. It is not necessary to make the patient and family professional health-care providers. It is necessary to give them the skills and knowledge they can use. When confronted with a patient and family who have read extensively about the patient's illness, the practitioner can act as a facilitator to ensure the needed skills and knowledge are present.

LEARNING ACTIVITIES

When trying to decide how best to teach the patient and family, the practitioner must carefully assess the climate for learning and understand how best to present different materials. Using the previously assessed needs, the practitioner must be able to develop a teaching plan that identifies the objectives of the process and the expected outcomes. When developing the plan, the practitioner is expected to identify whether the instruction will be delivered individually or in groups. He or she will need to decide the schedule, place, and duration of sessions that will allow for the maximum teaching/learning process within the constraints of normal life. It is also important for the practitioner to remember to present key points early, reinforce them often, and keep the material simple and stimulating. Finally, the practitioner must be able to integrate the knowledge into the lifestyle of the patient and the family or it will go unused and be forgotten quickly.

The climate for learning is continuously influenced by the emotions of the participants. Raymond Wlodkowski, in his 1985 book, *Enhancing Adult Motivation to Learn*, says, "Some psychologists have proposed that emotions are the 'chief movers' of behavior, and most psychologists accept the idea that thinking and feeling interact to mutually influence one another as well as to lead to changes in behavior" (Wlodkowski, 1985). The teaching process involves success and failure. It is important to clearly understand the emotional environment so that small setbacks will not sabotage the learning process. Fear and anxiety of failure may act as barriers. If the patient or family member has forgotten something, he or she may fear putting the patient in jeopardy. To reduce the anxiety of forgetting, the participant will try to rationalize an acceptable excuse for forgetting. However, the fear will still be a barrier. Even children are affected by the climate of fear, especially if they feel it in their parents. "In general, competence is the concept or major motivation factor that describes our innate desire to take the initiative and effectively act upon our environment rather than remaining passive and allowing the environment to control and determine our behavior" (Wlodkowski, 1985). The instructor must cultivate a climate that reinforces the concepts of competency and success.

To create the proper climate for learning, the instructor must stimulate discussion and the sharing of knowledge. June Dyche, in her 1988 book, *Educational Program Development for Employees in Health Care Agencies*, describes three climates for instruction: authoritarian, democratic, and laissez-faire. In the authoritarian climate all decisions are made by the instructor. This type of climate can be used for some teaching processes, especially when teaching young children, but it has limited success in generating self management skills (Dyche, 1988).

The democratic climate of learning has the most success, especially with adults. The instructor serves as a facilitator of knowledge but decisions are a group process with active participation by all in the education program. This is not a laissez-faire environment in which the participants make all decisions. A laissez-faire environment may be useful in some activities, but it usually leads to failure if used exclusively. The participants look to the instructor for guidance and information. If this is not forthcoming, the participants lose interest. The best educator uses all these educational climates effectively to ensure participation and success.

During the assessment of the readiness of the patient and the family to participate in the educational process, the practitioner obtains valuable insights into the type of learning activities and the type of teaching process that will succeed. Wlodkowski, in *Enhancing Adult Motivation to Learn*, states that the educator should, "make the learning goal as clear as possible. When learners understand exactly what they are to learn, confusion cannot detract from their expectancy to succeed" (Wlodkowski, 1985). When identifying objectives and expected outcomes for the patient and the family, the practitioner must understand the **cognitive, psychomotor,** and **affective domains** as classified by Bloom (1956) in his book *Taxonomy of Educational Objectives, Handbook I: Cognitive Domain.*

The cognitive or intellectual domain refers to where intellectual skills are obtained. This part of the learning activity addresses the need for information to be communicated and understood. Ideally, this kind of domain lends itself to verbal and written information. In a sense, knowledge and comprehension skills are communicated the strongest in the cognitive domain. However, while this domain is usually the easiest to plan for, it is the hardest to evaluate, and retention can be very short.

The psychomotor domain is the area health-care providers use a great deal. This domain includes many of the skills that patients and their families must master to lead to self-management. The psychomotor domain requires that certain motor skills be learned and evaluated by the practitioner. This domain can draw heavily on the intellectual domain. The patient and his or her family must understand the sequence of events or skills before trying to master them physically. Likewise, if there is a problem during the psychomotor learning of skills, it is usually because the patient or his or her family did not understand the cognitive skills completely.

The affective domain follows the other two domains. Once the intellectual skills are understood and the psychomotor skills are learned effectively, it is understood that, given the proper stimuli, the patient and the family will respond with the learned responses. Anyone who has tried to teach a patient understands that this is not always the case. Sometimes the patient or the family will respond differently than taught. Rice explains this behavior (Dantzker, 1995). The way in which different factors influence potential or actual responses is illustrated in Figure 15–3. The actual response may be affected by the attitudes of patients and their families or other factors like environment, resources, or

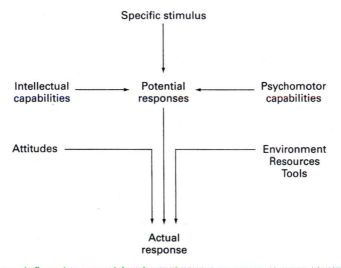

Figure 15–3 *Factors influencing potential and actual patient responses. (Source: Dantzker, MacIntyre, and Bakow,* Comprehensive Respiratory Care, *W. B. Saunders Company, 1995, p. 1209.)*

tools. For example, patients with asthma have been taught that when they feel the onset of an attack, they should stop and take their medicine. This is demonstrated many times for the health-care practitioner and is understood completely by the patient. However, some patients may find themselves in environments that would embarrass them when using their medicines, render them unable to afford their medications, cause them to forget their medicines, or believe they can make it through the attack. Because of these external forces, the patient's actual response may be diametrically opposed to the response taught and learned. Therefore, practitioners must understand that this does not reflect on their teaching. However, the practitioner must understand that this will probably happen and include examples of this kind of response in their teaching activities.

Deciding whether to teach patients individually or in groups is important when planning activities. Individual learning is probably more effective overall, but in today's health-care environment, it may be an unaffordable luxury. Therefore, the practitioner must understand group dynamics and be able to use them effectively.

When trying to determine the structure of the learning activities, it is necessary to understand where and when the sessions will occur. "If the environment is strange and frightening, the patient or health professional might well react in a fearful or angry manner. For many patients, a health-care facility can be an extremely threatening place" (Purtilo & Haddad, 1996). While the health-care professional may feel most at ease in the health-care facility, it is counterproductive if the patient and the family react negatively to the environment. The practitioner may feel just as threatened or uneasy in the patient's home. The important fact to remember is that the patient and the family must learn the skills outside health-care facility eventually to establish self-management skills.

The schedule and duration of the program are as important as the place of teaching. While time may seem endless to a child, the need for immediate gratification is important. A child lives more for the moment than for tomorrow. "Adults have more stable interests and a different perception of time. They are able to internalize long-range goals and work toward them over a period of time" (Kidd, 1977). Both the adult and child will lack a commitment to goals unless they have participated in the decision-making process. The practitioner must meet with all involved and develop a schedule that all will accept. These meetings sometimes appear to be negotiations and conflict resolution. However, if the schedule is too restrictive or the sessions too short or too long and the process is exhausting, learning will not occur.

Once the logistics of the teaching process have been worked out, the practitioner must plan the activities. The practitioner must learn to bring the material to the patient and family level and gradually bring the patient and family to a level of understanding that makes self-management possible. In addition, the practitioner must try to stimulate the patient and family to participate in the learning process. "Stimulation operates at many different levels. It varies according to what is done by the instructor and the degree of participation and quality of involvement that it influences within the learner" (Wlodkowski, 1985). The three goals of learner participation are attention, interest, and involvement. Attention is very close to the orientation or groping stage discussed previously. The group is uncertain about who they are and what they are supposed to do, but they are ready to acquire information. Stimulating the participants at this point means presenting the objectives and the expected outcomes clearly and having the group actively participate in the decision process. This is necessary to generate the interest that stimulates the learner to participate in the learning process. However, at this point the learner is passive. "There is listening, watching, feeling, reading, note taking, and so on, with a desire to comprehend and remember. This is recipient engagement where the amount of mental investment on the part of the learner remains modest" (Wlodkowski, 1985).

The participant must become actively involved in the learning process. "The learner is searching, evaluating, constructing, creating, and organizing the learning material into new and better ideas, memories, skills, understanding, solutions, or decisions. Considerable mental effort has been expended by the learner with varying amounts of emotional and physical energy exerted as well" (Wlodkowski, 1985). This closely relates to the problem-solving or cooperation stage stated previously. At this stage, the group works together and uses the group process to tackle harder and more complex problems. If the practitioner can stimulate the participants to reach the involvement stage, the learning process will be internalized and self-management skills will result.

TEACHING METHODOLOGIES

"The ultimate goal is to match learning methods with the needs of individuals and not implement a particular model of adult learning" (Dantzker, 1995). To succeed, the practitioner must be able to use many different forms of teaching methodologies. The most common methodology is verbal communication, but the practitioner must also understand and use nonverbal communication. Visual aids are vital in any teaching situation. These aids can include items like charts, graphs, flip charts, and illustrations. Handouts are commonly used to teach and reinforce, but the practitioner must know how to make them effective. Participation and demonstration are the cornerstone of teaching the skills necessary for self-management. Finally, the practitioner must understand how to use humor to facilitate learning.

Every practitioner understands the need for verbal communication. Most instruction is conducted by verbal communication. Verbal communication is instrumental in creating better understanding between patient and health-care professional, but it does not happen automatically. In fact, when patients fail to follow instructions, the health-care practitioner usually did not use adequate verbal communication (Purtilo & Haddad, 1996). Successful verbal communication requires the practitioner to present material correctly and have the proper attitude, tone, volume, and ability. It also requires the patient and/or family to listen effectively.

Material presentation is vital to patient and family understanding. Three key areas must be observed when presenting material. The first is vocabulary. As was stated before, "A health professional's failure to use appropriate vocabulary leads to several problems: (1) use of the wrong word, (2) omission of important ideas, and (3) long, rambling descriptions that confuse rather than enlighten" (Purtilo & Haddad, 1996). The practitioner must remember that the patient and family probably do not understand highly technical jargon unless the patient and family are also health-care providers. Knowing the audience and the level of understanding is important when selecting vocabulary. It is also important to have several different ways of describing aspects of the lesson should the patient and family fail to understand the first description. This is especially important when the practitioner is trying to communicate vital self-management skills. The practitioner must learn to translate the professional jargon into lay terms that will allow the patient and family to understand what is being communicated.

Clarity is also important. "A highly organized, technically correct, and very meaningful sentence loses its impact when poorly articulated or spoken too softly or hurriedly" (Purtilo & Haddad, 1996). Organization is important to presentation. "Failure to progress from one step to the next to reach a logical conclusion is usually caused by (1) a lack of understanding of the subject or of the steps in the procedure or (2) ironically, a too-thorough knowledge of the subject or procedure" (Purtilo & Haddad, 1996). Everyone has at one time tried vainly to comprehend the ideas of another who has not organized his or her thoughts before trying to explain. This process takes twice as long with less than half the understanding. When the practitioner is too knowledgeable, he or she may overlook certain facts that are vital to the patient and the family. No matter how practiced the practitioner, he or she must organize and practice the presentation before presenting it to the patient and family.

"Nonverbal communication is a complex and multifaceted phenomenon. Researchers have commonly divided the nonverbal communication area into five distinct categories: (1) **kinesics,** (2) **proxemics,** (3) **paralinguistics,** (4) touch, and (5) physical and environmental factors" (Northouse & Northouse, 1992). Kinesics is the use of body motion as a form of communication or language. These motions include gestures, facial expressions, and gaze. The practitioner must understand that different cultures may interpret kinesics differently than expected. Proxemics deals with personal space or comfort zone. Each person has a different comfort zone or personal space. The practitioner as well as the patient and family have this comfort zone. The practitioner must understand the differences between personal distance, social distance, and public distance and how each of these can affect the quality of learning. Paralinguistics refers to the physical characteristics of verbal communication and the role it plays in interpretation. It involves nonverbal communication to which health-care practitioners must be closely attuned.

Touch also is important in nonverbal communication. A message's meaning can be reinforced by touching correctly or eliminating inappropriate touching. The factors that influence touch are gender, sociocultural, type, location, and the nature of participants' relationship. Table 15–3 describes the various types of touches and the messages they convey. The practitioner must remember to, "use a form of touch that is appropriate to the particular situation . . . do not use a touch gesture that imposes more intimacy on a patient than he or she desires . . . observe the recipient's response to the touch" (Northouse & Northouse, 1992).

A picture is valuable when addressing patient and family education. A picture does not have to be a photograph. A picture can be a drawing, a chart, a graph, a demonstration, a pantomime, or some other graphic way of illustrating ideas. When the practitioner uses verbal communication, a picture, and demonstration in which the patient and family participate, the senses of hearing, sight, and touch are involved. The more senses that can be used during the educational process, the longer the information will be remembered.

"The basic reason for using handout material is to reinforce the content" (Dyche, 1988).

TABLE 15–3   **Messages conveyed by different types of touch**

Functional–professional	This type of touch usually involves task completion like touching a patient's arm to take a blood pressure or holding a patient's hand to assist him or her with ambulation. The professional use of this type of touch sends the message, "I will assist you."
Social–polite	This type of touch, exemplified by a handshake, is used to greet a new patient who has just been introduced. This type of touch characterizes a fairly superficial involvement between two people.
Friendship–warmth	This type of touch conveys a liking for the other person. If a patient tells a social worker a humorous story and the social worker laughs and squeezes the patient's arm, the social worker is using a type of touch that conveys the message, "I like you."
Love–intimacy	This type of touch signifies a close attachment between two people. It could be characterized by an enveloping hug between two people that transmits the message, "I care deeply for you."
Sexual arousal	This form of touch conveys physical attraction between two people and may be evident in a close physical embrace or stroking touch. This type of touch sends the message, "I am very attracted to you."

(Northouse, P., and Northouse, L., *Health Communications: Strategies for Health Professionals,* 2nd edition, © Appleton and Lange, 1992, p. 140. Reprinted with permission.)

Unless it is well-designed, a handout will only be another piece of written reading material. Handouts can be used to organize the material to facilitate note taking, or they can be used to summarize, highlight, and supplement the lesson information. Hanak developed an outline of suggestions for developing handouts for patient teaching aids (Table 15–4).

Vera Robinson in her book, *Humor and the Health Profession: The Therapeutic Use of Humor in Health Care*, says, "laughter creates the very air in which learning thrives" (1991). Humor can diffuse anxiety, help patients and families cope with stress, and help ideas flow.

> Humor can be used constructively in the teaching process. The use of humor is a mechanism which does not destroy one's self-image, but provides a way to criticize, show mistakes, and express values, yet save face for the individual and imply a loving relationship in doing so. It's all right. You made a mistake, just something to laugh about, to learn from. No harm done. You are not a terrible person, just human. (Robinson, 1991)

The practitioner must develop a sense of the humor the patient and family will tolerate. Some diseases and situations are not conducive to humor. However, practitioners will find they can use a personal humorous experience. "The teacher relating humorous experiences of his [her] own which often show 'boo-boos' and mistakes he [she] has made

---

TABLE 15–4   Guidelines for developing handouts for patient teaching

---

1. Briefly explain the objective of the handout.
2. Indicate why the information is necessary and when it is to be used.
3. List any supplies and equipment necessary to carry out the instructions.
4. Present information in a clear, concise, and logical sequence.
   a. Use short sentences and simple words.
   b. Avoid using jargon.
   c. Focus on key points and avoid unnecessary detail.
   d. Provide a brief explanation for each recommendation.
   e. Use list format when possible.
5. Select an appropriate printing style.
   a. Use easy-to-read type.
   b. Use boldface lettering, underlining, and asterisks to emphasize key points.
   c. Use spacing and/or symbols to separate and highlight individual sections.
6. If using illustrations or diagrams:
   a. Keep them simple and directly related to the written material.
   b. Provide clear, concise labels to clarify their purpose and meaning.
7. Evaluate the effectiveness of the handout with patients.
   a. Is the objective of the handout being met?
   b. What terms are unclear or confusing?
   c. What additional information is needed?
   d. Is there unnecessary information that can be deleted?
8. Make the necessary modifications.

(*Patient and Family Education,* Hanak, M., copyright 1986, Springer Publishing Company, Inc., New York, New York 10012. Used by permission.)

helps the student, who usually has unrealistic expectations of his [her] own performance, to relax and accept the learning process" (Robinson, 1991). With experience, the practitioner will understand when humor is helpful.

EVALUATION

Many programs forget the final important process in education, the evaluation. "The major purpose of evaluation in most educational situations is to find out how much change and growth have taken place as a result of educational experiences" (Wlodkowski, 1985). Many would assume evaluation comes at the end of the educational process. Although it is last in this section, evaluation should be performed through all phases of the educational process. Table 15–5 outlines the basic principles of the evaluation process. Dyche (1988) describes the three phases of evaluation as follows: **"Diagnostic evaluation** looks at the learner's ability and what is needed to learn. **Formative evaluation** occurs while a program is being conducted. **Summative evaluation** is the process of analyzing the results of a program when it has been completed" (Dyche, 1988). The formative and

---

TABLE 15–5   **Principles of evaluation**

---

1. Evaluation is an ongoing process that occurs in all phases of program development.
2. Decisions about evaluation are an integral part of the planning phase of any learning process.
3. Evaluation must be based on the objectives and expected outcomes for the program.
4. Evaluation is stated in terms of performance behaviors.
5. The scope of the evaluation process is predetermined.
6. Postsession follow-up is essential in that it relates the application of knowledge, skills, and attitudes to the job site.
7. Evaluation based on feedback techniques should lead to improved teaching techniques and learning. Negative feedback is better than no feedback.
8. The evaluation process is shared with all those involved in the learning experience (e.g., supervisors, learners, program designers/presenters).
9. More than one method should be used as an evaluation technique. Methods like pre- and post-tests, direct observations, interviewing techniques, written questionnaires, and checklists are essential for obtaining information regarding the learning process.

(Dyche, J., *Educational Program Development for Employees in Health Care Agencies*, Tri-Oak Educational Division, 1988. pp. 91–92. Reprinted with permission.)

summative evaluation can use a combination of verbal and written tests, return demonstrations, problem-solving exercises, checklists, and anecdotal records.

ASTHMA EDUCATION

While asthma's history can be traced back to 400 B.C., this disease has long been misunderstood and underestimated by the medical community. Asthma affects one in twenty Americans and was estimated in 1990 to cost over $6 billion per year in direct costs and lost productivity. The prevalence of asthma increased by 66 percent from 1979 to 1992. Asthma is most common in children under 18, and hospitalization for asthma has increased dramatically for children under 15. The most disconcerting statistic is that asthma deaths have increased 40 percent from 1980 to 1990. These deaths occur mostly in older age groups. African-Americans of both sexes are three times more likely to die from asthma than Caucasians.

The National Asthma Education and Prevention Program was developed to:

- raise awareness of patients, health professionals, and the public that asthma is a serious chronic disease;
- ensure the patient, the family, and the public recognize symptoms;
- ensure appropriate diagnosis by health professionals; and
- ensure effective control by encouraging a partnership among patients, physicians, and other health professionals through modern treatment and education programs.

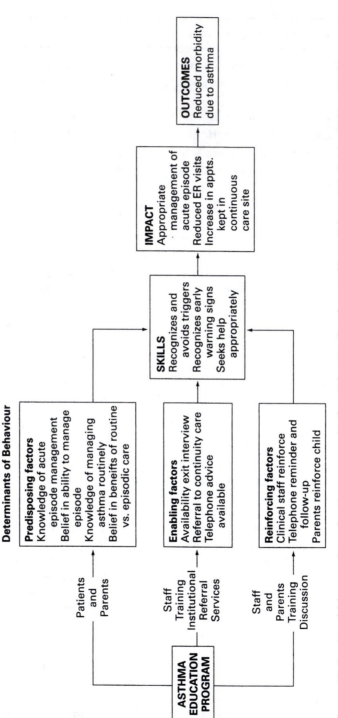

Figure 15–4 *A model for an asthma education program. (Asthma Education Supplement, Chest, Volume 106, October 1994, p. 187S.)*

The program lists patient and family education as an essential component of asthma management. It stresses that health-care providers must establish a partnership with the patient and the family, teach the essential content, and encourage adherence to a treatment plan that is basically controlled by the patient. The partnership must include open communication, an agreement of the goals and expectations of the treatment plan, joint development of a treatment plan, and encouragement of family efforts to help control the patient's asthma.

Asthma-education programs can be traced back to a study done at Johns Hopkins Hospital's emergency department. The model developed was named PRECEDE for **pre**disposing, **re**inforcing, and **e**nabling **c**onstructs in **e**ducational **d**iagnosis and **e**valuation. This model has formed the basis for many asthma-education programs. Figure 15–4 demonstrates such a model. As a result, many more educational programs have been developed and tested. The findings of the First National Conference on Asthma and Education in Canada were published in the October 1994 supplement to *Chest*. Combining these materials with the materials from the NIH can form an excellent asthma-education program.

PRACTITIONER READINESS TO TEACH AN ASTHMA-EDUCATION PROGRAM

Most asthma patients are treated by primary-care physicians who are usually unaware of the benefits of asthma education. General practitioners and doctors as a rule have thought that patient self-management is dangerous. Johanne Cote et al., in their *Chest* article, "Educating the Educators," stated that when surveyed, asthmatic patients also complained that physicians "spent an average of less than 30 minutes talking about their disease. Moreover, physicians often used vocabulary that patients do not understand." The authors' conclusions were, "physicians and specialized educators should work as a team to improve the knowledge and self-management skills of asthmatic patients" (1994).

To be effective educators, the practitioners "must be aware of current consensus on asthma treatment, management strategies, and particularly on how to teach asthmatics to determine the severity of asthma and modify therapy according to their assessment. In the rapidly evolving field of asthma treatment, educators should keep up to date with new therapies, devices, and approaches" (Cote et al., 1994). In 1991 a program that consisted of a full-day session of lectures, small-group discussions, and practical experience was developed in Quebec City to educate the educators (Table 15–6). Using questionnaires, the evaluation of the program showed that the knowledge of the participants increased from 61 percent before the session to over 85 percent after the session. This is one way in which practitioners can get the knowledge and specialized experience they need to be successful educators.

Because most areas do not have specialized programs for educating the educators, it is incumbent on the practitioner to find the information necessary to becoming fully knowledgeable in asthma. One of the most popular programs in the United States is the Open Airways programs developed by the American Lung Association. Although it is directed mainly toward elementary-age asthma patients and their families, this program also provides information for the practitioner teaching older patients. When the practitioner

---

TABLE 15–6   Example of a training program for asthma educators

---

1. Professionals involved in asthma education referred by their institutions
2. Initial training session (1 day)
    - Lectures and discussions on basic knowledge about
        Asthma pathophysiology
        Preventive measures
        Medication
        How to recognize asthma
        Asthma's etiologies and severity
        How to establish and maintain control of asthma with minimum medication
        Inhaler use
        Peak flow monitoring
        Risk factors
        How to treat exacerbations early and effectively with action plans
    - Pegagogical methods to provide asthmatics and their families wih effective self-management skills and relevant knowledge
    - Small workshop on case reports specifically developed to cover most aspects of asthma education and related problems
    - Before and after self-assessment questionnaire
    - Educational materials provided to the educator (e.g., demonstrators, plans of action, booklets)
3. One- to two-week sessions at experienced asthma clinics
4. Regular updates on asthma and its treatment (bulletin, network meetings, and educational activities)
5. Teaching assessment during accreditation visits to their centers

---

(Cote, J., et al., "Educating the Educators," *Chest,* October Supplement, Vol. 106, No. 4., 1994. Reprinted with permission.)

feels comfortable with his or her knowledge level, this confidence is transmitted to the patient and the family helping to forge the educational partnership.

PATIENT AND FAMILY READINESS TO LEARN ABOUT ASTHMA MANAGEMENT

To ensure the patient and family are receptive to the educational process, the practitioner must assess the impact of the illness on the patient's and family's lifestyle and their willingness to change. Even when the patient is physiologically ready to accept asthma education, recruitment into a program must occur when the patient and family are most receptive. Many education programs find recruitment and even initiation of the program in the emergency room gives the greatest chance for success. Having had to be treated for an acute episode allows the patient and family to realize the need for change. Beginning the educational process while still in the emergency room helps to initiate the patient and family to the benefits of asthma education.

However, certain barriers exist for the patient and family, including economic status, psychological factors, literacy level, ethnic background, and fear of the disease. In his *Chest* article, "Psychosocial Barriers to Asthma Education," Mark Fitzgerald states, "In our own study, it was especially disappointing that those subjects at highest risk, i.e., patients with asthma who were hospitalized and those with episodes of near-fatal asthma, were least likely to attend ambulatory-education programs" (1994). Fitzgerald goes on to say that the programs must target patients in the hospital setting. Many others agree that the patients most in need of education are those who have shown through hospital admission they do not have the self-management skills or support to control their disease.

In the article, "Prospective Study of Hospitalization for Asthma" in the *American Journal of Respiratory Critical Care Medicine*, Dominic Li et al. (1995) developed a simple screening method for identifying patients at risk of being hospitalized for asthma. Using the answers to five simple questions or results from common tests, a practitioner would be able to assess the risk factors and have a method for targeting the patient population most in need of patient and family education. These potential predictors are described in Table 15–7.

It is vital that the practitioner target the correct patient and family population, remove the barriers that would prevent the participation in the education program, and provide the initial education when the patient is either in the hospital due to an episode or has

---

TABLE 15–7 Definition of potential predictors of hospitalization for asthma

---

1. Prior hospitalization for asthma within the last year
    a. No
    b. Yes*

2. Respiratory impairment
    a. None (FEV$_1$ # 80%, FVC # 80% and FEV$_1$/FVC #75%)
    b. Mild (FEV$_1$ # 60–79%, FVC # 60–79% and FEV$_1$/FVC # 60–74%)
    c. Moderate* (FEV$_1$ # 41–59%, FVC # 51–59% and FEV$_1$/FVC # 41–59%)
    d. Severe* (FEV$_1$ < 40%, FVC < 50% and FEV$_1$/FVC < 40%)

3. Medication regimen
    a. Mild   = 1 medication as needed, or
                     > 1 medication as needed
    b. Moderate = 1 nonsteroid medication daily, or
                     1 nonsteroid medication daily plus medication as needed, or
                     2 to 3 nonsteroid medications daily, or
                     inhaled steroid daily and up to 2 other nonsteroid medications
    c. Severe* = 4 to 5 medications daily with or without inhaled steroid use, or
                     Systemic steroid as needed or short course, or
                     Systemic steroid every other day, or
                     Systemic steroid daily

---

continued

TABLE 15–7   continued

14. Overnight variability in peak expiratory flow (2-week observation period)
    a.   Nondipper (maximum overnight variability < 25%)
    b.   Dipper (maximum overnight variability 25–40%)
    c.   Severe dipper* (maximum overnight variability > 40%)

5.   Mean evening peak expiratory flow percent of predicted (2-week observation)
    a.   Mild (PEF % predicted > 80%)
    b.   Moderate (PEF % predicted 60–80%)
    c.   Severe* (PEF % predicted < 60%)

Count the number of starred (*) risk factors and use following scale:

0 risk factors	=	0% chance of hospitalization
1 risk factor	=	5% chance of hospitalization
2 risk factors	=	7% chance of hospitalization
3 risk factors	=	17% chance of hospitalization
4 risk factors	=	66% chance of hospitalization
5 risk factors	=	100% chance of hospitalization

Four or five risk factors or failure to use a peak flow meter can be used as entrance criteria for asthma-educational program.

(Li, D. et al., "Prospective Study of Hospitalization for Asthma," *American Journal of Respiratory Critical Care Medicine,* Vol. 151, 1995, p. 649. Reprinted with permission.)

sought medical advice due to worsening symptoms. Unfortunately, patients often do not heed advice until necessary. Once the patient and family understand the need for education, the practitioner can assess the needs of the patient and family and design a program that will allow as normal a lifestyle as possible.

LEARNING ACTIVITIES
FOR ASTHMA EDUCATION

The objective of asthma education is best stated in the Expert Panel Report from the National Asthma Education Program Guidelines for the Diagnosis and Management of Asthma: "Patient education involves helping patients understand asthma, learn and practice skills necessary to manage asthma, and be supported for adopting appropriate asthma management behaviors." To provide information to the patient is not enough. The practitioner must also encourage self-management skills and instill confidence in the patient and the family that they can control the patient's disease. Finally, the practitioner, patient, and family should agree on objectives and expected outcomes that center on the following essentials:

- the concept of developing a clinician-patient partnership;
- the assertion asthma is a chronic but controllable disease;
- the understanding that environmental control and medication play a role in controlling asthma;

- the belief that learning to measure lung function objectively is important;
- the contention that specific written guidelines for managing exacerbations must be developed; and
- the realization that it may be necessary to call for help.

Other objectives may include:

- successful communication with heath-care providers;
- knowledge of how to use health-care services;
- allaying patient fears of medications;
- general information on maintaining overall health and well-being; and
- local and national asthma resources.

The practitioner must assess the needs of the patient and family before discussing these objectives. If the patient and family already completely understand the role of environmental control, then this topic should be reinforced. Extensive education would probably be counterproductive because it would tend not to stimulate the patient or the family. Once they are mutually agreed upon, the objectives indicate the outcomes expected from the educational process (Wilson & Starr-Schneidkraut, 1994).

The climate for education, including whether to have individual or group sessions, when to schedule the sessions, where to hold instruction, and the duration of sessions, should also be mutually agreed upon by the practitioner, patient, and family. Patients are more receptive when they are calm. Although patients are usually receptive following an attack, follow-up sessions should be scheduled when their asthma is more stable (Boulet et al., 1994).

Patient-education programs appear to be most effective and have better attendance when they take place in the same location and at the same time as visits for treatment, evaluation, and follow-up. This appears to be true for hospital-based smoking cessation and asthma education programs. There is a concentration of learning resources and health-care professionals on site. These professionals can be trained to provide appropriate education to asthmatic patients. Patients treated in the emergency room or while hospitalized also constitute a captive and motivated audience (Newhouse, 1994).

However, high-risk groups like Hispanics or African Americans seem to be isolated from physicians and other health-care professionals. In their article, "Targeting High Risk Groups" in *Chest*, Edwin Fisher et al., (1994) said, "[African Americans] may be more influenced by informal networks of friends and family." This also seems to be the case with Hispanic asthmatics. The practitioner may be able to start the educational process in the hospital, but the bulk of the program may be more widely received in the community center or local church. In *Teach Your Patients About Asthma: A Clinician's Guide* (1992), the NIH provides ten teaching units that can be covered during regular office visits. However, the recommendation is to also consider scheduling educational visits after school for school-age children and in the early evenings or on Saturday mornings for working parents (p. vi).

The practitioner must be wary of trying to compress the educational program too much to fit the schedule of the patient, the family, or the practitioner. While it is necessary to be efficient, effective behavioral changes do not occur quickly and there

---

TABLE 15–8   Principles of behavior change and health education

Principle of educational diagnosis	Involves identifying the causes of behavior
Principle of hierarchy	States that there is a natural order in the sequence of factors influencing beahvior
Principle of cumulative learning	States that experiences must be planned in a sequence that considers the patient's learning experiences and concurrent incidental learning experiences or the opportunities to which patients may be exposed
Principle of participation	States that changes in behavior will be greater if patients have identified their needs for change and have actively selected a method or approach they believe will enable them to change
Principle of situational specificity	States that there is nothing inherently superior or inferior about any method of intervention or patient education but that the effectiveness and efficiency of any asthma management program depends on the circumstances and characteristics of the patient and/or the change agent (e.g., physician or nurse educator)
Principle of multiple methods	States that comprehension behavior-change programs should employ different methods or components in consideration of the interaction of person-specific and situation-specific factors
Principle of individualization	Individualizing or tailoring patient-education interventions applies the principle of participation, situational specificity, and cumulative learning in producing interventions that are both patient- and situation-relevant
Principle of relevance	States that the more relevant the contents and methods to the patient's (learner's) circumstances and interests, the more likely the learning and behavior process is to succeed
Principle of feedback	States that providing feedback allows the patient to adapt both the learning process and the resultant behavioral responses to his or her situation and pace
Principle of reinforcement	States that behavior that is rewarded tends to be repeated
Principle of facilitation	Involves the degree to which an intervention provides the means for patients to take action or reduces the barriers to action

(Adapted with permission from: Green, L., and Frankish, J., "Theories and Principles of Health Education Applied to Asthma," *Chest,* October Supplement, Vol. 106, No. 4, 1994, p. 222S–223S.)

---

must be enough time allotted to reach the expected outcomes. To change behavior, certain principles must be incorporated into the design and evaluation of asthma-prevention programs (Table 15–8). Changing behavior and educating asthmatic patients and families is best done calmly and unhurriedly so the knowledge can be integrated and internalized.

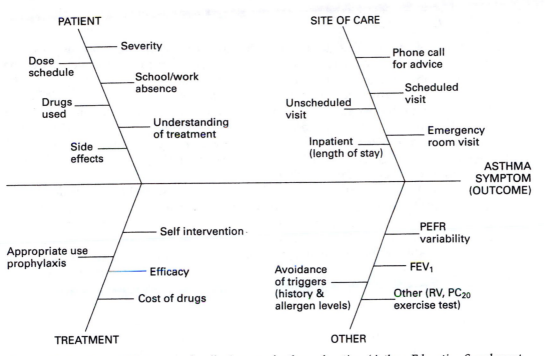

Figure 15–5 *Using CQI to assess the effectiveness of asthma education. (Asthma Education Supplement, Chest, Vol. 106, October 1994, p. 233S.)*

TEACHING METHODS AND EVALUATION OF ASTHMA EDUCATION

Many excellent, predesigned programs are available to the practitioner. Many have reproducible lesson plans and handouts. The practitioner should use effective components from all. The two free books from the National Asthma Education Program are an excellent start. They are *Guidelines for the Diagnosis and Management of Asthma* (1991) and *Teach Your Patients About Asthma: A Clinician's Guide* (1994). Each makes excellent suggestions for practical demonstrations and offers handouts and illustrations.

Asthma education has been proven to be a cost-effective, efficient way to prevent asthma patients from hospitalization. The effectiveness of the programs has been proven over all age groups and socioeconomic backgrounds. The evaluation of asthma education must be ongoing to ensure the best quality. In their *Chest* article, "Essential Ingredients for an Ideal Education Program for Children with Asthma and Their Families," Allan Becker et al. (1994) state:

> Usual accepted scientific techniques may not be the best approach for assessing asthma programs. The technique of continuous quality improvement has advantages as it lends itself to program development as well as evaluation. This could be applied to a specific program using a variety of parameters [Figure 15–5]. The use of continuous quality improvement will allow for modification of the program as it develops.

ROLES FOR THE RCP

Change is one of the few things practitioners can count on in the constantly evolving health-care system. This change affects not only providers but patients as well. By becoming educators and trainers, RCPs with their peers and, more importantly, with their patients, can take an active role in this change process. As trainers, RCPs must be completely familiar with the essentials of the training process as described in this chapter. The RCPS should know how to teach and to modify their teaching approaches to bring about the desired patient outcomes. This training process can also be applied to inservice or staff-development programs in which the focus is peer training and education (American Association for Respiratory Care [AARC], 1996b).

In 1996, the AARC published two CPGs on training the health-care professional to educate patients/caregivers and provide patient/caregiver training. These guidelines encompass elements like description of the process, identification of appropriate settings, limitations, assessment of need and outcomes, and identification of required resources. These CPGs enable RCPs to facilitate the patient's and/or caregiver's acquisition of knowledge, skills, understanding, and positive attitudes related to the patient's condition and related management. Consequently, with time and experience, the RCP will become a more effective trainer or educator (AARC, 1996a,b,c).

Specifically, RCPs can assume any training role when they have knowledge, experience, and the ability to relate this to a group of individuals (peers, patients and/or caregivers). Some areas in which RCPs are involved in patient training include:

- asthma-education programs;
- COPD support groups;
- pulmonary-rehabilitation programs;
- home care, including in-hospital training before patient discharge;
- bedside training in any aspect of respiratory care (e.g., breathing and coughing techniques, medication use, chest physiotherapy, and oxygen delivery);
- smoking-cessation or nicotine-intervention programs (group or individual);
- speakers' bureaus for charitable health organizations (ALS, AHA, American Cancer Society, and other similar organizations); and
- community health fairs and exhibitions.

The RCPs are experts in cardiopulmonary disorders and related respiratory care. As patient and caregiver educators, they can tremendously influence the public regarding the roles and responsibilities of the respiratory-care profession. Education and training on all levels are opportunities RCPs must not ignore.

SUMMARY

This chapter examined patient and family education. It presented the basic factors of patient and family education, like ensuring the practitioner is ready to educate, ensuring the patient and family are ready to be educated, determining the appropriate learning activities, using many teaching methodologies, and evaluating the success of the program. The National Asthma Education Program was used as an example of a nationally known, well-organized educational program. Patient and family education is vital to the continued well-being of all patients with chronic illness. It does not matter whether the practitioner is teaching a child with asthma, a teenager with cystic fibrosis, or an adult with emphysema as long as the practitioner remembers and applies the fundamentals of education.

Review Questions

1. How does a practitioner ensure he or she is ready to educate a patient and family?
2. Why may a patient and family not be ready to learn? How can barriers to learning be removed?
3. What are some of the learning activities RCPs can use in patient education?
4. How does the National Asthma Education Program exemplify preferred teaching methodologies?
5. What are the essential components of the training process?
6. In what specific ways or in which areas can the RCP function as patient educator?

References

American Association for Respiratory Care. (1996a, July). AARC clinical practice guideline: Providing patient and caregiver training. *Respiratory Care, 41*(7), 658–662.

American Association for Respiratory Care. (1996b, July). AARC clinical practice guideline: Providing patient and caregiver training, appendix—Essentials of the training process. *Respiratory Care, 41*(7), 663.

American Association for Respiratory Care. (1996c, July). AARC clinical practice guideline: Training the health-care professional for the role of patient and caregiver educator. *Respiratory Care, 41*(7), 654–657.

Barnes, G., & Chapman, K. (1994, October Supplement). Asthma education: The United Kingdom experience. *Chest, 106*(4), 216–218S.

Becker, A. et al. (1994, October Supplement). Essential ingredients for an ideal education program for children with asthma and their families. *Chest, 106*(4), 231–234S.

Boulet, L. et al. (1994, October Supplement). Asthma education. *Chest, 106*(4), 184–196S.

Cote, J. et al. (1994, October Supplement). Educating the educators. *Chest, 106*(4), 242–247S.

Dantzker, D. (Ed.). (1995). *Comprehensive respiratory care* (Chapter 60). Philadelphia, PA: W.B. Saunders Company.

Dantzker, D., MacIntyre, N., & Bakow, E. (1995). *Comprehensive respiratory care.* Philadelphia, PA: W.B. Saunders Company.

Dyche, J. (1988). *Educational program development for employees in health care agencies.* Murfreesboro, TN: Tri-Oak Educational Division.

Fisher, E. et al. (1994, October Supplement). Targeting high risk groups. *Chest, 106*(4), 248–259S.

Fitzgerald, M. (1994, October Supplement). Psychosocial barriers to asthma education. *Chest, 106*(4), 260–263S.

Green, L., & Frankish, J. (1994, October Supplement). Theories and principles of health education applied to asthma. *Chest, 106*(4), 219–230S.

Hanak, M. (1986). *Patient and family education.* New York, NY: Springer Publishing Company.

Kidd, J. (1977). *How adults learn.* New York, NY: Association Press.

Li, D. et. al. (1995). Prospective study of hospitalization for asthma. *American Journal of Respiratory Critical Care Medicine, 151,* 647–655.

Lorig, K. et al. (1994). *Living a healthy life with chronic conditions.* Palo Alto, CA: Bull Publishing Company.

National Asthma Education Program. (1991). *Guidelines for the diagnosis and management of asthma.* Bethesda, MD: National Institutes of Health.

National Asthma Education Program. (1994). *Guidelines for the diagnosis and management of asthma speaker's kit.* Bethesda, MD: National Institutes of Health.

National Asthma Education Program. (1992). *Teach your patients about asthma.* Bethesda, MD: National Institutes of Health.

Newhouse, M. (1994, October Supplement). Hospital-based asthma education. *Chest, 106*(4), 237–241S.

Northouse, P., & Northouse, L. (1992). *Health communications strategies for health professionals* (2nd ed.). Norwalk, CT: Appleton and Lange.

Purtilo, R., & Haddad, A. (1996). *Health professional and patient interaction* (5th ed.). Philadelphia, PA: W.B. Saunders Company.

Robinson, V. (1991). *Humor and the health professions* (2nd ed.). Thorofare, NJ: Slack Incorporated.

Webster's New World Dictionary of American English. Third College Edition. Victoria Newfeldt (editor). Simon & Schuster, Inc. New York, NY. 1988.

Wilson, S., & Starr-Schneidkraut, N. (1994, October Supplement). State of the art in asthma education: The US experience. *Chest, 106*(4), 197–205S.

Wlodkowski, R. (1985). *Enhancing adult motivation to learn.* San Francisco, CA: Jossey-Bass Publishers.

Suggested Readings

American Association for Respiratory Care. *Education section bulletins.*

Boulet, L., & Chapman, K. (1994, October Supplement). Asthma education: The Canadian experience. *Chest, 106*(4), 206–210S.

Campbell, M. et al. (1994, October Supplement). Consideration of public programs and techniques for public/community health education. *Chest, 106*(4), 274–278S.

Chapman, K. et al. (1994, October Supplement). Future research in asthma education. *Chest, 106*(4), 270–273S.

Elder, J.P., Geller, E.S., Hovell, M.F., & Mayer, J.A. (1994). *Motivating health behavior.* Albany, NY: Delmar Publishers, Inc.

Falvo, D.R. (1994). *Effective patient education: A guide to increased compliance.* Aspen, CO: Aspen Publishers, Inc.

Howell, J.H., Flaim, T., & Lum Lung, C. (1992, June). Patient education. *Pediatric Clinics of North America, 39*(6), 1343–1361.

Kolbe, J. et al. (1994, October Supplement). Influences on trends in asthma morbidity and mortality: The New Zealand experience. *Chest, 106*(4), 211–215S.

Krahn, M. (1994, October Supplement). Issues in the cost-effectiveness of asthma education. *Chest, 106*(4), 264–269S.

Lorig, K. (1992). *Patient education: A practical approach.* St. Louis, MO: Mosby-Year Book, Inc.

O'Donnell, M.P., & Harris, J.S. (1994). *Health promotion in the workplace.* Albany, NY: Delmar Publishers, Inc.

Owen, G. (1994, October Supplement). Consideration of program and techniques for general practice. *Chest, 106*(4), 235–236S.

GLOSSARY

accreditation Process by which a private, non-governmental agency recognizes that an institution or an organization meets specified standards of quality.

Accreditation Commission for Home Care (ACHC) One of the accrediting agencies that review and assess the operation of home-care providers.

Accreditation Council for Home Medical Services (ACHMS) Another accrediting agency established to review and assess the operation of home-care providers.

acuity A measure of the level and intensity of care a patient population mix requires; based on condition.

activities of daily living (ADL) A patient's routine activities that include self-care, personal hygiene, household chores, and ambulation.

aerobic Use of oxygen to produce energy.

affective domain Educational process that focuses on the learner's attitudes, impressions, and feelings.

airway resistance (R_{aw}) Force opposing the flow of gases during ventilation; results from obstruction or turbulence in the upper and lower airways.

alternate site Site of patient care, other than a hospital, that may be a skilled nursing facility, an extended-care facility, a rehabilitation hospital or center, or the home.

anaerobic threshold (AT) Onset of blood lactate accumulation that occurs as exercise intensity increases beyond the level that can be met by predominantly aerobic metabolism; also called *ventilatory threshold*.

arranged-for services Patient care services obtained through outside sources.

arterial desaturation Any decrease in the amount of oxygen bound to hemoglobin as oxyhemoglobin.

authoritarian Characterized by unquestioning obedience to authority rather than individual freedom of judgment and action.

basic home safety Fundamental aspects of a patient's home environment that create a nonhazardous setting conducive to the delivery of patient care.

breathing reserve Ventilatory capacity during physical exertion expressed as $1 - [V_{Emax}/MVV]$.

breathing retraining Physical activities designed to increase the strength and endurance of the respiratory muscles and promote their more efficient use.

calisthenics Athletic exercises to enhance flexibility and agility.

capitated care Patient care based on the payment of a fixed fee for a set period.

capitation Method of payment for health-care services in which the health-care provider pays a fixed fee for each person served in a set period; payment is on a per capita basis and has no relationship to the type of services performed or the number of services each patient receives.

capped rental Home-care equipment rented for a set period; when rental period ends, the patient owns the equipment and is responsible for its use and operation.

carbon dioxide production ($\dot{V}CO_2$) Amount of carbon dioxide produced per minute from the body's metabolic rate; normal value is approximately 200 ml/minute.

cardiac output Total amount of blood the heart is able to circulate per minute; normal adult value is 5 lpm.

cardiac rehabilitation Program of education and exercise that focuses on restoring cardiac patients to the highest possible functional capacity allowed by the cardiac impairment.

cardiopulmonary exercise (CPX) testing Diagnostic testing involving assessment of pulmonary and cardiac function during exercise.

caregiver Any nonprofessional individual, including family members, who delivers care to homebound patients.

care map Reflects a patient's response to an action or an intervention while identifying time frames in which further actions may be taken.

carve-out Ability to establish a position in an area of responsibility based on knowledge, skill, and/or expertise.

case management A CPT evaluation and management service in which the attending physician or agent coordinates the care given a patient by other health-care providers and/or community organizations.

certificate of medical necessity (CMN) Form that authorizes payment by Medicare for health-care services rendered to qualified beneficiaries.

certificate of need Authorization granted by state departments of health for the expansion of health-care facilities, patient beds, and other related levels of care.

clinical associates Unlicensed personnel who provide basic levels of patient care under the supervision of licensed health-care practitioners.

clinical practice guidelines (CPGs) Standards for various modalities of respiratory care developed by the American Association for Respiratory Care (AARC).

clinical (critical) pathways Flowcharts illustrating key events or decisions that lead to the successful care and treatment of patients.

closed-format programs Pulmonary rehabilitation programs that have set starting and completion dates.

cognitive domain Domain that involves the process of knowing or perceiving.

Community Health Accreditation Program (CHAP) Accrediting agency that reviews and assesses the operation of HME providers.

compliance To act in accordance with a request.

comprehensive outpatient rehabilitation facilities (CORFs) Pulmonary-rehabilitation programs that meet a certain criteria as prescribed by Medicare for the implementation of physical reconditioning in chronic lung patients.

comprehensive pulmonary rehabilitation Extensive coverage of the education and physical reconditioning components of pulmonary rehabilitation.

constructive dependence Situation in which a patient works to develop skills and abilities through a positive partnership with the practitioner.

continuing care Continuity of care that follows a patient from hospital admission to appropriate discharge, including care delivered at alternate sites.

continuous positive airway pressure (CPAP) Method of ventilatory support whereby the patient breathes spontaneously without mechanical assistance against threshold resistance, with pressure above atmospheric maintained at the airway throughout breathing.

continuous quality improvement (CQI) Management tool that evaluates process and strives to constantly improve outcomes.

continuum of care Uninterrupted or seamless patient care from one care site to another care site resulting in overall continuity.

copayment Coinsurance or the amount a patient is responsible for after insurance payment has been made.

COPD disability scales Rating scales that categorize the level of dyspnea and inactivity resulting from chronic lung disease.

cor pulmonale Right-sided heart failure due to pulmonary hypertension that results from acute or chronic pulmonary disease.

cost-based contract Government payments to an HMO based on actual incurred costs.

critical pathway protocols Standards and procedures used in making key patient-care decisions.

cross-training Health-care practitioners who receive training in various levels of patient care.

current procedural terminology (CPT) coding Medical procedure coding system maintained and published by the American Medical Association (AMA).

deadspace to tidal volume ratio (V_D/V_T) Comparison of the respired gas volume that does not participate in gas exchange to a tidal breath.

decentralization To break up the centralization of authority.

democratic The process of considering and treating others as equals.

descriptor Explanation of a procedure or service that accompanies a CPT code.

detraining effect Loss of physical conditioning that results when patients cannot continue their exercise prescriptions.

diagnosis related groups (DRGs) System of coding used by the Health Care Financing Administration (HCFA) to set prospective reimbursement schedules for patients according to their diagnoses.

diagnostic evaluation Assessment based on testing criteria.

discharge plan Strategy formulated by a multidisciplinary health-care team to place a patient in an appropriate alternate-care site, including the home.

discharge planning Process of formulating a discharge-plan strategy.

disease-management program Comprehensive plan of care for specific disease entities.

disease specific Treatment or care that is based on the nature of a patient's disease, disorder, or underlying impairment.

downsizing Hospital structuring that results in the merging or elimination of specific departments and/or services.

durable medical equipment (DME) Nondisposable medical devices.

durable medical equipment, prosthetics, orthotics and supplies (DMEPOS) Nondisposable home medical equipment and appliances for physical rehabilitation.

durable medical equipment regional carriers (DMERCs) The four Medicare intermediaries, based on region, that reimburse providers for home-care equipment and services.

dyspnea indices *See functional status scales.*

employer health plans Health-care coverage provided by an individual's place of employment.

ergometer Apparatus designed to measure the amount of work performed by an animal or a human.

ethics Standards of conduct and moral judgment.

exclusive provider organizations (EPOs) A closed-panel PPO plan in which enrollees receive no benefits if they opt to receive care from a provider who is not in the EPO.

exercise intolerance Inability of a patient to endure physical activity and stress.

exercise prescription Amount and intensity of exercise recommended for patients in rehabilitation and physical-reconditioning programs.

extended-care facilities One type of subacute-care site that provides long-term patient care.

extended-care services Spectrum of services and care provided at extended-care facilities.

finders fees Illegal payment to any individual for patient referrals.

formative evaluation Assessment that occurs while the program is being conducted.

functional status Ability of a patient to perform routine activities without discomfort.

functional status scales System of rating a patient's ability to perform specific activities.

gatekeeper Primary physician or other health-care professional assigned by the insurer to review the medical management of plan enrollees.

glossopharyngeal ("frog") breathing Method of breathing used in quadraplegics that involves using the lips, mouth, and tongue to swallow air to effect breathing and cough.

gradational (incremental) Gradual increases in that level of intensity that are used commonly in cardiopulmonary exercise testing.

grandfathering Accepting preexisting conditions or situations after the passage of a ruling or law.

group support Individuals (peers or patients) form a network of mutual support based on common experiences or afflictions.

HCFA common procedure coding system (HCPCS) The HCFA common procedural coding system used for reporting outpatient health-care services provided to Medicare beneficiaries.

Health Care Financing Administration (HCFA) Federal administrative agency charged with primary responsibility for Medicare and the federal portion of the Medicaid programs.

health-care reform Process of revamping the health-care delivery system.

Health Security Act Legislation proposed as part of national health-care reform that would provide individuals with health-care coverage; debated but never passed.

health maintenance organizations (HMOs) Care delivery programs that have their own point-of-service sites; referral decisions can be made at the different sites or by a gatekeeper.

heart rate reserve Reflects cardiac capacity during physical exertion; expressed as $1 - [(HR_{max} - HR_{resting}/HR_{pred.max} - HR_{resting})]$.

high-technology home care Home care that involves complex equipment like mechanical ventilators and infusion therapy pumps.

holistic Philosophy whereby the person is viewed in totality as a mental, physical, and emotional being interacting with the environment.

homebound patient Any patient who receives health-care services in the home.

home health agency (HHA) Public agency or private organization that is engaged primarily in providing skilled nursing care and other therapeutic services.

home health care Provision of health services in the home to aged, disabled, sick, or convalescent who do not need institutional care.

home medical equipment (HME) Newer term for durable medical equipment.

Home Oxygen Services Coalition (HOSC) Dedicated group of manufacturers, providers, and practitioners who are involved in the delivery of and reimbursement for home oxygen therapy.

homogenous patient characteristics Similar patient traits or qualities.

hospital restructuring The process of reexamining and redefining every hospital department by role and function in an effort to increase the efficiency within an institution.

hypoxic drive Subnormal levels of oxygen in the blood which act as the stimulus for ventilation.

iatrogenic Caused by treatment or diagnostic procedures.

incident to physician services Services or supplies furnished as part of a physician's professional services in the course of diagnosis or treatment.

independent practice associations (IPAs) Group of individual health-care providers who join to provide prepaid health care to individuals or groups who purchase coverage; closed-panel HMO with no common facilities.

inspiratory (flow-resistive) breathing Same as inspiratory muscle training that uses techniques to improve the condition of respiratory muscles.

inspiratory muscle training (IMT) Breathing retraining techniques that employ resistance during inspiration to enhance respiratory muscle conditioning.

insurance co-payment Provision in an insurance policy requiring the policyholder or patient to pay a specified dollar amount or a percentage of the allowed fee for medical services.

integrated delivery systems (IDS) Combine the resources of physicians, hospitals, and other services to provide continuing and coordinated care to a defined portion of enrolled beneficiaries; associated with health-care plans. Also known as integrated health care delivery systems.

integrated health networks Consolidation of health-care plans to provide more cost-effective delivery of health-care services.

International Classification of Diseases, 9th Revision, Clinical Modification (ICD-9-CM) Coding mechanism for classifying disease entities.

isokinetic Physical exercises that use movement and resistance to develop muscle tone and strength.

isometric exercises Physical exercises in which there is resistance but no movement.

isotonic See *aerobic*.

Joint Commission on Accreditation of Healthcare Organizations (JCAHO) Private, nonprofit organization that evaluates and accredits hospitals and other health-care organizations and facilities.

kinesics Use of body motion as a form of communication, same as *body language*.

lactic acidosis Reduction in blood pH resulting from a buildup of lactate in the blood stemming from anaerobic metabolism.

laissez-faire "Hands-off" policy followed by governments, organizations, or agencies. A process where all the decisions are made by the participants.

left ventricular filling pressure Pressure in the left ventricle of the heart during diastole.

left ventricular function Ejection fraction of the left side of the heart.

legal credentialing Involves governmental regulation of a profession through licensure, state credentialing, or title protection.

length of stay (LOS) Amount of time in days a patient spends in a specific health-care setting.

long-term oxygen therapy (LTOT) Supplemental oxygen therapy used by a patient to relieve hypoxemia and/or cardiovascular sequelae and does not necessarily imply continuous use.

maintenance program Rehabilitation activities aimed at maintaining a patient's level of physical conditioning.

managed care System for operating an insurance program by controlling the utilization of services with a system that assigns patients to case managers who are responsible for prospective and retrospective review of the physician's treatment plans and patient discharge planning.

managed-care organizations (MCOs) Organizations like HMOs that provide health-care coverage.

management by objectives (MBO) System of management that involves identification of measurable objectives followed by outcomes assessments using those objectives.

management service organization (MSO) Separate legal entities similar to service bureaus that provide practice-management services to physicians, hospitals, or physician-hospital organizations; a form of an integrated health-care delivery system that emerged as a way to contract with managed-care organizations more effectively.

maximum oxygen consumption ($\dot{V}O_{2max}$) Maximum amount of oxygen consumed during strenuous physical activity.

medical savings accounts Method of obtaining health-care coverage through an account in which benefits are kept.

medical subacute Patients who are not acutely ill.

Medicare—Part A Benefits covering inpatient hospital and skilled nursing facility services, hospice care, home health care, and blood transfusions.

Medicare—Part B Benefits covering outpatient hospital and health-care provider services.

Medisave Concept in which private insurance companies can charge deductibles as high as $10,000 to beneficiaries who switch to a catastrophic-only Medicare plan.

membrane oxygenator A system of oxygen delivery that uses a thick membrane to separate gases according to their diffusion rates thereby increasing the amount of oxygen delivered. Same as an oxygen enricher.

(MET) metabolic equivalent of energy expenditure or oxygen consumption One MET equals approximately 3.5 ml of oxygen consumption per kilogram of body weight per minute.

metered dose inhalers (MDI) A handheld canister of medication that is activated by the patient.

modifier Qualifier that is used when a service or a procedure has been altered or when billing for procedures that are separate but necessary.

molecular sieve Aluminum sodium phosphate or zeolite used in oxygen concentrators to separate nitrogen atoms from room air thus increasing the concentration of oxygen delivered.

multicompetency Practitioners with various patient-care skills.

multidisciplinary team Group of a number of different health-care disciplines or professions.

multiskilling Similar to multicompetency in which practitioners have mastered various skills and abilities.

muscle oxygen extraction Amount of oxygen muscles required to perform physical activities.

National Committee for Quality Assurance (NCQA) Body that accredits managed-care organizations.

National Technical Expert Panel (NTEP) Select group of specialists who examine medical or technical equipment for evaluation.

negative pressure ventilation (NPV) Application of subatmospheric pressure to the airway during the expiratory phase of positive pressure ventilation.

nocturnal oxygen therapy trial (NOTT) Supplemental oxygen therapy administered at night to patients to relieve hypoxemia and/or cardiovascular sequelae, such as pulmonary hypertension.

noninvasive positive pressure ventilation (NIPPV) Positive pressure ventilation applied with a mask.

O₂ pulse Amount of oxygen consumption per heartbeat.

open-ended programs Pulmonary-rehabilitation programs with no specified end date.

organ specific Care or treatment that focuses on a disease related to the dysfunction of a specific organ system.

orientation or groping stage Initial stage in which a newly formed group seeks identity and purpose.

outcome oriented Focuses on results or outcomes.

outcomes assessment Evaluating results of an educational program.

over dependence Situation in which a patient relies too much on the practitioner.

overload Concept that dictates muscles must be forced or pushed beyond a certain level to produce a training effect.

oxygen concentrators System of oxygen delivery that uses devices to filter out nitrogen and concentrate oxygen for patient delivery.

oxygen-conserving devices Appliances or systems that extend the amount of oxygen available for patient use.

oxygen consumption (V̇O₂) Amount of oxygen consumed, in ml/minute, as a result of body metabolism; normal value at rest approximates 250 ml/minute.

oxygen enricher A system of oxygen delivery that uses a thick membrane to separate gases according to their diffusion rates thereby increasing the amount of oxygen delivered. Same as a membrane oxygenator.

paralinguistics Physical characteristics of verbal communication and the resulting impact on interpretation.

patient acuity The level of severity of a patient's condition based on the level of care provided.

patient attrition Loss of patients due to a number of variables or circumstances.

patient care associates (PCAs) Unlicensed individuals responsible for basic levels of care delivered under the supervision of a licensed practitioner.

patient care technicians (PCTs) See *patient*

patient care technicians (PCTs) See *patient care associates (PCAs)*.

patient-driven protocols Method of delivering patient care based on established standards.

patient-focused (patient-centered) care Delivery of care aimed specifically at patients and their related conditions and needs.

patient inducement Enticements, incentives, or motives that result in patient participation or activity.

patient-treatment or care plans Strategy for delivering patient care that involves therapy and related assessment.

peer credentialing Professional recognition of a designated level of competency through either documented experience and/or an examination process.

per member per month (PMPM) Fixed capitation payment to a health-care provider from an HMO on a per-member-per-month basis.

Pew Foundation Health Professions Commission Program of the Pew Charitable Trusts that routinely publishes documents on the status of health-care-practitioner training in the United States and other related issues.

physical reconditioning Process of improving a patient's level of fitness through a program of exercise and physical activity.

physician hospital organizations (PHOs) Groups being formed in many parts of the country to provide vertically integrated health-care services; a group of hospitals and a group of doctors form a network of provider services for someone who will buy those services.

physician information sheet (PHYIS) HCFA form designed for the prescribing physician to assist providers in obtaining payment for patient equipment or services under Medicare.

plan of care Strategy for the delivering patient care that involves therapy and related assessment; see *patient treatment or care plans*.

pneumotachometer Transducer designed to measure the flow of respiratory gases, usually by measuring pressure differences across a tube of known resistance.

point of service (POS) Health-care enrollment programs that use different points of service; referral decisions can be made at the different sites or by a gatekeeper.

polysomnography Management and recording of variations in airflow and diaphragmatic activity during sleep; used in the diagnosis of sleep apnea.

positive pressure ventilator Mechanical application and maintenance of pressure above atmospheric at the airway.

postacute care See *subacute care.*

PRECEDE Acronym for an asthma program model of predisposing, reinforcing and enabling constructs in educational diagnosis and evaluation.

preferred provider organization (PPO) Prepaid managed care, open panel, non-HMO affiliated plan that provides more patient management than is available under regular fee-for-service medical insurance plans and contracts to provide medical care to PPO patients for a special reduced rate.

problem-solving or cooperation stage Constructive stage of the patient-education process.

prospective payment system (PPS) Predetermined method of payment based on diagnostic related groups (DRGs) regardless of the amount of care or services.

proxemics Study of personal space or comfort zone.

psychomotor domain Educational domain that focuses on the performance of certain skills or motor functions.

pulmonary hypertension Condition characterized by abnormally high pulmonary artery pressures (e.g., mean pulmonary artery pressures over 22 mmHg).

pulmonary rehabilitation Program of education and exercise that focuses on restoring chronic respiratory patients to the highest possible functional capacity allowed by the pulmonary impairment.

pulse oximetry Noninvasive estimation of arterial oxyhemoglobin saturation based on the combined principles of photoplethysmography and spectrophotometry.

pump failure Inability to ventilate properly due to neuromuscular dysfunction.

quality assurance (QA) Process of determining that procedures are performed to certain prescribed standards and employing corrective measures when deficiencies are identified.

ramp Process of gradually increasing intensity as during cardiopulmonary exercise testing.

rating of perceived exertion (RPE) Scales used to determine a patient's level of dyspnea with certain intensities of activity.

reengineering (restructuring) Process of examining and implementing changes within a hospital's organization and operation.

rehabilitation Restoring the individual to the fullest medical, mental, emotional, social, and vocational potential of which he/she is capable.

rehabilitative subacute care Involves patient and family education, patient retraining, and pulmonary rehabilitation.

respiratory home care Delivery of respiratory equipment and related services in the home.

respiratory quotient (RQ) Ratio of carbon dioxide production to oxygen consumption; normal value is 0.8 at rest.

restructured Changes that occur within an institution as a result of reengineering.

reversibility Process of losing physical conditioning through inactivity; see *detraining effect.*

right atrial pressures Pressure in the right atrium during diastole.

rights and responsibilities Full disclosure of information pertaining to home care equipment rental and/or purchase by a patient from a home-care provider.

risk-based contract Payments made by the government to the HMO in the form of a flat fee for each beneficiary.

rubrics Formulations that are common to diagnostic coding as per *ICD-9-CM.*

scope of practice Identifies set of procedures that can be legally performed by a profession.

seamless care Patient care that is continuous despite changes in care settings.

self-dependence Patient has the skills and abilities to confidently address or control situations.

Six-Point Plan Implemented by HCFA to change the ways in which home-care equipment was paid for or reimbursed.

skilled nursing facilities (SNFs) Subacute-care site that provides 24-hour nursing care.

specificity of training Exercise programs designed to have patients achieve specific goals and objectives based on the concept that exercising muscles is only beneficial to the targeted group.

step desaturation Reduction in blood oxygen as a result of increasing levels of exercise or physical activity.

standard precautions Infection-control measures that prevent the spread of infection in blood, body fluids, secretions, excretions, mucous membranes, and nonintact skin.

subacute care Comprehensive inpatient care designed for patients who do not depend on high technology monitoring or complex diagnostic procedures.

summative evaluation Assessment conducted at the conclusion of an educational program.

sustained maximum inspiration (SMI) Therapeutic breathing maneuver in which patients are coached to inspire from the resting expiratory level to their inspiratory capacity (IC), with an end-inspiratory pause.

target heart rate Heart rate at which a patient exercises to achieve maximum physical and cardiovascular conditioning.

telemetry Any method of monitoring patients at a distance using electronic signals.

therapist-driven protocols (TDPs) Method of delivering patient care based on established standards; see *patient-driven protocols.*

third-party reimbursement Payment made by an insurance company, friend, attorney, or other to a health-care provider to pay for medical expenses incurred by a patient.

threshold loading Method of inspiratory resistance breathing that requires patients to generate a pressure to overcome a set threshold.

total quality management (TQM) Specific management tool that focuses on process and ways to improve outcomes.

total-body workouts Physical exercise that involves the upper and lower body simultaneously.

traditional indemnity Customary payment by certain insurance carriers for health-care services or benefits received.

transfer agreement Arrangement between a hospital and a subacute-care facility to augment the continuity of patient care.

transtracheal oxygen therapy (TTOT) Method of delivering oxygen to a patient that employs a surgical opening in the trachea through which a small catheter is inserted.

unique physician identification number (UPIN) Identification number assigned to physicians that is required on certificates of medical necessity (CMNs) and other prescription forms.

unlicensed assistive personnel (UAP) Unlicensed individuals who provide basic levels of patient care under a licensed practitioner; see *patient care technician* or *clinical associates.*

utilization management Supervision of patient care based on care and services needed and delivered; with utilization review is becoming part of case management.

utilization review Analysis of the care and services delivered to a patient with regard to patient condition and status.

ventilator-assisted individuals (VAI) Individuals who depend on ventilatory support.

ventilatory isocapnic hyperpnea Breathing retraining technique in which patients sustain high levels of ventilation for approximately 15 minutes, two to three times daily, using a breathing circuit with fixed carbon dioxide and oxygen concentrations.

ventilatory muscle endurance Ability of the respiratory muscles to provide adequate levels of ventilation during physical exertion.

written confirmation of a verbal order (WCVO) Form home-care providers use as a cover letter to a certificate of medical necessity (CMN).

written confirmation of a physician's order (WCPO) HCFA form used as a cover letter to a certificate of medical necessity (CMN).

INDEX